Health Issues
for Minority
Adolescents

Child, Youth, and Family Services

Health Issues for Minority Adolescents

Edited by
Marjorie Kagawa-Singer,
Phyllis A. Katz,
Dalmas A. Taylor, and
Judith H. M. Vanderryn

University of Nebraska Press
Lincoln and London

Manufactured in the United States of America

⊖ The paper in this book meets
the minimum requirements of American National
Standard for Information Sciences –
Permanence of Paper for Printed Library Materials,
ANSI Z39.48-1984.

Library of Congress Cataloging-in-Publication Data
Health issues for minor-
ity adolescents / edited by Marjorie Kagawa-Singer . . .
[et al.].   p.   cm. —
(Child, youth, and family services) Includes biblio-
graphical references and index.
ISBN 0-8032-2732-9 (cloth : alk. paper) 1. Minority
teenagers—Medical care—
United States.   2. Minority teenagers—Health and
hygiene—United States.
I. Kagawa-Singer, Marjorie, 1947–
II. Series.   RJ102.H39   1996
362.1'08'693—dc20   95-41942   CIP

Contents

Foreword vii
Gary B. Melton

Preface xiii
Ruby Takanishi and Elena O. Nightingale

Introduction xix
Marjorie Kagawa-Singer

1. Poverty and Adolescent Health 1
LaRue Allen and Christina M. Mitchell

2. Health and Related Services Available to Black Adolescents 36
Dalmas A. Taylor and Phyllis A. Katz

3. The Health of Latino Youth:
Challenges for Disease Prevention 80
Hortensia Amaro, Miriam Messinger, and Richard Cervantes

4. American Indian Adolescent Health 116
Candace M. Fleming, Spero M. Manson, and Lois Bergeisen

5. Health Issues of Asian Pacific American Adolescents 142
Nolan Zane and Stanley Sue

6. Health and Related Services for
Native Hawaiian Adolescents 168
Lawrence Miike

7. The Federal Government's Role in Improving
the Health of Poor and Ethnic-Minority Adolescents 188
Denise Dougherty and Kerry B. Kemp

8. Policy Recommendations for Ethnic-Minority
Adolescent Health Issues: A Paradigm Shift 217
Nancy Lois Ruth Anderson and Marjorie Kagawa-Singer

List of Contributors 243

Author Index 249

Subject Index 262

Foreword

Calling the 1994 election not a "drive-by shooting" but instead an "anxiety attack," columnist Ellen Goodman began 1995 by nominating the Angry White Man for 1994 man of the year (Goodman, 1995b). She noted the increasingly marked gender and ethnic differences in voting patterns and the anger that seemed to accompany them. Attacks on candidates, especially incumbents, became more and more personal and vitriolic and ad hominem charges were accompanied and followed by mean-spirited proposals for new public policies.

Voters in some states indicated their desire to transform professionals who provide services to children and families into de facto part-time Border Patrol agents legally charged with reporting illegal immigrants, and moves to dismantle affirmative-action programs for disadvantaged groups have become common. The new congressional leadership made elimination of social and economic benefits even to families of legal immigrants a cornerstone of its agenda. Compounding the injury, some congressional leaders framed such policies as means to strengthen the resources available to parents for their children's support (see Goodman, 1995a).

Although the claim that increasingly miserly social policies are "pro-child" is disingenuous, it does respond to the anxiety underlying the anger driving contemporary policies. As Goodman (1995b) noted, White males increasingly face "a bad case of the jitters": "Jitters about the new world economy and our old jobs, jitters about our kids, our futures, and the frayed connections between people who call themselves Americans"

(Goodman, 1995b, p. 9A). In a society in which only a small proportion of the population has been experiencing an increase in its real income (see Lindsey, 1994), the traditional role of family provider is increasingly difficult for White males—and other, historically less privileged groups—to meet.

This economic stress is compounded by decreases in social connectedness—the informal support of neighbor for neighbor that has traditionally been a marker of American culture (Melton, 1993b, 1995; Putnam, 1995a, 1995b). Not only do many parents struggle to keep their children nourished and safe, but too often they also do so alone. The politics of anger reflect an age of not only anxiety but also alienation, as Americans report ever-greater fear and ever-weaker trust (Putnam, 1995a, 1995b).

These social, economic, and psychological changes coincide with extraordinary demographic changes. For example, the proportion of American children born abroad now is the same as it was at the beginning of the twentieth century, the time of the famous wave of immigration from Europe (Lewit & Baker, 1994). The current wave is much more diverse, with new immigrants arriving primarily from Asia and Latin America and often escaping not only grinding poverty but also political persecution and war. The population growth among ethnic minorities as a result of immigration is magnified by higher birth rates among minority groups within the United States and therefore substantially greater natural population growth than among European Americans. Within a generation, the United States is expected to become a "majority of minorities" (Lewit & Baker, 1994), a change that has already taken place among children in California (Melton, 1993a).

The United States was built on diversity, but it has long struggled to cope with the challenges that heterogeneity brings. Although the richness of American culture—probably including the ethic of neighborliness itself—emanates from this diversity, most of the shameful moments in U.S. history have been episodes, often stretching across decades and even centuries, of degradation of minorities: slavery, segregation, forced movement, and confiscation of property.

Fortunately, such overt discrimination and outright subjugation of minorities are largely things of the past. It is not difficult, however, to demonstrate subtle discrimination by people who believe themselves not to be prejudiced (see, e.g., Crosby, Bromley, & Saxe, 1980; Dovidio & Gaertner,

1981; Frey & Gaertner, 1986; McConahay, 1983). As the contributors to this book repeatedly note, ethnic-minority families often are at a disadvantage in socioeconomic and, therefore, health status. Moreover, for ethnic-minority youth, "social morbidity" is translated disproportionately into incarceration and foster care (see, e.g., Federle & Chesney-Lind, 1992). Discrimination may intensify as a result of the current political movement toward limitation of benefits to the "deserving" poor and the fear-based tendency to group the world into "them" and "us" as real income stagnates or drops.

Just as society at large must guard against relatively subtle manifestations of racism, researchers need to move beyond simple descriptions of ethnic-group differences in prevalence rates of one problem or another to understand the phenomena underlying such differences. Similarly, program developers need to go beyond sloganeering about cultural sensitivity or competence to care in determining specific ways in which health and social services might be matched to cultural experiences or norms—in effect, to do segmented marketing of services (see U.S. Advisory Board on Child Abuse and Neglect, 1993).

For example, as efforts are being made to design universal systems of home visitation to support families of young children, research is needed to explore the meaning of home visitation for groups with different experiences of government involvement, varying norms of privacy, and perhaps differences in psychological boundaries within the home. Similarly, as well illustrated by New Zealand's experience in implementing family-group conferences (drawing on Maori culture) for resolution of problems of juvenile delinquency and child maltreatment, much can be learned by close examination of practices among ethnic minorities that may be useful in dealing with issues in the society as a whole (Melton, 1992).

In short, society has far to go in building healthy environments for its youth, especially those in ethnic minorities. Scholarship also has far to go if it is to be useful in constructing service systems responsive to the needs of minority youth and their families and built on the strengths of their communities. Marjorie Kagawa-Singer and her colleagues provide a comprehensive overview of knowledge about the health needs of ethnic-minority adolescents and the state of the art in services responding to such needs. They are to be congratulated for their scholarship, especially at such a critical historical point. I am proud to add this volume to the Child, Youth, and

Family Services Series. I hope that it will stimulate a new generation of careful research that will serve as the foundation for establishing and implementing programs and policies that will facilitate development of youth in a society respectful of personal integrity, including cultural identity.

GARY B. MELTON
Series Editor

References

Crosby, F., Bromley, S., & Saxe, L. (1980). Recent unobtrusive studies of black and white discrimination and prejudice: A literature review. *Psychological Bulletin, 87,* 546–563.

Dovidio, J. F., & Gaertner, S. L. (1981). The effects of race, status, and ability on helping behavior. *Social Psychology Quarterly, 44,* 192–203.

Federle, K. H., & Chesney-Lind, M. (1992). Special issues in juvenile justice: Gender, race, and ethnicity. In I. M. Schwartz (Ed.), *Juvenile justice and public policy: Toward a national agenda* (pp. 165–195). New York: Lexington.

Frey, D. L., & Gaertner, S. (1986). Helping and the avoidance of inappropriate interracial behavior: A strategy that perpetuates a nonprejudiced self-image. *Journal of Personality and Social Psychology, 50,* 1083–1090.

Goodman, E. (1995a, March 3). Gramm pushes his pro-kid line. *Arizona Republic,* p. B15.

Goodman, E. (1995b, January 2). Men: "We ARE angry!" *Charlotte Observer,* p. 9A.

Lewit, E. M., & Baker, L. G. (1994). Race and ethnicity: Changes for children. *Future of Children, 4* (3), 134–144.

Lindsey, D. (1994). *The welfare of children.* New York: Oxford University Press.

McConahay, J. B. (1983). Modern racism and modern discrimination: The effects of race, racial attitudes, and context on simulated hiring decisions. *Personality and Social Psychology Bulletin, 9,* 551–558.

Melton, G. B. (1992). *Foreign innovation and dispute resolutions in matters related to juvenile justice and child protection.* Report to the Judicial Council of California, 20/20 Vision Project Committee on Family Relations.

Melton, G. B. (1993a). Children, families, and the courts in the twenty-first century. *Southern California Law Review, 66,* 1993–2047.

Melton, G. B. (1993b). Is there a place for children in the new world order? *Notre Dame Journal of Law, Ethics, and Public Policy, 7,* 491–532.

Melton, G. B. (1995, March). *Beyond symbolism: Family policy for a renaissance.* Roberta A. Morris Memorial Lecture presented at the University of Nebraska–Lincoln.

Putnam, R. D. (1995a). Bowling alone: America's declining social capital. *Journal of Democracy, 6* (1), 65–78.

Putnam, R. (1995b). Bowling alone, revisited. *Responsive Community, 5* (2), 18–33.

U.S. Advisory Board on Child Abuse and Neglect. (1993). *Neighbors helping neighbors: A new national strategy for the protection of children.* Washington DC: U.S. Government Printing Office.

Preface

Ruby Takanishi and Elena O. Nightingale

In the year 2020, one third of the nation's new workers is projected to be youth from ethnic minorities (Quality Education For Minorities Project, 1990). Their physical and mental health will be critical to our country's social and economic well-being. This workforce is likely to be smaller overall, and minority workers are also likely to be in poor health and inadequately educated if we continue on our present course. Nonetheless, all these workers will be called on to support the health care and Social Security costs of a larger, vulnerable, and elderly population (Hayes-Bautista, Schink, & Chapa, 1988). At the same time, the United States will find itself competing among several equals in a global economy. This convergence of factors—an aging population and changed economic conditions—requires our urgent attention to ensure that all minority adolescents become healthy, productive adults.

Yet the health status of minority adolescents is only beginning to receive the serious attention it deserves. When thirty-seven members of the U.S. Congress asked that its nonpartisan Office of Technology Assessment (OTA) report to them about the health status and needs of American adolescents, a major part of that request was for a strong focus on the health of ethnic-minority adolescents. Indeed, one of the first papers released during the course of the OTA study documented the unmet mental-health needs of American Indian adolescents (U.S. Congress, Office of Technology Assessment, 1990).

As a collaborator in the OTA study, Carnegie Corporation of New York continued its tradition of commitment to the education and healthy development of all children and youth, especially those from poor and from minority families. Thus, OTA commissioned, and Carnegie Corporation supported, the preparation of seven papers synthesizing what is currently known about the health of adolescents from different minority groups and about effective approaches to enhancing their health. A workshop on issues related to the delivery of health services to minority adolescents was also held during the course of the OTA study.

This volume brings together many of these papers on the health of minority adolescents from different ethnic-minority groups. Together they point to unevenness in the knowledge base about health status and the factors that enhance healthy development in each group. For some ethnic-minority groups, specifically Asian-Americans and Latinos, our knowledge base is extremely sparse. For other groups, such as African-Americans, more progress has been made. Even in those cases for which reasonably reliable health statistics exist, we lack tested explanations for observed differences. In the absence of knowledge about contributing factors, health indicators become associated with ethnicity and, regardless of the problem, are often implicated in assigning blame to the individual or group.

We fully recognize that the health needs of adolescents cannot wait for definitive studies. Thus, we believe it is worthwhile to share these papers widely. They synthesize the current knowledge about healthy development and will be an important resource for professional practice and policy development. Together they constitute and are being used as starting points for further research that can better inform approaches to health promotion and disease prevention among adolescents from understudied ethnic-minority backgrounds.

Much has been said about the "unique needs" of adolescents from ethnic-minority groups. The current wisdom is that "generic" approaches and interventions must be modified to account for these differences. While acknowledging the diversity within and among the groups, we should not fail to recognize that there are common goals for healthy development. We want all adolescents to be sound of body and mind, to be free of abuse of drugs, alcohol, tobacco, and other substances, to deal with sexual issues with knowledge and maturity, to learn about health risks, and to protect themselves from intentional and unintentional injuries, including those from violence. Unfortunately, the pathways to such good outcomes—whether genetic, cultural, economic, gender related, environmental, or in some combination—remain elusive.

The incompleteness of our knowledge about the healthy development of ethnic-minority adolescents can lead to erroneous assumptions and possibly damaging neglect. Even on the prevalence of certain health problems, we lack basic information on variations among ethnic groups (Elliott & Feldman, 1990). For example, eating disorders are commonly thought to be a condition found almost solely among middle- and upper-class White adolescent girls. However, in one study African-American low-income adolescents also report eating disorders that require attention (Balentine et al., 1991). This example points to the importance of skepticism toward widely held assumptions, elevated to "facts," in the absence of good information about both strengths and problems among adolescents from different ethnic groups.

Several highly encouraging federal initiatives in research and intervention for adolescent health are being launched by the National Institutes of Health (NIH), specifically to agencies including the National Institute of Mental Health (NIMH), the National Institute for Child Health and Human Development (NICHD), and the National Institute for Nursing Research (NINR). These initiatives were partially stimulated by the OTA study, which highlighted the neglect of research on adolescent health, as well as by congressional concern, augmented by the OTA report, about ways to improve health among minority adolescents.

In 1991, the NIH awarded initial grants to establish centers on adolescent health research focused on understanding the factors related to a variety of adolescent health problems, as a basis for planning interventions on a sound scientific foundation. In 1992, the NICHD launched initiatives on understanding normal development among minority adolescents and on research and evaluation of prevention and treatment interventions for minority adolescents. The NINR supported another initiative on adolescent health promotion, building on a Carnegie Corporation volume on that subject (Millstein, Petersen, & Nightingale, 1993). — Text - I have copied.

The OTA staff, particularly Denise Dougherty, the project director for the study *Adolescent Health*, deserves our profound appreciation for overseeing the publication of that three-volume study (U.S. Congress, Office of Technology Assessment, 1991a, 1991b, 1991c). As a result of the OTA study, Congress passed legislation to establish an Office of Adolescent Health within the U.S. Department of Health and Human Services (U.S. Congress, House of Representatives, 1992). These legislative and federal agency activities are highly encouraging for placing the health of minority adolescents higher on the national agenda.

Adolescent Health provided the first broad, national examination of the health status, needs, and approaches to prevention and treatment of health problems during the adolescent years (U.S. Congress, Office of Technology Assessment, 1991a, 1991b, 1991c). It will remain a valuable resource for many years to come. However, the OTA was unable to distribute every commissioned paper, another key resource for professionals and researchers. In response, the Carnegie Council on Adolescent Development assisted in the distribution of a paper on legal and ethical issues in decisions about health care by adolescents (Gittler, Quigley-Rick, & Saks, 1990). We are most grateful to Marjorie Kagawa-Singer, Phyllis Katz, Dalmas Taylor, and Judith Vanderryn for taking on the considerable task of editing this group of commissioned papers on the health of ethnic-minority adolescents. Kagawa-Singer and Nancy Anderson provide an integrative chapter on cross-cutting issues in the delivery of services to such adolescents. This volume makes a much-needed contribution to a crucial area in which some progress in knowledge building and professional practice is beginning.

All American adolescents are at risk of damaging their health now or of establishing patterns of behavior that will adversely affect their adult years (Hamburg, 1992). All indications are that minority adolescents are at greater risk, because of their ethnic-minority status and disproportionate representation in poor socioeconomic circumstances. The precise contributions of ethnicity, education, and social class, independently and in concert, remain controversial and unknown. We hope this volume will contribute to the improvement of the quality of the health services that minority adolescents experience and to the enhancement of our knowledge about creating conditions that result in better health for all of them. Their future health and well-being, and ours, are crucially linked.

References

Balentine, M., Stitt, K., Bonner, J., & Clark, L. (1991). Self-reported eating disorders of black, low-income adolescents: Behavior, body weight perceptions, and methods of dieting. *Journal of School Health, 61*, 392–396.

Elliott, G. R., & Feldman, S. S. (1990). Capturing the adolescent experience. In G. R. Elliott & S. S. Feldman (Eds.), *At the threshold: The developing adolescent* (pp. 1–13). Cambridge: Harvard University Press.

Gittler, J., Quigley-Rick, M., & Saks, M. J. (1990). *Adolescent health care decision making: The law and public policy*. Washington DC: Carnegie Council on Adolescent Development.

Hamburg, D. A. (1992). *Today's children: Creating a future for a generation in crisis*. New York: Times.

Hayes-Bautista, D. E., Schink, W. O., & Chapa, J. (1988). *The burden of support: Young Latinos in an aging society*. Stanford, CA: Stanford University Press.

Millstein, S. G., Petersen, A. C., & Nightingale, E. O. (Eds.). (1993). *Promoting the health of adolescents: New directions for the twenty-first century*. New York: Oxford University Press.

Quality Education for Minorities Project (1990). *Education that works: An action plan for the education of minorities*. Cambridge MA: Quality Education for Minorities Project.

U.S. Congress, House of Representatives (1992, October). *Preventive health amendments of 1992*. (Conference Report No. 102-1019). Washington DC: U.S. House of Representatives.

U.S. Congress, Office of Technology Assessment (1990). *Indian adolescent mental health*. (OTA-H-446). Washington DC: U.S. Government Printing Office.

U.S. Congress, Office of Technology Assessment (1991a). *Adolescent health—Volume I: Summary and policy options*. (OTA-H-468). Washington DC: U.S. Government Printing Office.

U.S. Congress, Office of Technology Assessment (1991b). *Adolescent health—Volume II: Background and the effectiveness of selected prevention and treatment services*. (OTA-H-466). Washington DC: U.S. Government Printing Office.

U.S. Congress, Office of Technology Assessment (1991c). *Adolescent health—Volume III: Cross-cutting issues in the delivery of health and related services* (OTA-H-467). Washington DC: U.S. Government Printing Office.

Introduction

Marjorie Kagawa-Singer

The overall adolescent population in the United States has grown rapidly over the past fifteen years, and within this group, the percentage of racial and ethnic minorities is increasing. By 1995, a third of U.S. students will be from minority groups, and such students will make up a majority of high school graduates in Hawaii, New Mexico, California, Mississippi, and the District of Columbia. Yet compared with those of children, adults, and the geriatric population, the health needs of adolescents in the United States have received relatively little attention.

Growing evidence indicates that the health problems of U.S. adolescents have reached critical levels, particularly with regard to ethnic-minority youth who have little access to appropriate health care. Available evidence suggests that roughly 5.3 million adolescents live in poverty and that 9 million Black, Latino, Asian, Native American, and other marginalized racial/ethnic-minority adolescents are at a disproportionately high risk for some health problems and experience these health problems at disproportionate rates. Unfortunately, many adolescents are without health insurance or must deal with health care providers who are incompetent and unwilling to treat adolescents or with unreasonable legal requirements for parental consent or notification. Poor and ethnic-minority adolescents, moreover, confront other barriers (e.g., financial, cultural, linguistic) that go beyond what most other U.S. adolescents (face Bergeison, 1989; Liu & Yu, 1985; Miike, 1989; Ooms & Herendeen, 1990).

This volume is the first effort to collate and synthesize the theoretical and programmatic knowledge currently available on the health needs of poor and ethnic-minority adolescents. Information herein provides a base from which researchers, health professionals, program planners, and policy-makers can assess the effectiveness of existing health programs and identify areas for future development. We also hope that physicians, nurses, psychologists, social workers, teachers, and counselors who work daily with adolescents will find this information useful.

Each of the chapters in this volume documents the health status of specific adolescent populations and addresses barriers to optimal health care. The first chapter in this sequence discusses the effect of poverty as a major health-risk factor. The next five chapters describe health issues associated with specific ethnic group aggregates: Black, Latino, American Indians, Asian and Pacific Islanders, and Native Hawaiians. Each chapter provides data covering the following areas: statistics and demographics of the population described; prevalence of physical, mental/emotional, and social health problems; strengths and buffering effects of ethnic identity; potential or documented areas of conflict with dominant, middle-class cultural values and behaviors; consideration of how the combined effects of socio-economic and cultural influences can be analyzed to address the above-mentioned problems; identification and description of successful programs that meet the needs of the identified groups; and recommendations and implications for program development, evaluation, and research within each community and within the federal government.

The last two chapters provide a general overview for adolescent health. Chapter eight gives a current description of the many federal agencies that allot funds for adolescents—often at cross-purposes—and a picture of the bureaucracy that community groups and state and local agencies must navigate to provide health services, thus clearly documenting the overlap and competition among federally funded agencies and programs.

The final chapter summarizes the volume and recasts adolescence and ethnicity within a cross-cultural framework. Adolescent minority health programs often suffer from a "deficit theory" mentality of assistance, which overlooks and/or misunderstands the support and strength available in a multicultural society. Each culture sets rules that enable its youth to enter their adult roles successfully. But ethnic-minority youth are often forced to choose, at a personal cost, between their ethnic values and those of the dominant White Euro-American ethos. This chapter suggests that such choices may not be necessary. Supporting individual cultural affinities might be more effective than acquiescing to monocultural demands, and such a course would foster a positive transition to adulthood with respect and honor for one's own heritage and that of others in our ever-growing multicultural society.

Before we can design strategies to solve the problems of adolescent health, we must first adequately define them. It cannot be stressed strongly enough that all the authors in this volume had considerable difficulty in obtaining statistics that would document the empirical picture of the problems adolescents experience in dysfunctional situations.

Ages designated in data sources as "adolescent" vary considerably, if they are noted at all, and even gender classification was missing from many of the data sources. Comparison across databases becomes problematic with these omissions. The error of misclassification of ethnicity also compounded the issue of measurement. For example, in the National Health Interview Survey, 32.2% of self-reported Asians and 70% of self-reported American Indians were classified as "White" or "Black" by interviewers (Hahn, 1992).

Often in national registries, such as the Surveillance, Epidemiology and End Results (SEER) program of the National Cancer Institute, data are collected regionally and then generalized to national populations. This method creates several problems, exemplified by interpretation of data on Native Americans from the SEER. Native American data are collected from New Mexico. Most American Indians live elsewhere, however, and this population consists of more than 500 tribes, each with its own culture. Tribes in the Southwest are not representative of the American Indian population in the entire United States. In other registry data in individual states, the error rate in classification of American Indians is unacceptable (ranging from less than 10% to 100%; Burhansstipanov & Dressler, 1993). The person filling in the form classifies the individual by surname, and many American Indians with Spanish surnames are classified as Hispanic. Without accurate baseline data, it is difficult to document the extent of problems in specific minority groups or to evaluate the actual outcomes of demonstration projects or new federal programs. Kemp and Dougherty's chapter (in this volume) highlights this obstacle to accurate evaluation.

Two additional areas that must be addressed in designing any future adolescent health research are gender differences and the interdependence of socioeconomic factors and culture. Gender socialization has a major effect on identity formation and may create special problems for ethnic-minority youth as Amaro, Messinger, and Cervantes's chapter (in this volume) on Latino youth shows. Each culture prescribes different coping strategies and sanctions different modes of expressing distress for males and females (Chung & Kagawa-Singer, 1994). The literature on gender issues for adolescents is growing and is covered in depth elsewhere (see Russo, 1990; Wyatt, 1991).

The synergistic effects of social class and ethnicity on identity formation and behavior modeling are inextricably entwined. The effects of ethnicity and social status on attitudes and health behaviors form the whole environment in which an adolescent lives, and one aspect cannot be extricated from the other. Thus, ethnicity must be seen as a marker of behaviors and beliefs within a social context and not as a risk factor in and of itself.

The forces of social class and ethnicity inform the viewer's perception of issues as well. The behavior and perception of the viewer is formed and constrained by his or her own cultural lens. The refraction of this lens is formed according to learned, culturally molded beliefs and attitudes.

Attention to the interaction of gender, ethnicity, and social class must be included in any future study of minority adolescent health to inform accurately both the design of the study and the validity of its findings. Identifying the unique contribution of social class and ethnicity on attitudes and behavior is at the present one of the primary conundrums of researchers on minority health. Study of the multidimensional reality created by the cultural paradigm described in the last chapter of this volume requires a fundamental restructuring of research designs. Funding agencies and review panels attempting to meet the needs of minority adolescents will have to become more informed about these requirements if effective programs are to be developed.

Aside from its negative consequences, adolescence, as stated at the outset, has received relatively little research or service interest as a discreet developmental stage of life. Yet this period of life harbors great strengths: abstract thinking, idealism, energy, and unbridled enthusiasm (Konner, 1991). The adolescent's impassioned embrace of causes and ideals beyond the limited self appears to be a cross-cultural universal. Historically, young people have played a key role in rebellions and revolutions, not just because they naively accept radical theories but also because developmentally, as late adolescents, they are fiercely idealistic and unconventional.

Most cultures form, channel, and mold this high energy and enthusiasm in its youth, preparing them to assume adult responsibilities. If the youth assumes the adult role, each culture supplies in exchange the three basic needs of life: a sense of security, self-worth, and belonging (Kagawa-Singer, 1994). Security entails physical safety, food, and shelter. Self-worth gives a sense of importance and value; and belonging is having the sense of being an integral, productive, and contributing member of one's social group. When adolescents fulfill a needed and valued position within their social network of family, kin, and friends, they find security and self-worth and learn they are not alone, not useless or powerless (Carnegie Commission, 1989; Doi, 1985; Weisman, 1984). Each culture defines the ideal individual within its reality (Heelas & Lock, 1981). When an individual is faced with membership in two or more cultures, portions of these identities may overlap, but there will also be areas of conflict. Moreover, if the individual feels that he or she must make an either/or choice in identity, too often the resulting psychological and social state is one of rejection, embarrassment, or both.

Belonging is essential to human health. Previous studies on infants and young children have shown a "failure to thrive" in physical and mental development without physical and psychological nurturance (Droter, 1991; Phelps, 1991). More recent gerontology work indicates similar needs for the elderly (Berkman, Foster, & Campion, 1989); high death rates occur when elderly are placed in nursing homes, compared with rates when the individual remains at home. Even caring for pets by the residents seems to ameliorate the ill effects of a lack of loving physical contact (Netting, Wilson, & New, 1987).

Human beings are motivated to develop behaviors that ensure they will have security, self-worth, and belonging, and human groups have used culture to provide the sanctioned and meaningful ways to meet these needs. Even the most simplistic cost-benefit analysis indicates that preparatory behavior requiring sacrifices for a nebulous or negative future is not cost-effective (Johnson, 1978). Ethnic-minority and poor youth who see their options limited in this society may harbor a reluctance to accept the responsibilities of adulthood. Too often, the energy of adolescence is dissipated by a lack of hope and turned instead into rage and despair. As one youth stated, "I'm only waiting to die or get locked up"; sadly, this youth's attitude is becoming more common in the inner cities (Boyle, 1991;

do AA & A have more fatalistic view of the future?

Tuckson, 1993). Self-destructive behaviors, including drug use, may be relatively rational reflections of a need for immediate gratification or for escape from fears and anxieties created by limited visions of a future and a sense of powerlessness to change that reality.

This despair over the future may also be expressed by an indifference to self-care. Preventive health practices hold little relevance when survival is precarious. Distressingly, when inner-city youth were asked the question, "How long do you think you'll live?" the mean response was 19 (Boyle, 1991; Kessler, 1990). Black mothers of Head Start children in a program in the South Central section of Los Angeles were identified as practicing few preventive health behaviors for themselves or their children. When asked how many had lost a family member to violence in the last two years, 25% of them raised their hands (Sanders-Phillips, 1989). The problem is growing.

Unless social forces or environmental conditions are addressed, the despair registered by these youth pose an almost-insurmountable barrier to preventive health practices (Palank, 1991). Programs directed toward dental health, prenatal care, or safe-sex practices have little relevance to their lives and subsequently little effect on actual behavior.

The authors of this volume call for a new paradigm, one that will enable youth to value the strengths of their ethnic identities and synthesize them with strengths of the Euro-American society rather than degrade one or the other. This paradigm shift entails moving from a monocultural to a multicultural base for U.S. society.

The authors of this volume identified six recommendations to promote quality health-care delivery for ethnic teenagers. First, adolescence must be recognized as a discreet developmental period with unique health needs. As noted by Taylor and Katz (in this volume), risk behaviors, like all learned behaviors, are not random (Jessor, 1984). They are purposive and goal directed and fulfill multiple goals. We must understand adolescents' motivations if we are to design more effective and relevant prevention and treatment programs.

Second, more health research must be conducted on adolescents in general and on minority adolescents in particular to discover the determinants of negative physical- and mental-health behaviors and to identify those cultural values and behavioral patterns that promote or mitigate these negative behaviors.

Third, researchers and providers must appreciate the tremendous differences that exist both between and within the broad racial categories. As is shown in several chapters in this volume, intragroup and individual differences often exceed between-group differences, and researchers and providers must be educated to assess and incorporate these differences into their work.

Fourth, affordable and accessible services should be provided by bilingual and bicultural staff who are trained and skilled in working with adolescents. Community health workers from the ethnic groups involved should be paid at salary levels competitive enough to attract these providers.

Fifth, establishing culturally responsive, multiservice centers that would provide a variety of physical- and mental-health and social services may improve utilization and effectiveness of care. For example, the school-based clinic is one successful model cited by each author to provide ambulatory care to the adolescent population. In 1991, the Office of Technology Assessment, through the adolescent-health study from which these papers emanated, found that school-based health centers would be the best approach to overcome the barriers to health care that adolescents face (U.S. Congress, Office of Technology Assessments, 1991a, 1991b, 1991c). Some proponents of school-based clinics also recommend linking these clinics to community health centers, local hospitals, and health agencies to ensure the comprehensiveness of the program, provide services to adolescents not in school, and make available evening, weekend, and school-holiday coverage.

The sixth and last recommendation is for aggressive efforts to develop prevention and education programs targeted at adolescents to promote health practices and knowledge of health problems and their consequences. These services should be made available, culturally appropriate, congruent, and responsive to the specific group being addressed.

Each chapter stresses that the challenge to everyone who works with the youth of America is to transform the present infrastructure of health-care services for adolescents into one that truly respects and incorporates the richness within the diversity of our youth and within the currently isolated efforts of many good programs. Adolescents will soon be adults. Unless they desire and are prepared to assume the privileges and responsibilities of adulthood, the problems of homelessness, joblessness, self-destructive behavior, and emotional distress will continue on their present course. The adolescent period constitutes a critical time for educators, researchers, and policymakers to make a difference.

The authors in this volume are all knowledgeable researchers and practitioners in minority adolescent health and bring a wealth of expertise and experience to their chapters. This book should be a valuable addition for adolescent health-care professionals, teachers, researchers, and program planners at the local, state, and federal levels. It documents the multifaceted aspects of teenage health. It recasts the stage of adolescence within a cultural context that clearly stresses the necessity to coordinate existing programs and to use and to create, through a holistic, integrated, multifaceted perspective, innovative programs that would support our youth during their adolescence.

Practitioners are currently hampered by an inability to attend to the contextual nature of ethnic-minority health problems. Funding and personnel are limited to efforts focusing on single problems with less attention paid to the total lifestyle and milieu of these teens (Palank, 1991). Thus, their efforts are too often predestined to be inadequate. Discussion of these key variables should provide needed information for policymakers and developers of health programs for adolescents to reduce teenage morbidity and mortality and increase the number of adolescents who will become competent and productive citizens of our society. For the survival of our nation, it is imperative that we address these issues now.

References

Bergeison, L. (1989, December). *Physical health of Indian adolescents.* Contract paper prepared for the Office of Technology Assessment, U.S. Congress, Washington DC.

Berkman, B., Foster, L. W., & Campion, E. (1989). Failure to thrive: Paradigm for the frail elder. *Gerontologist, 29* (5), 654–659.

Boyle, G. J. (1991, November 19) Waiting to die or get locked up. *Los Angeles Times.*

Burhansstipanov, L., & Dressler, C. M. (1993). *Native American monograph no.1: Documentation of the cancer research needs of American Indians and Alaska Natives.* National Cancer Institute. NIH Publication No.93-3603.

Carnegie Commission (1989, June). *Turning points: Preparing youth for the 21st century.*

Chung, R.-C. Y., & Kagawa-Singer, M. (1995). Gender differences in symptom presentation. (Submitted).

Doi, T. (1985). *The anatomy of self: The individual versus society*. Tokyo: Kodansha International.

Droter, D. (1991). The family context of nonorganic failure to thrive. *American Journal of Orthopsychiatry, 61* (1), 23–34.

Hahn, R. A. (1992). The state of federal health statistics on racial and ethnic groups. *JAMA, 267* (2), 270.

Heelas, P., & Lock, A. (1981). *Indigenous psychologies: The anthropology of the self*. London: Academic Press.

Jessor, R. (1984). *Adolescent problem drinking: Psychological aspects and developmental outcomes*. Paper presented at the meeting of the Carnegie Conference on Unhealthful Risk-Taking Behavior Among Adolescents. Stanford, California.

Johnson, A. W. (1978). *Quantification in cultural anthropology: An introduction to research design* (pp. 141–157). Stanford CA: Stanford University Press.

Kagawa-Singer, M. (1994). *Cross-cultural concepts of quality of life*. Unpublished manuscript.

Kessler, S. (1990). The mysteries program: Educating adolescents for today's world. *Holistic Education, 3* (4), 10–19.

Konner, M. (1991). *Childhood*. Boston: Little, Brown.

Liu, W. T., & Yu, E. S. H. (1985). Ethnicity, mental health, and the urban delivery system. In J. W. Moore & L. W. Moldonado (Eds.), *Urban ethnicity in the United States: New immigrants and old minorities* (pp. 211–247). Beverly Hills CA: Sage.

Miike, L. (1989). *Health and related services for Native Hawaiian adolescents*. Contract paper prepared for the Office of Technology Assessment, U.S. Congress, Washington DC.

Netting, F. E., Wilson, C. C., & New, J. C. (1987). The human-animal bond: Implications for practice. *Social Work, 32* (1), 60–64.

Ooms, T., & Herendeen, T. O. (1990, July 20). *Evolving state policies on teen pregnancy and parenthood: What more can the Feds do to help?* Background briefing report of the Family Impact Seminar, sponsored by the American Association for Marriage and Family Therapy Research and Education Foundation, Washington DC.

Palank, C. L. (1991). Determinants of health-promotive behavior. A review of current research. *Nursing Clinics of North America, 26* (4), 815–832.

Phelps, L. (1991). Non-organic failure-to-thrive: Origins and psychoeducational implications. *School Psychology Review 20* (3), 417–427.

Russo, N. F. (1990). Overview: Forging research priorities for women's mental health. *American Psychologist, 45* (3), 368–373.

Sanders-Phillips, K. (1989). Lecture in Human Response to Illness course, University of California Los Angeles School of Nursing.

Tuckson, R. V. (1993). Keynote. *Cancer, ethnicity, and caring.* Fourth Cancer Patient Education Conference, National Cancer Institute, and the Five Southern California Comprehensive Cancer Centers, Pasadena, California. April 2–3.

U.S. Congress, Office of Technology Assessment (1991a). *Adolescent health. Volume 1: Summary and policy options.* (OTA-H-468). Washington DC: U.S. Government Printing Office.

U.S. Congress, Office of Technology Assessment (1991b). *Adolescent health. Volume 2: Background and the effectiveness of selected prevention and treatment services.* (OTA-H-466). Washington DC: U.S. Government Printing Office.

U.S. Congress, Office of Technology Assessment (1991c). *Adolescent health. Volume 3: Crosscutting issues in the delivery of health and related services.* (OTA-H-467). Washington DC: U.S. Government Printing Office.

Weisman, A. D. (1984). *The coping capacity.* New York: Human Sciences.

Wyatt, G. E. (1991). Examining ethnicity versus race in AIDS related sex research. *Social Science and Medicine, 33* (3), 37–45.

I

Poverty and Adolescent Health

LaRue Allen and Christina M. Mitchell

An adolescent lacking money in the United States is at increased risk for getting sick, having no medical care, and dying young (Miller & Coulter, 1984). Researchers have repeatedly documented a relation between economic hardship and aggregate measures of illness, both physical (Adler et al., 1994) and mental (Aldwin & Revenson, 1986). This chapter reviews the literature on the effects of poverty on adolescent health.

This review, however, is frustrated in several ways by the lack of adequate data. First, comparatively little attention is paid to adolescent health at all. Second, official statistical reports on health indicators vary in their definition of adolescence. Some reports combine ages 0–18; ages 15–19 from one agency can only be compared with ages 14–21 from another. Third, research on adolescents frequently ignores social class or uses race as a proxy for social class.

The Poverty Problem

DEFINITION OF POVERTY

The official poverty level is adjusted to family size and inflation but not to the increasing standard of living in the United States (Schiller, 1989) or to geographic differences in the cost of living. In 1992, the poverty threshold for a family of four was $14,335, compared with a median income of $44,615 for a family of the same size (U.S. Bureau of the Census, 1993a).

Poverty is categorized as "short-term," "persistent," or "underclass." Two thirds of poor children are in the short-term category, experiencing poverty for no more than four years over a fifteen-year period (U.S. Congress, Committee on Ways and Means, 1985). One poor child in seven, however, spends at least ten of fifteen years in poverty (i.e., persistently poor). About 90% of persistently poor children are Black, live in female-headed households, and are disproportionately from rural homes. Fewer than 9% of the poor children in 1980 were members of the "underclass" (Bane & Ellwood, 1989): a group characterized by low level of skills, long-term unemployment, deviant behavior, and residency in urban areas of highly concentrated poverty (Wilson, 1987).

CAUSES OF POVERTY

Since the 1940s, a number of social programs have been instituted to counteract the impact of sudden economic hardship or chronic unemployment. Many Americans believe that the "safety net" of such programs (such as Aid to Families with Dependent Children [AFDC], Medicaid, food stamps, and unemployment benefits) has solved the poverty problem in our country and that true poverty is rare. Many believe that the poor remain so because they lack the motivation or ability to improve themselves (W. T. Grant Foundation Commission on Work, Family and Citizenship, 1988).

In fact, large gaps exist in the safety net of support for poor families. For example, Moen (1983) found that many unemployed workers were ineligible for benefits either because they were in occupations not covered by such programs (e.g., domestic work) or because they had already used up their benefits through long-term unemployment. Fully half of all families with unemployed heads of household in 1975 received no income support from either AFDC or unemployment benefits.

The leading structural causes of poverty are differential educational opportunities and access to employment, wage structures, unemployment rates, retirement, and disability. Family structure is also a significant determinant of economic well-being (Ellwood, 1988). When poverty occurs within a two-parent family, it is relatively short-term. However, short-term poverty can become persistent when family stress and discord lead to increased numbers of high-risk, single-parent homes (Bane & Ellwood, 1989). In families with only one parent, usually the mother, earning potential is low, child-support payments from fathers are almost nonexistent, and benefits from public-assistance programs are meager (Garfinkel & McLanahan, 1986).

Measuring Adolescent Poverty

Although the number of poor adolescents is increasing (Blum, 1987), demographic and health statistics on the adolescent age group alone (i.e., ages 10–18) are, as previously noted, difficult to find. In 1974, children (birth–18 years old) surpassed the aged as the poorest group of U.S. citizens, with a continuing decline in economic conditions relative to all other age groups since then (U.S. Bureau of the Census, 1993b). Currently, one of every five children in the United States lives in families that earn less than the national poverty level (U.S. Bureau of the Census, 1989). In 1988, 8.27 million adolescents ages 10–18 were poor (i.e., living below the poverty level) or near poor (i.e., living in families with incomes between 100 and 149% of the poverty level; Dougherty & Kemp, in this volume).

Children in female-headed households were almost four times more likely to be poor (57%) than those with both a mother and father in the home (15.1%; U.S. Congress, Office of Technology Assessment, 1991c). Even with two working parents, Black children are still more likely to be poor than White children with only a father in the workforce (U.S. Congress, Committee on Ways and Means, 1985).

Fewer than half of all impoverished children live in urban areas: nearly 30% live in rural areas, and 28% live in suburban areas (Bane & Ellwood, 1989). Children's chances of being poor also vary by ethnicity: minority children are disproportionately represented among the poor. In 1986, for example, the rate of poverty for Black children increased three times as much as that of White children (Sandefur, 1988).

Poverty as a Construct in Research on Adolescent Behavior

The construct of poverty, or of socioeconomic status (SES) in general, has been ignored by and large in research on adolescent behaviors, despite its obvious and growing importance in the United States. Meuller and Parcel (1981) reported that, when SES is reported in the empirical literature, most researchers rely on "impressionistic criteria" (such as the apparent SES of the neighborhood or school) to indicate the construct. The official poverty level is rarely used. Furthermore, Mitchell et al. (1993) reviewed the literature on the etiology of adolescent delinquency and depression, noting that more than half of all studies reviewed reported no information on SES.

This glaring neglect may reflect problems in determining economic status. Measures such as the Hollingshead-Redlich four-factor index (Hollingshead, 1975) or indices of household prestige (Nock & Rossi, 1979) are too often designed for use with traditional family structures. Thus, guidance is difficult to find for determining SES in nontraditional families. Furthermore, many youths do not know the details of their family's economic situation. For example, a teenager may know that his or her mother works in a bank but not her title or income.

Research on the effects of poverty on health is hampered by the frequent failure to include this measure in health research. It should also be noted that this review reflects a common but as yet untested assumption throughout the literature, that problem and positive behaviors in adolescents are independent of each other (Mitchell et al., 1993). Individual categories of adolescent behaviors are thus treated as distinct; for example, depression is conceptualized separately from delinquency, substance abuse, or adolescent pregnancy.

Poverty and Health Problems of Adolescents

Children and adolescents living in poverty suffer negative health effects. Walker and her colleagues (Walker et al., 1982) asked youth in grades 9–12 in an inner-city high school about their health concerns and problems, health status, and utilization of health services. Poor adolescents had more health worries, greater desires for more help with problems such as headaches, and social problems such as racial discrimination and relationships with parents than did private-school students. Poor youth were most likely to seek help for dental problems, acne, and health worries; private-school youth ranked depression or sadness, tiredness, and acne highest. These findings corroborated an earlier triethnic study of youth in Galveston, Texas (Parcel, Nader, & Meyer, 1977).

NUTRITION

In the late 1960s and again in the 1980s, national attention focused on the relation between poverty and malnutrition for millions of Americans. Despite such help as the Supplemental Food Program for Women, Infants, and Children (WIC; Graham, 1985), malnutrition, obesity (Sullivan & Carter, 1985), and other dietary problems among poor adolescents and their families remain a pressing national problem.

In a sample of 9,000 socioeconomically disadvantaged children in Baltimore, there was a 33% prevalence of signs of malnutrition such as deficiency levels of vitamin A, carotene, total protein, and serum albumin (Hepner & Maiden, 1971). Adolescents ages 11–18 had the poorest nutrition of all age groups in several studies (Koh & Caples, 1979). Plots of various nutritional intake indices by age suggest that borderline nutritional status becomes overt malnutrition with the stress of rapid adolescent growth (U.S. Congress, Office of Technology Assessment, 1991b). Thus, adolescents might be at a greater risk for malnutrition if their SES dictated poor nutritional status as younger children.

Jones and colleagues (1985) analyzed data from the National Health and Nutrition Examination Surveys (HANES) I (1971–1975) and II (1976–1980) to examine the relation between poverty and child growth. Middle-income 12–17-year-olds were significantly taller and weighed more than poor youth. The differences between poor and nonpoor decreased over time. This change may be a reflection of the large increase in social programs that occurred between the two test periods. These included the quadrupling of enrollment in the food stamp program from HANES I to HANES II. Nonetheless, poor children remained smaller—a condition that may be a sign of increased risk for malnutrition.

DENTAL HEALTH

Data demonstrating socioeconomic differences in dental health for adolescents are hard to find. The percentages of adolescents receiving dental care increases with family income, even with no group differences in perception of the need to see a dentist (Nikias, Fink, & Shapiro, 1989). In 1988, 46 states and the District of Columbia reported that only 26% of Medicaid recipients under 18 had at least one dental service of some kind performed (American Dental Association, 1988). A recent study found that six of seven state Medicaid programs covered professionally applied topic fluoride as a dental benefit. State reporting practices preclude determining how many teenagers have used such preventive care (U.S. Congress, Office of Technology Assessment, 1991b).

UNINTENTIONAL INJURIES, VIOLENCE, SUICIDE, AND ABUSE

Injuries are the leading cause of death among adolescents (Blum, 1987). In 1987, unintentional injuries were responsible for more than half of all deaths to adolescents between ages 10 and 19 (U.S. Congress, Office of Technology Assessment, 1991b).

Unintentional Injuries

About 75% of the fatal injuries to adolescents are caused by automobile accidents (U.S. Congress, Office of Technology Assessment, 1991b). Fire and burn rates, another important cause of unintentional injury for this age group, were negatively related to a community's median family income. Finally, death rates due to accidental firearm injuries tend to be among the highest in poor areas and in rural areas (Paulson, 1988).

Intentional Injuries

Acts of violence that are meant to harm the self or others are a major cause of death and injury among adolescents. In a hospital population of 87,022 persons ages 0–19, intentional injuries accounted for 3.4% of all injuries. In this sample, the rate of intentional injury was directly related to the level of poverty in the victim's community (Guyer et al., 1989).

Homicide and assaults are the second leading cause of deaths among adolescents. Poverty and its correlates—including joblessness, family dysfunction, community disorganization, and density—are implicated as significant correlates of violent acts (Wilson, 1987). When one controls for SES, even the apparently dramatic differences in assaultive injuries among ethnic groups become less significant (Hammond & Yung, 1993).

Guns are a major factor in the rates of violence in urban communities. In 1989, guns were responsible for 81% of the homicides in which adolescents ages 15–19 were victims. Many youth are being shot by other youth. In a sample of high school youth, 4% had carried a gun during the previous month. Another survey of ten inner-city high schools in five cities revealed that 20% of the students had been threatened with a gun and 12% had actually been shot at (Sheley, McGee, & Wright, 1992). Clearly the prevention of gun-related crimes is a major public-health concern.

Suicide

Suicide is currently the third leading cause of death among adolescents, accounting for 14% of all deaths. In 1987, 5,121 of the 29,453 recorded suicides were by youth (Garland & Zigler, 1993). Among children between the ages of 5 and 14, as many as 12,000 may be hospitalized for self-injurious behavior. These numbers may in fact underrepresent the actual problem by a factor of two or three, given the widespread underreporting of the problem—whether for religious reasons, to protect life-insurance payments, or out of concern for the family (Garland & Zigler, 1993).

Adolescents who attempt suicide are likely to show one of several risk factors, all of which occur more often among socioeconomically disadvantaged youth. These include greater numbers of negative life events, fewer social supports, higher incidence of family violence (Pfeffer, 1989), greater incidence of running away from home, more unwanted pregnancies, and fewer personal resources for coping with a more stressful environment (Blumenthal, 1988). Mental-health and substance-abuse problems are also risk factors for adolescent suicide (U.S. Congress, Office of Technology Assessment, 1991b).

Living away from home in a correctional facility (Cantor, 1989) or group home is an additional risk factor more likely to occur among socioeconomically disadvantaged youth (American Academy of Pediatrics Committee on Adolescence, 1988). In a survey of 2,792 adolescents ages 13–18 who attended free clinics in ten large cities, severe poverty increased the risk of suicidal thoughts by a factor of two to three (Robins, 1989).

Abuse

Abuse of adolescents that results in physical or emotional injury is less likely to be reported to officials than is abuse of infants or children (Hampton & Newberger, 1985). Although reports of abuse of infants and young children tend to be concentrated among low-income groups and may be correlated with the stress of economic hardships, adolescent abuse may instead represent a failure in interpersonal relationships (Garbarino & Gilliam, 1980).

Families of adolescents suffering short-term abuse are more often middle income, more settled, and stable (Blum & Runyan, 1980). Conversely, the smaller proportion of adolescents suffering long-term abuse—abuse that begins in childhood and continues into adolescence—are more often from families of relative poverty, marital instability, and residential mobility (Galambos & Dixon, 1984).

ADOLESCENT SEXUALITY
Sexual Behavior

According to the National Survey of Family Growth, 15–19-year-olds are becoming sexually active at increasingly early ages (U.S. Congress, Office of Technology Assessment, 1991b). One third of males and 20% of females have had sexual intercourse before age 15 (Rickert, Jay, & Gottlieb, 1990).

An important question about sexuality and other health-risky behaviors is whether the correlates, precursors, and outcomes of a given behavior can

7

be anticipated. Data from the Chicago Woodlawn Project suggest that peers are an important influence on sexual activity. Students were more likely to have intercourse when they were in a homogenous peer group that is sexually active (Furstenberg et al., 1987).

Moreover, follow-up interviews with youth from the Woodlawn Project revealed that, among low-income Black males, those involved in substance abuse, assault, and sexual activity differed little from those males involved only in sexual activity. For girls, however, developmental antecedents for the sex-only females were distinct from those of the no-problem females. They came from families characterized by teenage motherhood and low maternal education with backgrounds that were limited in the opportunities that may provide alternatives to early childbearing. Thus, sexual activity that does not co-occur with other risky behaviors seems to have a different meaning for males and females, perhaps consistent with the societal view that premarital sexual activity is forbidden to females but more acceptable for males. Adolescents were also more likely to engage in sexual intercourse as population density increased (Franklin, 1988).

These contextual variables are more likely to exist among the poor. Poor adolescents are more likely to initiate sexual activity at an early age. Some have argued that adolescents' anticipated or aspired-to social class is more predictive of their pattern of sexual behavior than their parents' social class (U.S. Congress, Office of Technology Assessment, 1991b) while others have argued for the importance of both factors (Scott-Jones & White, 1990).

Sexual abuse during childhood and adolescence may also shed light on gender differences. For instance, both Black and White women who report sexual abuse involving contact (e.g., fondling) engaged in high-risk sexual behavior at an earlier age (Wyatt, 1988, 1989). Moreover, a large proportion of pregnancies in these young adolescent girls were the result of sexual abuse as well (Wyatt, 1988, 1989).

Pregnancy

In 1990, births to teenage mothers were 12.8% of all births. Overall, 40% of Whites and 60% of Blacks become pregnant at least once by age 20 (National Center for Health Statistics, 1993). Poverty and teen pregnancy are inextricably intertwined. Adolescent parenthood triggers a series of related events that heighten a new family's likelihood of being poor: greater medical risks during pregnancy; increases in single parenthood; inadequate child support from an absent father; larger family size; truncated education; lower lifetime earnings; and welfare dependency (Hogan, Astone, & Kitagawa, 1985; U.S. Congress, Committee on Ways and Means, 1985). Not only does becoming an adolescent parent heighten a woman's chances of being poor, but being poor is related to a heightened likelihood of becoming pregnant as a teenager (Franklin, 1988).

CONTRACEPTION

Parental social class is positively correlated with use of contraception for both Black and White females, although Blacks are generally less likely to use contraception during their first experience with sex (U.S. Congress, Office of Technology Assessment, 1991b; Taylor & Katz, in this volume). Social class, however, does not appear to explain differences in contraceptive use among Latinos, in contrast to Blacks and Whites (Amaro, Messinger, & Cervantes, in this volume).

Sexually Transmitted Diseases

The prevalence of sexually transmitted diseases (STDs) among adolescents appears quite low compared with older age groups. However, when prevalence is computed as the percentage of sexually active adolescents with STDs, 15–19-year-olds exhibit the highest rates of STDs (such as gonorrhea and syphilis) as well as the highest rates of hospitalization for pelvic inflammatory disease (Brooks-Gunn, Boyer, & Hein, 1988). The most prevalent STD for all ages, chlamydia infection, is most common among youth ages 15–19 years (Rickert et al., 1990). It is estimated that one quarter of all adolescents will contract an STD other than AIDS before graduating from high school.

The most life-threatening STD is AIDS. Currently, the number of cases of AIDS in adolescents ages 13–21 is low (percentage of all reported cases); these numbers, however, have been doubling annually (Brooks-Gunn et al., 1988). In fact, adolescents and young adults make up one of the fastest-growing categories of AIDS cases (Walter & Vaughan, 1993), and AIDS has become the sixth leading cause of death for 15–24-year-olds (U.S. Congress, Office of Technology Assessment, 1991b). One can infer from both the long incubation period of the disease and the high rates found among young adults that many initial HIV infections actually occur during adolescence (Slap et al., 1991).

Adolescents, like adults, acquire AIDS through exchange of bodily fluids with an infected person, contact with contaminated blood products, and

9

intravenous drug use (Millstein & Litt, 1990). Thirty percent of adolescents contract the disease through homosexual contact, compared with 60% for adults. Intravenous drug use accounts for 16% of adolescent cases and 28% among adults. Adolescents with hemophilia have an inordinate rate of infection (30.6%) compared with adults (0.8%).

Runaways and homeless teens, among the poorest groups, have extraordinarily high levels of HIV infection compared with other adolescents. Estimates range from an overall of 3.4% (U.S. Congress, Office of Technology Assessment, 1991b) to 5.3% in New York City and 8.2% in San Francisco (Rotheram-Borus et al., 1991). The reported occurrences of all STDs are highest for persons of lowest SES; occurrence is higher for those in urban settings than for those living in suburban or rural areas and is much higher for Blacks and Latinos than for other groups (Holmes, Karon, & Kreiss, 1990). A number of phenomena in inner-city indigent populations may also interact to accelerate transmission in these areas: prostitution and early onset of sexual intercourse; unsafe practices involving intravenous drug use; and increasing use of drugs such as crack cocaine that promote high-risk sexual behavior and the exchange of sex for drugs (Holmes et al., 1990). An indirect effect of poverty can be hypothesized by the greater proportion of HIV-infected teens who are members of racial/ethnic-minority groups.

In Boston and San Francisco, ethnicity was an important predictor of knowledge about AIDS among adolescents: a greater percentage of Whites than Blacks and Latinos were aware that the virus is not casually transmitted (Strunin, 1991). In Chicago, however, both Whites and Blacks were more knowledgeable than Latinos. In this study, 90% of Blacks, 92% of Latinos, but only 28% of Whites indicated concern about contracting the virus. More Black and Latino adolescents reported having changed their sexual and contraceptive behaviors to prevent infection, but most were still not using effective methods. The dearth of safe-sex behavior among adolescents constitutes an urgent public-health concern.

MENTAL HEALTH
General Rates of Mental Disorder
The relation between low social class and higher rates of mental disorder in adults is one of the most firmly established findings in psychiatric epidemiology (Allen & Britt, 1983). Substantial differences also occur in where,

how, and how long treatment is provided to members of different social classes (Hollingshead & Redlich, 1958).

Epidemiological data replicating this relation among youth are scarce. Because of the lack of consensus regarding the definition of youth disorders (Bromet & Schulberg, 1989), researchers and diagnosticians experience difficulty in distinguishing transient, developmentally appropriate changes in behavior from clinical disorders that warrant treatment (Allen & Majidi-Ahi, 1989). Furthermore, the sheer amount of research attention devoted to adolescent disorders is far less than that spent on adults or children (Kazdin, 1993).

In a review of thirty-five studies of the epidemiology of childhood psychopathology, Gould, Wunsch-Hitzig, and Dohrenwend (1981) found that studies in poor, Black, urban communities reported the highest rates of disorder. Costello (1989) also found that low SES was consistently related to a greater likelihood of having mental-health problems, reporting overall prevalence rates ranging from 17.6% to 25% in samples of adolescents. Epidemiological studies report that the most common disorders are attention deficit disorder, oppositional defiant disorder, conduct disorder, and separation anxiety disorder (Costello, 1989). Similarly, parents of socioeconomically disadvantaged 13–18-year-olds in a different study complained of school grades, attendance, and household behavior problems such as fighting with siblings, in descending order of frequency (Hawley et al., 1984).

Single-parent families, which are more likely to be poorer, reported three times the number of behavioral problems as did two-parent families (Wilson, 1987). Adolescents from families with low incomes also have higher rates of depressive moods (Wells, Deykin, & Klerman, 1985). Depression during adolescence has been of special interest in recent years because of the rapid increase in the rates of adolescent self-injury and suicide, which may be related to depression. An estimated 15% of patients with a severe depressive disorder of at least one month's duration commit suicide.

Substance Use and Abuse

Many Americans believe that families of lower SES produce a disproportionate share of substance-using youth (Fawzy et al., 1987). One explanation—that of social adjustment—is that the use of illegal substances reflects an adolescent's problems in dealing with the pressures of daily life

(Dembo et al., 1979). Thus, it is believed that adolescents living in poverty attempt to compensate for the deficiencies accompanying poverty by using or abusing both licit and illicit substances (Fawzy et al., 1987).

A second explanation—a social-crisis perspective—holds that, in settings in which teens experience few opportunities for legitimate access to goals, variations in substance use can be explained primarily by differences in social class. Issues such as the cost and availability of particular drugs, current popularity of drug usage, and socialization of drug use are critical in understanding substance use among poor adolescents (Dembo et al., 1979).

Researchers examining the popular belief that poorer youth are heavier substance users have reported mixed results. Marston et al. (1988) compared adolescents who reported no use of nicotine, alcohol, or other drugs with those who reported using at least one substance. They found no differences in educational or employment levels between nonusers and users. Blount and Dembo (1984) explored teenagers' perceptions of the "toughness" of their neighborhoods and the level of drug use. Although no meaningful differences emerged for alcohol use, those living in neighborhoods they believed to be tougher and to have higher levels of drug use were more likely to have used marijuana. Teenagers from lower-SES families are also more likely to smoke cigarettes (Evans & Raines, 1982).

As noted, available statistics rarely include measures of SES. Vega et al. (1993) did not include any indicator of family- or neighborhood-income levels in their study of the differences in drug use among different racial or ethnic groups in the greater Miami area. General lifetime use rates of 5% for illicit drugs, 37% for alcohol, and 21% for tobacco use were found. Significant differences existed in the pattern of risk factors across racial or ethnic groups, underlining the importance of directly examining cultural and socioeconomic variation in drug use.

Delinquency

Delinquency can be defined as reporting by a youth of delinquent activities or as the number of official contacts by a youth with the juvenile-justice system. A number of researchers have pointed out the lack of relation between social class and self-reported delinquency (e.g., Hindelang, Hirschi, & Weis, 1981). Differences in SES appear in archival statistics, however, leading some to suggest a bias in the juvenile-justice system against adolescents from lower socioeconomic levels (e.g., Westendorp et al., 1986; Taylor & Katz, in this volume). The consistency and strength of the relation between community-level poverty and officially recorded delinquency are beyond dispute (Hindelang et al., 1981; Joe, 1987). This association can overestimate individual differences in behavior. Reinarman and Fagan (1988) found no significant relations between *self-reported* delinquency and any community variables and suggested that perhaps poorer neighborhoods were simply more heavily patrolled, leaving their adolescents more vulnerable to arrest. The authors also noted that those being rearrested for multiple crimes were disproportionately located in neighborhoods with higher chronic unemployment, a greater proportion of female-headed households, lowest median incomes, and greater household density.

Serving Poor Adolescents: Utilization and Its Discontents

Barriers to service utilization begin with the nature of adolescence as a developmental stage and with the context in which many adolescents live. Contextual issues may include the financial constraints of poverty as well as the diverse social and cultural attitudes toward seeking help among racial and ethnic subgroups of the poor. The motivations, home life, or habitual health behaviors of socioeconomically disadvantaged youth are largely a mystery to health professionals. Little research or even thoughtful discussion can be found in the literature on the barriers to services experienced by adolescents living in poverty.

PHYSICAL HEALTH CARE
Utilization

The 1980 National Medical Care Utilization and Expenditure Survey showed that rates of care use and patterns of expenditure for health care differed dramatically according to poverty status (Butler et al., 1985). In this national probability sample of parents reporting on more than 5,000 children and youth, poor youth had fewer visits and received less preventive care when rates were adjusted for need and quality of care received.

Among adolescents, the number without public or private health insurance increased from 4.6 million to 4.7 million from 1988 to 1989 (U.S. Congress, Office of Technology Assessment, 1991a). Poverty is the most

13

important determinant of health-insurance status, with 30% of the poor or near poor without insurance while only 5% of adolescents in families at 300% of the poverty level or above were uninsured.

Medicaid has made health care significantly more accessible to the poor; however, it has not afforded equal access. Medicaid has stimulated the expansion of services from public agencies without increasing the participation of poor children in private services. As many as 50% of physicians refuse to accept Medicaid assignment, and many areas have no available practitioners at all.

A five-city study of the impact of Medicaid on use of health services found that a high proportion of children and the poor were covered and that Medicaid coverage was associated with increased utilization of health services (Okada & Wan, 1980). Increased use of Medicaid did not, however, close the gap between utilization rates of the poor and national averages. Not all of the eligible poor are actually covered by Medicaid (McManus & Davidson, 1982). Eligibility requirements for Medicaid changed between 1975 and 1983, leading to a reduction of the proportion of poor Americans covered, from 63% to 46% (Blendon et al., 1986; Dougherty & Kemp, this volume).

Neighborhood-based community health centers (CHCs) were developed to help address the lack of access among the poor (Pless & Haggerty, 1985). Community health centers have attracted a disproportionately high number of children (ages 0–17). These populations shifted from using hospital clinics and emergency rooms to use of the CHCs, in part because of the decrease in travel time to these centers (Okada & Wan, 1980).

In a national demonstration project in the early 1980s, the Robert Wood Johnson Foundation funded twenty teaching hospitals to implement programs of community-based, comprehensive services to high-risk youth and to train physicians to work with this population (Lear, Foster, & Wylie, 1985). In the first two years of operation, 64% of the patients were between the ages of 15 and 19, and 15% were ages 10–14. Insufficient availability of health-care workers and recent trends in funding cuts have eroded further development of this project (U.S. Congress, Office of Technology Assessment, 1991a).

Barriers to Access

Underuse appears to explain at least part of the differences in health status between poor and nonpoor adolescents in this country (Pauly, 1971). In rural areas, availability of professionally staffed mental- and physical-health services is limited. Private physicians are frequently the only source of services and are scarce; only 20% of all physicians—few of whom are specialists—practice in rural areas (U.S. Congress, Office of Technology Assessment, 1991c).

Cost is a barrier, and many physicians do not accept Medicaid. Moreover, the logistics involved in traveling to more populous areas for treatment, such as time, cost, and actual means, are sometimes insurmountable (U.S. Congress, Office of Technology Assessment, 1991c). Distance was inversely related to use of a public hospital for poor Blacks, but poor Whites were unwilling to use the public hospital, no matter how close it was to their residences (Goering & Coe, 1970).

Despite data showing that low-income urban population reported medical care as a high priority, socioeconomically disadvantaged youth rarely encounter medical professionals who understand their backgrounds, cultures, or attitudes toward health and illness (Fielding & Nelson, 1973). Among disadvantaged American Indian and Mexican American youth in the Southwest, for example, use of health-care services was not determined by economic factors alone. In fact, much of the care that was offered for free went unused. Barriers cited by the 14–21-year-old youth included anticipation of condescending attitudes from physicians, transportation problems, and culturally determined acceptance of illness as inevitable (Walter & Leahy, 1983). These barriers to utilization often result in poor adolescents receiving crisis- rather than prevention-oriented care.

NUTRITION

Few studies discuss service approaches to improving nutrition. However, Dillon (1975) presented a one-year nutrition intervention program in a socioeconomically disadvantaged area of Chicago staffed by family health workers recruited from the neighborhood. The project demonstrated that a community-based program could be implemented on a reasonable budget to provide outreach to other public service agencies for coordination of services for clients, home visits, nutritional education, and dietary counseling.

Poor children are eligible for reduced-cost or free breakfast and lunch in school. Given the high fat content of the model menu though, it seems unlikely that exposure to these meals would improve nutritional knowledge or habits (U.S. Congress, Office of Technology Assessment, 1991b).

DENTAL HEALTH CARE

At the completion of a five-year intervention program in which University of Kentucky dental students implemented a community-wide program of education and treatment, both the caries attack rate and the extraction of diseased permanent teeth had been reduced among 11- to 13-year-olds (Heiss et al., 1973).

Only about half (54%) of those treated in the first year returned for continued care in the second, with continuous participation at 41% in the third year dropping to 21% by the fourth year. The independent spirit and self-reliance of rural populations may be an explanation for their refusal to continue to accept what they perceived as handouts (U.S. Congress, Office of Technology Assessment, 1991b).

INJURIES

Suicide

A survey of 396 community programs serving suicidal adolescents revealed that a skewed income distribution was the most common special characteristic among populations served by these agencies. Fourteen percent (55 programs) were in areas of high poverty or unemployment or both (Simmons, Comstock, & Franklin, 1989), and thirteen programs reported serving high concentrations of both wealthy and poor clients.

Adolescent Abuse

While the United States has done far too little to serve abused infants and young children, even less has been done for abused adolescents. By all accounts, the level of unmet need is staggering, regardless of SES (Straus & Gelles, 1990). Social class clearly influences the treatment of an abused adolescent, however. Abused poor adolescents encounter the juvenile-justice system more often than do adolescents from higher SES levels—most often as status offenders. Status offenses include a variety of behaviors that are illegal only because of a youth's age, such as drinking alcohol or running away from home. Although running away is a status offense, it may also be a rational response to emotional or physical abuse of adolescents within their home when they lack other resources (Bolton, Reich, & Gutierres, 1977, cited in Garbarino & Gilliam, 1980).

Another reason abused teenagers tend to be labeled status offenders lies in petitions filed on youth as "persons in need of supervision" (PINS). The system, as it currently operates, is heavily weighted in favor of the parents. For example, even if an officer of the juvenile court believes such a PINS petition is unfounded or unnecessary, a parent can still legally insist that it be filed. When a youth runs away because of abuse in the home, a social worker can seek legal action either on the teenager as a runaway or on the parent as an abuser. Unfortunately, the greater ease of filing petitions on youths means that workers often elect to prosecute the youth victim rather than the parent abuser. As a result, adolescents are more likely than children to appear in juvenile or family court and to be institutionalized as a result of abuse. Once teenagers are institutionalized, they too often become vulnerable to other forms of mistreatment from fellow residents or staff (Garbarino & Gilliam, 1980).

Institutions are not the only option for out-of-home placements. In fact, the protective service system places more adolescents in foster care than in any other placements. Placements are difficult to arrange—and even harder to maintain—for teenagers; when adolescents are not happy, they can easily run away or otherwise undermine any nonsecure placement. Community-based group homes are another alternative and are typically considered to be a good way to care for teenagers. Unfortunately, because of lack of money and pervasive community resistance, too few group homes are available to provide secure and developmentally enhancing care for all the youth who would benefit by living in one.

Class issues abound in abuse of adolescents. The lower the family's income, the more reluctant the community has been to assist low-income families by creating low-cost, high-quality community-based intervention settings such as group homes and the greater the rate of court referrals (Garbarino & Gilliam, 1980). Furthermore, the poor in general have less access to traditional psychiatric services; they are therefore less able to get professional help for their problems.

In sum, poverty appears to both cause problems and subsequently prevent their successful resolution. Social-service and juvenile-justice systems may react less favorably to victims from these families than they do to more affluent youths.

Recently, laws have been enacted requiring the reporting of even the slightest suspicion of child or adolescent abuse by a wide variety of service providers—teachers, nurses, social workers, and physicians. Yet the lack of resources to pay for treatment sabotages any appropriate help. The hazards and ethical problems of increasing overall reporting without the programmatic resources to provide effective and developmentally appropriate help cannot be denied.

ADOLESCENT SEXUALITY

Pregnancy Prevention

The most direct approach to the prevention of teen pregnancies is to convince adolescents not to have sexual intercourse in the first place. In 1985, the Department of Health and Human Services' Adolescent Family Life Program, through the Office of Adolescent Pregnancy Prevention, spent approximately $3 million for programs attempting to prevent teenage sexual intercourse through enhancing parents' ability to educate their children about sexual matters and to encourage them not to have intercourse. Sexuality-education programs such as these have been found to increase girls' knowledge about sexuality without increasing their sexual activity. The impact on adolescent pregnancy itself, however, seems to be clearest only when delivered in tandem with accessible clinic services, such as school-based clinics (U.S. Congress, Office of Technology Assessment, 1991b).

A second approach to pregnancy prevention, and the one most discussed in the research literature, attempts to lower the likelihood of unprotected sexual intercourse by increasing utilization of contraception by sexually active teenagers. Social-class differences emerge in the practice of contraception. For example, Hogan et al. (1985) reported that 41% of the adolescent females from higher SES utilized some form of contraception at their first experience of sexual intercourse, compared with only 17% of those from the lower SES. A similar pattern held for adolescent males. Adolescents from higher-SES families were roughly 83% more likely than lower-SES teenagers to have practiced contraception at first intercourse.

Poverty appears to be related to regular contraception practices as well. Emans et al. (1987) found that, overall, an older, White adolescent living with married parents and with health care provided by a private physician was more likely to follow a contraceptive regimen than was an inner-city adolescent female from a single-parent household who received her health care in an inner-city clinic funded by Medicaid. Numerous studies have shown that higher levels of educational achievement, clear educational goals, and positive attitudes toward education appear to make nonmarital births less likely for both Black and White females (Emans et al., 1987; Franklin, 1988). Hogan et al. (1985) found, however, that high career aspirations may become an important motivation for contraceptive use only in situations in which future aspirations are encouraged by others in the community.

Barriers to Access

Barriers to the utilization of contraception to prevent pregnancy abound for teenagers in the United States. Major obstacles may occur in the use of nonprescription methods (e.g., condoms, spermicidal foam, contraceptive sponge). First, condoms are too often not displayed openly in stores. Instead, an adolescent must request them from a store clerk. The potential or ensuing embarrassment can be prohibitive for adolescents. Second, any user of these methods must be relatively familiar and comfortable with their genitalia to use these methods effectively; adolescents are not likely to be either.

For those choosing prescription methods of contraception, barriers can appear in several areas. First, adolescent-utilization issues include the lack of special outreach and aggressive follow-up to ensure compliance with the required regimen of contraception. In addition, many teenagers avoid physicians and clinics because they believe (rightly or wrongly) that parental consent is required. Second, aspects of the clinics can be barriers. Too few clinics exist, and of those that do, too few have after-school, evening, and weekend hours. Staff who are untrained in working with adolescents can make service use difficult, and the expense of prescription methods and the required medical visits may make their use unlikely (Chamie et al., 1982).

Finally, *all* contraceptive methods currently available in the United States present barriers to adolescents, since all are developmentally inappropriate for this age group. Every contraceptive requires high levels of motivation, careful planning, and vigilant responsibility to be utilized effectively. Given the often disruptive and chaotic environment accompanying those living in poverty, contraceptive techniques such as those now available are undeniably difficult for poor adolescents to use effectively and consistently.

TREATMENT AND PREVENTION OF STDS

Utilization

The HIV epidemic has eluded both cure and vaccine. As a result, preventing initial infection is the only method available today for controlling the spread of HIV (U.S. Congress, Office of Technology Assessment, 1991b).

While the specific behaviors required for effective prevention are quite straightforward, convincing teenagers to implement and maintain such preventive techniques is not (Martin, 1990). Education aimed at behavior changes has become the linchpin of the prevention efforts, with school-based AIDS-prevention classes currently the most common intervention. Although some school-based programs have reported significant increases in students' knowledge about AIDS transmission and prevention, few can demonstrate changes in students' reports of risk behaviors; none can make the critical leap to actual lowered levels of infection (Walter & Vaughan, 1993). Success in HIV prevention—especially in inner-city environments—requires helping teens to make and vigilantly maintain specific behavior changes, often with very little forgiveness for error or lapses. This reality presents "a challenge virtually unprecedented in the behavioral sciences" (Kelly et al., 1993, p. 1024).

Education-based prevention efforts alone are a dangerously passive approach to prevention of such a deadly problem (U.S. Congress, Office of Technology Assessment, 1991b). Little is known about how interventions can and should be adapted to account effectively for differing developmental processes, such as cognitive levels or social skills (Kelly et al., 1993). Moreover, adolescents as a whole are an extremely heterogeneous group; preventive interventions need to use different goals and approaches depending on the subgroup targeted (U.S. Congress, Office of Technology Assessment, 1991b). For example, young gay and lesbian teenagers experience cognitive, social, and emotional isolation as major factors leading to their high-risk behavior; socialization and counseling programs would be appropriate for preventive efforts. For runaway and homeless youth, though, daily survival is the primary motivation driving their risk behaviors; services must include such basics as food, clothing, education, and medical care (Martin, 1990).

Barriers to Access

For adolescents both to change behaviors that put them at risk for infection and to continue these safe behaviors, they must actually perceive that they could become infected. Yet in light of the estimated ten-year latency period between HIV infection and AIDS diagnosis, few adolescents today know or even casually encounter another adolescent who has AIDS. With so little concrete experience with AIDS, adolescents often do not weigh pertinent, albeit distant risks in making preventive decisions (U.S. Congress, Office of Technology Assessment, 1991b). Abstinence is one way to avoid STDS; effective use of condoms is a second approach. When adolescents *use* contraception, condoms are actually one of the most commonly used methods, although condom use does not begin until many months after becoming sexually active (U.S. Congress, Office of Technology Assessment, 1991b). A number of powerful barriers—both perceived and real—to the consistent use of condoms exist (U.S. Congress, Office of Technology Assessment, 1991b). Jemmott and colleagues (Jemmott et al., 1992) implemented a 105-minute intervention for Black female inner-city adolescents, using videos, exercises, and games. They found that self-efficacy in using condoms was significantly higher for women in the social-cognition condition than in the "information only" or general "health promotion" conditions. These results, though promising, should be interpreted cautiously, since the sample was a small, clinical sample and no follow-up data were reported.

Another potential barrier to condom use may be adolescents' beliefs that their friends are less supportive of condom use than they themselves are. In fact, discrepancies between teenagers' knowledge and actual behavior is commonly noted. One widely cited explanation for this disjunction focuses on teenagers' difficulties in resisting peer pressure and limited identification with adult role models who serve as primary health educators (U.S. Congress, Office of Technology Assessment, 1991b). Thus, peer counseling may offer an effective alternative to traditional health education. For example, Slap et al. (1991) reported that an HIV peer education program for urban adolescent girls resulted in positive changes in protective sexual behavior. Researchers had to rely on teenagers' reports of behavior changes, and the follow-up period was only two to six weeks.

Thus far, we have discussed only aspects of adolescent behaviors themselves that create barriers to seeking or succeeding in intervention programs. Community-level barriers exist as well. For instance, most fiscal support for HIV prevention efforts has been directed to adolescents in schools. As a result, those youth who are more marginally attached to school—or who have left school completely—are totally ignored. Furthermore, state and local boards of education have control over the precise scope and content of HIV and STD preventive messages in the schools. In too many communities, a combination of political and religious forces works actively to restrict the overarching messages to the teaching of total abstinence as the only safe behavior. Yet given the large numbers of sexually active adolescents, such approaches are at best inadequate and at worst unethical and dangerous. Increased utilization of community-based organizations (CBOs) in place of current reliance on school systems offers one avenue for improvement. While not totally independent of community pressures, CBOs are usually not under the direct control of bureaucracies such as local boards of education. In addition, CBOs typically are in better positions to reach youth who are more marginal, such as school dropouts or "pushouts" (U.S. Congress, Office of Technology Assessment, 1991b).

MENTAL HEALTH

It has been estimated that only 1.2 million of the 5.6 to 6.8 million U.S. adolescents who are in need of mental-health services receive them (U.S. Congress, Office of Technology Assessment, 1991b). Mental-health insurance coverage has more limitations, such as higher copayments, annual and lifetime benefits limitations, and higher deductibles than coverage for physical health. Thus, cost is a major barrier to utilization of mental-health service (U.S. Congress, Office of Technology Assessment, 1989).

A number of other difficulties accompany emotional problems for poor, minority adolescents (Cross, Bazron, & Dennis, 1989). For example, Indian children are much more likely than White children to go without treatment or to be removed geographically from their families and home nations to receive treatment. A Spanish-speaking Latino child is likely to be assessed in a language other than his or her native tongue. Compared with troubled White teenagers, Black teenagers are more likely to be placed in the juvenile-justice system than to receive services through the mental-health system. Thus, even teenagers and families seeking help may find themselves receiving little or no appropriate care.

Substance Use and Abuse

A few studies have looked at issues involved in treatment provision for poor adolescents abusing substances. Friedman and Glickman (1986) focused on a group of adolescents receiving treatment for substance abuse, 39% of whom were in lower- or working-class families. They found no relation between SES and treatment success. Treatment success did vary with the provision of developmentally appropriate components such as work skills, educational assistance, and birth-control services. In fact, the presence of such components had a stronger relation to treatment success than did any specific individual therapy methods utilized. Approximately half of all adolescent participants left the programs or were terminated before completing treatment.

Chitwood and Chitwood (1981) compared characteristics of participants attending a metropolitan drug-abuse program to those appearing in a hospital emergency room for treatment of problems related to substance use. Those in the substance-use treatment program came from families of higher social-class levels than did the emergency room patients. More important, more of the emergency room patients were under 18. These findings support the conclusion that substance-using adolescents living in poverty may be seriously underserved by treatment programs.

Delinquency

The primary treatment for an officially adjudicated delinquent is either formal or informal probation or some form of incarceration. Shanok et al. (1983) compared delinquent and nondelinquent psychiatric inpatients; Lewis et al. (1980) compared violent adolescents referred either to a state training school or a state hospital psychiatric unit. Unfortunately, the influence of poverty on such treatment decisions cannot be examined, since the vast majority in these samples (not surprisingly) came from the lowest socioeconomic classes. Westendorp et al. (1986), however, compared a sample drawn from several samples of mental-health treatment programs and one drawn from placements mandated by the juvenile-justice system. Of the four demographic variables utilized—social class and ages of mother, father, and subject—none were significantly different between the two systems.

Promise for the Future: Services That Poor Adolescents Will Use

This chapter has repeatedly shown that the rates of many health problems are higher among poor adolescents than among their nonpoor counterparts. A variety of barriers to using and receiving services have been delineated, but little empirical work has focused on the utilization of health services by poor adolescents. Thus, we have little firm knowledge on which to base plans for a better future. Exceptions to this trend were found and are reported here.

One study of inner-city sixth-grade asthma patients found that a youth's choice of emergency room or private physician care for asthma was unrelated to SES (Mak et al., 1982). The authors speculated that this lack of a relation may have been due to the restricted range of SES in their sample.

In use of dental services, however, Reisine (1987) reported that, as the level of education (a proxy for SES) increased, utilization also increased. Health-insurance coverage and welfare care were also significant predictors of utilization. Dental insurance increased service utilization above national norms for most sociodemographic groups, with the primary beneficiaries being children from low-income families and/or those whose parents had little formal education (Grembowski, Conrad, & Milgrom, 1985).

Resnick, Blum, and Hedin (1980) surveyed adolescents about their attitudes toward health-care provision. Teenagers reported concerns that included providers perceived as cold, aloof, and inconsiderate of teenagers, limited financial resources, and issues of confidentiality. Health clinics for adolescents, on the other hand, were perceived to be staffed by caring and compassionate service providers, with low or flexible payments and clear statements about the confidentiality of the service provision.

Kisker (1984) found that nonmetropolitan clinics were generally more effective in delivering services (e.g., teenagers reported less delay in seeking services, higher retention rates, and greater satisfaction) than were metropolitan clinics. Thus, inner-city areas may be especially in need of extra help for teens. She also found that more convenient hours and a wider range of services resulted in less delay in adolescents' initially seeking contraception, while longer travel time resulted in a greater delay.

In general, the opening of school-linked health centers—currently located primarily in low-income areas—presents a hopeful new approach to the delivery of symptomatic and preventive health-care services to youth (Kirby, 1985). In fact, by 1985, nearly fifty communities were supporting or planning such clinics (Kenney, 1986)—an increase of 300% in less than one year (Foley, 1985). Yet, while school-based clinics have existed for more than a decade, few thorough evaluations have been conducted (Dryfoos, 1985). Those that have been carried out have focused primarily on the impact of the total package or "black box" of the school-based clinic on simple and basic outcomes, such as lowering the mean delay time of adolescents in seeking contraception, delay of first intercourse, and decreasing teen pregnancies (Kirby, 1985). However, not all programs have examined

24

the same outcomes, making comparisons or general recommendations extremely difficult (Brooks-Gunn et al., 1988). In addition, effects on overall health have not been systematically documented.

Although school-based interventions are critical, we need to go beyond the school building to serve hard-to-reach teenagers—runaways, chronic truants, dropouts, drug users, or youth living in extreme poverty. For such youth, community-based interventions are clearly needed. Anecdotal information about two community-based service approaches, both found in New York City, illustrates the studies needed.

The Argus community in the South Bronx offers a program that attempts to help troubled youth connect with the community through jobs. This program works with youth who frequently have few educational skills, little job training, and no work history. The staff help participants obtain and hold on to jobs in the "real" (e.g., nonsubsidized) world. The program consists of a job-readiness program tailored to the needs and strengths of each participant along with efforts to persuade private-sector employers to take a chance on the inexperienced Argus applicants. A self-evaluation in 1980 reported that the overall rate of successful placement outcomes for Argus enrollees was 67% for more than 100 trainees (Sturz, 1983).

The Door is a multiservice program established in 1972 in lower Manhattan. The Door is a freestanding clinic that takes a smorgasbord approach to engaging adolescents in health-promoting behaviors. Youth can come in for any of its services—tutoring, counseling, recreation, or mental-health counseling. The Door staff emphasize ready access to services for youth, meeting them on their own terms and providing a range of "identity exploring" activities. Many support services are simultaneously available. Staff reported that participants who were surveyed had participated in an average of 5.3 services (Rapoport, 1987).

Conclusion

Adolescents in poverty are a population at risk for developing multiple negative health outcomes. Their need for services is greater than average, while their access to usable services is inadequate.

The harm of inappropriate services is heightened when they are overlaid onto the often chaotic and unpredictable environments in which many poor adolescents live. Economic concerns plague the poor adolescent in seeking help; services that require either insurance or cash payments are shunned by or are unavailable to poor adolescents. Geographic barriers can be sizable for adolescents in poor communities; expensive, inadequate, or undependable transportation systems discourage teenagers from attending available clinics. Racism and cultural barriers are rarely acknowledged and addressed in service plans, and societal problems prevent adolescents living in poverty from seeking appropriate preventive care. Concerns with low wages, joblessness, and difficulties involved in establishing desirable futures compete with teenagers' interests in seeking care on anything other than a crisis-oriented basis.

It should be noted that many, if not most, teenagers living in poverty appear to survive their childhoods and are able to pull themselves out of poverty (U.S. Congress, Office of Technology Assessment, 1991c). Research on the predictors of this resilience among adolescents from disadvantaged backgrounds such as impoverished homes and neighborhoods is now receiving increasing attention from researchers. It appears that having access to supportive individuals and networks combined with the cognitive and social abilities to use these resources helps adolescents overcome adverse circumstances. In addition, since so many poor adolescents are from ethnic-minority groups, there is increasing consensus that health services would be improved if they were not just culturally *sensitive*—that is, aware of the diversity of important cultural differences—but also culturally *competent* and able to capitalize on the strengths and naturally occurring helping processes extant in various cultures (Institute of Medicine, 1994; U.S. Congress, Office of Technology Assessment, 1991a).

Meaningful policy solutions to the problems of health-care access for poor children will not succeed without incorporating concern for these economic, social, and cultural context issues. The emergence of innovative multiservice arenas, such as school-linked health centers, and the continued survival of successful programs such as Argus and the Door, along with renewed policy interest in providing adequate health care to all, provide hope that we will see improved health care for those adolescents most in need.

References

Adler, N., Boyce, T. Chesney, M. A., Cohen, S., Folkman, S., Kahn, R. L., & Syme, S. L. (1994). Socioeconomic status and health. *American Psychologist, 49,* 15–24.

Aldwin, C. M., & Revenson, T. A. (1986). Vulnerability to economic stress. *American Journal of Community Psychology*, *14*, 161–175.

Allen, L., & Britt, D. (1983). Social class, mental health and mental illness. In R. D. Felner, L. Jason, J. Moritsugu, & S. Farber (Eds.), *Preventive psychology: Theory, research and practice* (pp. 149–161). New York: Pergamon.

Allen, L., & Majidi-Ahi, S. (1989). Black American children. In J. T. Gibbs & L. N. Huang (Eds.), *Children of color: Psychological interventions with minority youth* (pp. 148–178). San Francisco: Jossey Bass.

American Academy of Pediatrics Committee on Adolescence (1988). Suicide and suicide attempts in adolescents and young adults. *Pediatrics*, *81*, 322–324.

American Dental Association, Council on Dental Care Programs. (1988). *Dental programs in Medicaid: 1988* survey. Chicago: American Dental Association.

Bane, M. I., & Ellwood, D. T. (1989). One fifth of the nation's children: Why are they poor? *Science*, *245*, 1047–1053.

Blendon, R., Aiken, L., Freeman, H., Kirkman-Liff, B., & Murphy, I. (1986). Uncompensated care by hospitals or public insurance for the poor: Does it make a difference? *New England Journal of Medicine*, *314*, 1160–1163.

Blount, W. R., & Dembo, R. (1984). The effect of perceived neighborhood setting on self-reported tobacco, alcohol, and marijuana use among inner-city minority junior high school youth. *International Journal of the Addictions*, *19*, 175–198.

Blum, R. W. (1987). Contemporary threats to adolescent health in the United States. *Journal of the American Medical Association*, *257*, 3390–3395.

Blum, R. W., & Runyan, C. (1980). Adolescent abuse: The dimensions of the problem. *Journal of Adolescent Health Care*, *1*, 121–126.

Blumenthal, S. (1988). A guide to risk factors, assessment, and treatment of suicidal patients. *Medical Clinics of North America*, *72*, 937–939.

Bromet, W., & Schulberg, H. (1989). Special problem populations: The chronically mentally ill, elderly, children, minorities, and substance abusers. In D. A. Rochefort (Ed.), *Handbook on mental health policy in the United States* (pp. 67–85). New York: Greenwood.

Brooks-Gunn, J., Boyer, C. B., & Hein, K. (1988). Preventing HIV infection and AIDS in children and adolescents. *American Psychologist*, *43*, 958–964.

Butler, J., Winter, W., Singer, J., & Wenger, M. (1985). Medical care use and expenditure among children and youth in the United States: Analysis of a national probability sample. *Pediatrics, 76*, 495–507.

Cantor, P. (1989). Intervention strategies: Environmental risk reduction for youth suicide. In *Report of the Secretary's Task Force on Youth Suicide. Volume 3: Prevention and interventions in youth suicide* (pp. 285–293) (DHHS Pub. No. 89-1622). Washington DC: Superintendent of Documents, U.S. Government Printing Office.

Chamie, M., Eisman, S., Forrest, J. D., Orr, M. T., & Torres, A. (1982). Factors affecting adolescents' use of family planning clinics. *Family Planning Perspectives, 14,* 126–139.

Chitwood, D. D., & Chitwood, J. S. (1981). Treatment program clients and emergency room patients: A comparison of two drug-using samples. *International Journal of the Addictions, 16,* 911–925.

Costello, E. J. (1989). Developments in child psychiatric epidemiology. *Journal of the American Academy of Child and Adolescent Psychiatry, 28,* 36–84.

Cross, T., Bazron, B., & Dennis, K. (1989). *Toward a culturally competent system of care: A monograph on effective services for minority children who are severely emotionally disturbed.* Washington DC: CASSP Technical Assistance Center, Georgetown University.

Dembo, R., Burgos, W., DesJarlais, D., & Schmeidler, J. (1979). Ethnicity and drug use among urban junior high school youths. *International Journal of the Addictions, 14,* 557–568.

Dillon, H. (1975). Improvement of the quality of life through a food and nutrition project. *Perspectives in Practice, 67,* 129–131.

Dryfoos, J. (1985). School-based health clinics: A new approach to preventing adolescent pregnancy? *Family Planning Perspectives, 10,* 223–235.

Ellwood, D. T. (1988). *Poor support: Poverty in the American family.* New York: Basic Books.

Emans, S. J., Grace, E., Woods, E. R., Smith, D. E., Klein, K., & Merola, J. (1987). Adolescents' compliance with the use of oral contraceptives. *Journal of the American Medical Association, 257,* 3377–3381.

Evans, R. I., & Raines, B. E. (1982). Control and prevention of smoking in adolescents: A psychosocial perspective. In T. J. Coates, A. C. Petersen, & C. Perry (Eds.), *Promoting adolescent health: A dialogue on research and practice* (pp. 101–136). New York: Academic Press.

Fawzy, F. I., Coombs, R. H., Simon, J. M., & Bowman-Terrell, M. (1987). Family composition, socioeconomic status, and adolescent substance use. *Addictive Behavior, 12,* 79–83.

Fielding, J., & Nelson, S. (1973). Health care for the economically disadvantaged adolescent. *Pediatric Clinics of North America, 20,* 975–988.

Foley, J. (1985). Preventing teenage pregnancy: Health experts turn to a school-based approach. *Youth Policy, 7,* 1–6.

Franklin, D. L. (1988). Race, class, and adolescent pregnancy: An ecological analysis. *American Journal of Orthopsychiatry, 58,* 339–354.

Friedman, A. S., & Glickman, N. W. (1986). Program characteristics for successful treatment of adolescent drug abuse. *Journal of Nervous and Mental Disease, 174,* 669–679.

Furstenberg, F. F., Morgan, S. P., Moore, K. A., & Peterson, J. L. (1987). Race differences in the timing of adolescent intercourse. *American Sociological Review, 52,* 511–518.

Galambos, N. L., & Dixon, R. A. (1984). Adolescent abuse and the development of personal sense of control. *Child Abuse and Neglect, 8,* 285–293.

Garbarino, J., & Gilliam, G. (1980). *Understanding abusive families.* Lexington MA: Heath.

Garfinkel, I., & McLanahan, S. S. (1986). *Single mothers and their children.* Washington DC: Urban Institute.

Garland, A. F., & Zigler, E. (1993). Adolescent suicide prevention: Current research and social policy implications. *American Psychologist, 48,* 169–182.

Goering, J., & Coe, R. (1970). Cultural versus situational explanations of the medical behavior of the poor. *Social Science Quarterly, 51,* 309–319.

Gould, M., Wunsch-Hitzig, R., & Dohrenwend, B. S. (1981). Estimating the prevalence of childhood psychopathology. *Journal of the American Academy of Child Psychiatry, 20,* 462–476.

Graham, G. (1985). Poverty, hunger, malnutrition, prematurity, and infant mortality in the United States. *Pediatrics, 75,* 117–125.

Grembowski, D., Conrad, D., & Milgrom, P. (1985). Utilization of dental services in the United States and an insured population. *American Journal of Public Health, 75,* 87–89.

Guyer, B., Lescohier, I., Gallagher, S. S., Hausman, A., & Azzara, C. V. (1989). Intentional injuries among children and adolescents in Massachusetts. *New England Journal of Medicine, 321,* 1584–1589.

Hammond, W. R., & Yung, B. (1993). Psychology's roles in the public health response to assaultive violence among young African-American men. *American Psychology, 48,* 142–154.

Hampton, R. L., & Newberger, E. H. (1985). Child abuse incidence and reporting by hospitals: Significance of severity, class, and race. *American Journal of Public Health, 75,* 56–59.

Hawley, L., Shear, C., Stark, A., & Goodman, P. (1984). Resident and parental perceptions of adolescent problems and family communications in a low socioeconomic population. *Journal of Family Practice, 19,* 652–655.

Heiss, A. L., Mullins, M. R., Hill, C. J., & Crawford, J. H. (1973). Meeting the dental treatment needs of indigent rural children. *Health Sciences Reports, 88,* 591–600.

Hepner, R., & Maiden, N. (1971). Growth rate, nutrient intake and "mothering" as determinants of malnutrition in disadvantaged children. *Nutrition Reviews, 29,* 219–223.

Hindelang, M. J., Hirschi, T., & Weis, J. G. (1981). *Measuring delinquency.* Beverly Hills CA: Sage.

Hogan, D. P., Astone, N. M., & Kitagawa, E. M. (1985). Social and environmental factors influencing contraceptive use among Black adolescents. *Family Planning Perspectives, 17,* 165–169.

Hollingshead, A. B. (1975). *Four factor index of social status.* Unpublished manuscript, Yale University, New Haven CT.

Hollingshead, A. B., & Redlich, F. C. (1958). *Social class and mental illness.* New York: Wiley.

Holmes, K. K., Karon, J. M., & Kreiss, L. (1990). The increasing frequency of heterosexually acquired AIDS in the United State, 1983–88. *American Journal of Public Health, 81,* 858–862.

Institute of Medicine. (1994). *Reducing risks for mental disorders: Frontiers for preventive intervention research.* Washington DC: National Academy.

Jemmott, J. B., Jemmott, L. S., Spears, H., Hewitt, N., & Cluz-Collins, M. (1992). Self-efficacy, hedonistic expectancies and condom-use intentions among inner-city Black adolescent women: A social cognitive approach to AIDS risk behavior. *Journal of Adolescent Health, 13,* 512–519.

Joe, T. (1987). Economic inequality: The picture in Black and White. *Crime and Delinquency, 33,* 287–299.

Jones, D. Y., Nesheim, M. C., & Hibicht, J. P. (1985). Influence on child growth associated with poverty in the 1970's: An examination of HANES I and HANES II cross-sectional surveys. *American Journal of Clinical Nutrition, 42,* 714–724.

Kazdin, A. E. (1993). Adolescent mental health: Prevention and treatment programs. *American Psychologist. 48* (2): 127–141.

Kelly, J. A., Murphy, D. A., Sikkema, K. J., & Kalichman, S. C. (1993). Psychological interventions to prevent HIV infection are urgently needed: New priorities for behavioral research in the second decade of AIDS. *American Psychologist, 48,* 1023–1034.

Kenney, A. M. (1986). School-based clinics: A national conference. *Family Planning Perspectives, 18,* 44–46.

Kirby, D. (1985). *School-based health clinics: An emerging approach to improving adolescent health and addressing teenage pregnancy.* Washington DC: Center for Populations.

Kisker, E. E. (1984). The effectiveness of family planning clinics in serving adolescents. *Family Planning Perspectives, 16,* 212–218.

Koh, E., & Caples, V. (1979). Frequency of selection of food groups by low-income families in southwestern Mississippi. *Journal of the American Dietetic Association, 74,* 660–664.

Lear, J., Foster, H., & Wylie, W. G. (1985). Development of community-based health services for adolescents at risk for sociomedical problems. *Journal of Medical Education, 60,* 777–785.

Lewis, D. O., Shanok, S. S., Cohen, R. J., Kligfeld, M., & Frisone, G. (1980). Race bias in the diagnosis and disposition of violent adolescents. *American Journal of Psychiatry, 137,* 1211–1216.

Mak, H., Johnston, P., Abbey, P., & Talamo, R. C. (1982). Prevalence of asthma and health service utilization of asthmatic children in an inner city. *Journal of Allergy and Clinical Immunology, 70,* 367–372.

Marston, A. R., Jacobs, D. F., Singer, R. D., Widaman, K. R., & Little, T. D. (1988). Adolescents who apparently are invulnerable to drug, alcohol, and nicotine use. *Adolescence, 23* (91), 593–598.

Martin, A. D. (1990). Prevention education for adolescents. In G. R. Anderson (Ed.), *Courage to care: Responding to the crisis of children with AIDS* (pp.259–269). Washington DC: Child Welfare League of America.

McManus, M. A., & Davidson, S. M. (1982). *Medicaid and children: A policy analysis.* Evanston IL: American Academy of Pediatrics.

Miller, C., & Coulter, E. (1984). The world economic crisis and the children: A United States case study. *World Development, 12,* 339–364.

Millstein, S. G., & Litt, I. F. (1990). Adolescent health. In S. S. Feldman & G. R. Elliot (Eds.), *At the threshold: The developing adolescent* (pp.431–456). Cambridge: Harvard University Press.

Mitchell, C. M., Seidman, E. S., Aber, J. L., & Allen, L. (1993). *Adolescent depression and delinquency: Untested assumptions about demography, organization and development.* Unpublished manuscript, New York University, New York.

Moen, P. (1983). Unemployment, public policy, and families: Forecasts for the 1980's. *Journal of Marriage and the Family, 45,* 751–760.

Mueller, C. W., & Parcel, R. L. (1981). Measures of socioeconomic status: Alternatives and recommendations. *Child Development, 52,* 13–30.

National Center for Health Statistics. (1993). Advance report of final natality statistics, 1990. *Monthly Vital Statistics Report, 41* (9) (Suppl.)

Nikias, M., Fink, R., & Shapiro, S. (1989). Comparisons of poverty and non-poverty groups on dental status, needs, and practices. *Journal of Public Health Dentistry, 35,* 237–259.

Nock, S. L., & Rossi, P. H. (1979). Household types and social standing. *Social Forces, 57,* 1325–1345.

Okada, L., & Wan, T. (1980). Impact of community health centers and Medicaid on the use of health services. *Public Health Reports, 95,* 520–534.

Parcel, G., Nader, P., & Meyer, M. (1977). Adolescent health concerns, problems, and patterns of utilization in a tri-ethnic urban population. *Pediatrics, 60,* 157–164.

Paulson, J. A. (1988). The epidemiology of injuries in adolescents. *Pediatric Annals, 17,* 84–96.

Pauly, M. (1971). An analysis of government health insurance plans for poor families. *Public Policy, 19,* 489–521.

Pfeffer, C. (1989). Family characteristics and support systems as risk factors for youth suicidal behavior. In *Report of the Secretary's Task Force on Youth Suicide. Volume 2: Risk factors for youth suicide* (pp. 71–87) (DHHS Pub. No. 89-1622). Washington DC: Superintendent of Documents, U.S. Government Printing Office.

Pless, I. B., & Haggerty, R. J. (1985). Child health: Research in action. In R. N. Rapoport (Ed.), *Children, youth, and families: The action-research relationship* (pp. 206–235). Cambridge: Cambridge University Press.

Rapoport, R. N. (1987). *New interventions for children and youth: Action-research approaches.* Cambridge: Cambridge University Press.

Reinarman, C., & Fagan, J. (1988). Social organization and differential association: A research note from a longitudinal study of violent juvenile offenders. *Crime and Delinquency, 34,* 307–327.

Reisine, S. (1987). A path analysis of the utilization of dental services. *Community Dental and Oral Epidemiology, 15,* 119–124.

Resnick, M., Blum, R. W., & Hedin, D. (1980). The appropriateness of health services for adolescents. *Journal for Adolescent Health Care, 1,* 137–141.

Rickert, V. I., Jay, M. S., & Gottlieb, A. A. (1990). Adolescent wellness: Facilitating compliance in social morbidities. *Adolescent Medicine, 74,* 1135–1148.

Robins, L. (1989). Suicide attempts in teen-aged medical patients. In *Report of the Secretary's Task Force on Youth Suicide. Volume 4: Strategies for the prevention of youth suicide* (pp.94–114) (DHHS Pub. No.891622). Washington DC: Superintendent of Documents, U.S. Government Printing Office.

Rotheram-Borus, M. J., Koopman, C., Haignere, C., & Davies, M. (1991). Reducing HIV sexual risk behaviors among runaway adolescents. *Journal of the American Medical Association, 266*, 1237–1241.

Sandefur, G. D. (1988). Blacks, Hispanics, American Indians, and poverty—and what worked. In F. R. Harris & R. W. Wilkins (Eds.), *Quiet riots: Race and poverty in the United States* (pp.46–74). New York: Pantheon.

Schiller, B. R. (1989). *The economics of poverty and discrimination.* Englewood Cliffs NJ: Prentice Hall.

Scott-Jones, D., & White, A. B. (1990). Correlates of sexual activity in early adolescence. *Journal of Early Adolescence, 10*, 221–238.

Shanok, S. S., Surendar, C. M., Ninan, O. P., Guggenheim, P., Weinstein, H., & Lewis, D. O. (1983). A comparison of delinquent and nondelinquent adolescent psychiatric inpatients. *American Journal of Psychiatry, 140*, 582–585.

Sheley, J. F., McGee, Z. T., & Wright, L. D. (1992). Gun-related violence in and around inner-city schools. *American Journal of Diseases of Children, 146*, 677–682.

Simmons, J., Comstock, B., & Franklin, L. (1989). Prevention/intervention programs for suicidal adolescents. In *Report of the Secretary's Task Force on Youth Suicide. Volume 3: Prevention and interventions in youth suicide* (pp.80–92). (DHHS Pub. No.89-1622). Washington DC: Superintendent of Documents, U.S. Government Printing Office.

Slap, G. B., Plotkin, S. L., Khalid, H., Michelman, D. F., & Forke, C. M. (1991). A human immunodeficiency virus peer education program for adolescent females. *Journal of Adolescent Health, 12*, 434–442.

Straus, M. A., & Gelles, R. J. (1990). *Physical violence in American families.* New Brunswick NJ: Transaction.

Strunin, L. (1991). Adolescents' perceptions of risk for HIV infection: Implications for future research. *Social Science and Medicine, 32*, 221–228.

Sturz, E. L. (1983). *Widening circles.* New York: Harper & Row.

Sullivan, J., & Carter, J. (1985). A nutrition-physical fitness intervention program for low-income black parents. *Journal of the National Medical Association, 77*, 39–43.

U.S. Bureau of the Census. (1989). *Statistical abstract of the United States: 1989* (190th ed.). Washington DC: U.S. Government Printing Office.

U.S. Bureau of the Census. (1993a). Money income of households, families, and persons in the United States: 1992. *Current Population Reports*, Series P60-184. Washington DC: U.S. Government Printing Office.

U.S. Bureau of the Census. (1993b). Poverty in the United States: 1992. *Current Population Reports*, Series P60-185. Washington DC: U.S. Government Printing Office.

U.S. Congress. Committee on Ways and Means. (1985). *Children in poverty*. Washington DC: U.S. Government Printing Office.

U.S. Congress. Office of Technology Assessment. (1989). *Adolescent health insurance status: Analyses of trends in coverage and preliminary estimates of the effects of an employer mandate and Medicaid expansion on the uninsured—Background paper.* (OTA-BP-H-56). Washington DC: U.S. Government Printing Office.

U.S. Congress. Office of Technology Assessment. (1991a). *Adolescent health. Volume 1: Summary and policy options.* (OTA-H-468). Washington DC: U.S. Government Printing Office.

U.S. Congress, Office of Technology Assessment (1991b). *Adolescent health. Volume 2: Background and the effectiveness of selected prevention and treatment services.* (OTA-H-466). Washington DC: U.S. Government Printing Office.

U.S. Congress. Office of Technology Assessment. (1991c). *Adolescent health. Volume 3: Crosscutting issues in the delivery of health and related services.* (OTA-H-467). Washington DC: U.S. Government Printing Office.

Vega, W. A., Zimmerman, R. S., Warheit, G. J., Apospori, E., & Gill, A. G. (1993). Risk factors for early adolescent drug use in four ethnic and racial groups. *American Journal of Public Health, 83* (2), 185–189.

Walker, D. K., Cross, A. W., Heyman, P. W., Ruch-Ross, H., Benson, P., & Tuthill, J. W. (1982). Comparisons between inner-city and private school adolescents' perceptions of health problems. *Journal of Adolescent Health Care, 3,* 82–90.

Walter, H. J., & Vaughan, R. D. (1993). AIDS risk reduction among a multiethnic sample of urban high school students. *Journal of the American Medical Association, 270,* 725–730.

Walter, J., & Leahy, W. (1983). Demand for medical services by deprived urban youth in North and South America. *American Economist, 27,* 29–33.

Wells, V., Deykin, E., & Klerman, G. (1985). Risk factors for depression in adolescence. *Psychiatric Developments, 3,* 83–108.

Westendorp, F., Brink, K. L., Roberson, M. K., & Ortiz, I. E. (1986). Variables which differentiate placement of adolescents into juvenile justice or mental health systems. *Adolescence, 21* (81), 23–37.

Wilson, W. L. (1987). *The truly disadvantaged*. Chicago: University of Chicago Press.

W. T. Grant Commission on Work, Family and Citizenship (1988). *The forgotten half: Pathways to success for America's youth and young families.* Washington DC: W. T. Grant Foundation.

Wyatt, G. E. (1988). The relationship between child sexual abuse and adolescent sexual functioning in Afro-American and White American women. *Annals of the New York Academy of Sciences, 528,* 111–122.

Wyatt, G. E. (1989). Reexamining factors predicting Afro-American and White American women's age at first coitus. *Archives of Sexual Behavior, 18,* 271–298.

2

Health and Related Services Available to Black Adolescents

Dalmas A. Taylor and Phyllis A. Katz

Advances in medicine have led to health improvements for all Americans, but the gap between ethnic minorities and Whites still exists. More than 80% of excess deaths among all minorities are accounted for by cancer; cardiovascular diseases; chemical dependency; diabetes; homicide, suicide, and unintentional injuries; infant mortality and low birthweight; and AIDS. Blacks, who represented the single largest minority group in the country in 1990, are disproportionately at risk in the health problem areas compared with Whites. How can we understand these findings, and how are youth being affected by them? This chapter reviews information needed to begin answering these questions.

The history of Black Americans in the United States is synonymous with disadvantage that continues to manifest itself in earlier ages of death and more illnesses. This chapter examines the barriers to prevention and treatment of health problems among Black adolescents (youth between 10 and 18 years of age) even though the data are incomplete.

This chapter is divided into three sections: consideration of how cultural factors interact with health issues; specifics about the major health issues of Black adolescents; and issues of service delivery. In this latter section, we also provide information on possible alternatives to traditional treatment modalities that are often oriented toward White, middle-class, and adult clientele.

Cultural Factors and Black Adolescent Health

POPULATION CHARACTERISTICS

In 1990, there were 4.5 million Black adolescents (between ages 10 and 19) living in the United States. According to census statistics of the early

1990s, the median age of all Blacks was 28.1, compared with a national median of 32.9. In 1991, more than 30% of Blacks lived in families earning less than the poverty line, and 39.5% of children under the age of 18 lived in poverty. This already-shocking figure was substantially higher for the 44% of Black youths living in female-headed families. The median income for Black families in 1991 was $21,548, compared with $37,783 for White families. Among Black female-headed homes, however, the median income was $11,414, whereas intact Black families had a median income of $33,307. Poverty among Blacks is thus highly related to single-female parent status. As is true for all families, economic stability among Black families is more readily found in homes in which both parents are present.

It should be noted that, while many Black Americans live in ghettos (approximately 30% are urban and poor), more than 70% do not. A substantial proportion of poverty-level families live outside metropolitan areas. Moreover, middle-income Black families ($15,000–$35,000 income in 1991) constitute 32% of all Black families, and 12% of all Black families in that year had annual incomes of more than $50,000. Clearly, the issues of health problems and service delivery differ markedly for these various income and geographical groups. Most research studies, however, do not provide sufficient data to differentiate them.

The Black population is heterogeneous in background as well as in income level. A number of subpopulations, each with a special history and unique cultural focus, add to the ethnic diversity in the United States. Minority status in itself may render these groups more vulnerable to health problems, while historical and sociocultural elements influence their psychological adaptation and psychopathology. An examination of the ecological systems and coping strategies of these subpopulations may elucidate their relation to both health and treatment approaches, particularly in the area of mental health.

For example, there is an increasingly large population of Blacks in the United States whose roots trace to English-speaking Caribbean peoples (West Indies). Economies of these countries are based largely on individual farming, skilled and unskilled labor, and tourism. Attending secondary school is relatively rare. Hence, the experiences of these immigrants do not parallel that of Blacks born in the United States. Furthermore, unlike in the United States, Black middle-class individuals in the West Indies are dominant in politics and the government; there is no overt discrimination against Blacks as a whole. Yet poverty is a way of life for most, and light skin color is more valued than dark skin color.

These conditions contribute to poor self-esteem and inferiority complexes among poor Black adolescents in Caribbean countries and have been found to contribute to considerable social disintegration (e.g., high illegitimacy rates, inadequate socialization; see Allen, 1988). Such conditions have consequences for the mental health of emigrants to the United States from these countries. The effects are quite different, however, for the poor and the middle class. West Indians who come to the United States from highly skilled middle-class and professional families do not come with the same problems as those from poor families; they are usually highly motivated to achieve wealth, status, and security. Their aspirations may serve to shield them to some extent from the horrors of American racism. They nonetheless experience a new type of discrimination from American Whites—and Blacks. Their resultant ambitions, homesickness, loneliness, and culture shock significantly affect stress level and mental health. This limited discussion of one Black subpopulation only illustrates the manner in which mass relocation, social disintegration, and economic control and oppression can affect the health status of Black immigrants. The history and demography of these groups, while different from native-born Blacks, nonetheless result in increased family trauma and morbidity, with perhaps dfferent patterns of illness. These differing mosaics of cultural patterns and their effects on health status suggest that the heterogeneity of the Black population needs to be considered more frequently by researchers.

Census data indicate that the Black population is increasing relative to Whites, from approximately 10% in 1900 to 12.1% in 1990. Projections indicate that, by the year 2000, the Black population will increase to 13.3% — well over 35 million. The group is also becoming increasingly urban. At the turn of the century, greater than 90% of all Blacks lived on southern farms. By 1990 only 53% of the Black population remained in the South. This movement from the rural South to the urban North produced mixed blessings. Greater economic opportunities existed in the North, but the greater urbanization brought with it ghetto circumstances. Many northern Blacks now live in large cities in predominately Black neighborhoods. The pathology associated with urban ghettos appears to be a product of both physical isolation and economic distress (Comer & Hill, 1985).

The ecological environments (urban ghettos) in which many Black adolescents and their families live are characterized by irregular employment, or what Wilson (1988) referred to as "structural unemployment," women depending largely on welfare assistance to survive, and rampant crime and social disorder. Black teenagers have been hit harder by downward economic swings. They have higher rates of unemployment than any group in the workforce, 42% in 1992 compared with 18% among White teenagers (U.S. Bureau of the Census, 1993). Unemployment creates stressful situations for laid-off workers and their families, and stress has long been recognized as a major contributor to various physical and mental disorders. Other stressful factors such as racism and discrimination, unfulfilled rising expectations, life in the inner city, limited opportunities, and cultural conflict create special risk for Black adolescents in the United States, and these factors probably erode their capacity to resist illness.

PATHWAYS TO ADAPTIVE BEHAVIOR

While Blacks are often overrepresented in the various disease categories, they are not uniformly at risk in all categories. Black adolescents are unlikely to commit suicide, for example, and although they have higher rates of homicide, they are less likely to die from motor-vehicle injuries than Whites. They also have lower rates of alcohol and illicit drug use than Whites (National Institute on Drug Abuse, 1987). Thus, we believe that an examination of the context and precursors of adaptive behavior for Blacks could be more informative than the cataloguing of maladaptive behaviors. There are not many examples of the former approach.

Ogbu (1985), using a cultural-ecological model, catalogued a host of adaptive behaviors among inner-city Blacks. Citing a "Black cultural imperative," Ogbu argued that clues about how Blacks in urban centers acquire instrumental competencies lie in an examination of inner-city social organizations and childrearing techniques. Although such an examination is beyond the scope of this chapter, we concur with Ogbu that inner-city Black Americans and White middle-class Americans do not share the same effective environment, even within the same city. Several different theoretical approaches have focused on this "effective environment," and two are described below.

Social-Ecological Approach

Bronfenbrenner (1979) has elaborated the construct of an ecological system, within which the range of adaptation can be examined and understood. His descriptive categories are applicable to a full range of adolescent-environment interactions. This model is helpful in organizing the pernicious social, political, and economic dynamics that generate stress in the lives of Black youths and their families and is useful in describing the coping and successful adaptation of many Black youths.

The model delineates four kinds of system variables. Microsystems include those daily interactions with family members, peers, school teachers, and others who have a direct impact on the child. Interactions between and among elements of the microsystem that affect the child more indirectly are referred to as mesosystems (e.g., interactions between family and school). Exosystems refer to those formal settings (agencies) within the child's environment where decisions occur that will directly affect the child or his or her microsystems, even without direct contact. The most comprehensive system in Bronfenbrenner's framework, and perhaps the most important, is the macrosystem. This system comprises the pervasive values and mores in institutional (exosystem) settings.

The social ecology of Black youth, therefore, is characterized by a common culture derived from the macrosystemic devaluation of Black people. Pervasive macrosystem values such as prejudice and racism that permeate American institutions can contribute to the stress experienced by its victims and have pernicious direct and indirect effects throughout the ecological environment of children, adolescents, and adults. Such stress may readily manifest itself in psychological and behavioral disorders.

These various ecological systems (together with the relevant data) provide a context within which to understand the disorders affecting Black adolescents. They also highlight the complexity of the barriers experienced in the search for traditional remedies—and the alternative strategies that can lead to adaptive outcomes. For example, at the exosystem level, the only mental-health facility in the Black community may have too few therapists because of an unfair allocation of resources from the city, and Black parents may fail in their attempts to address this problem with White city officials (mesosystem level) because of racial prejudices and insensitivity (macrosystem level). At the microsystem level the Black adolescent seeking an alternative to the overcrowded mental-health clinic may be frustrated by his or her difficulty in commuting to another part of town where facilities are less crowded because of an inability to pay for transportation. He or she may arrive successfully at another clinic only to be turned away because of a residential requirement. A similar sequence of events could be replicated across a variety of experiences and institutions in Black communities. It is thus important to understand the cumulative effects associated with such frustrating experiences. The second approach helps in this task.

Survival Strategies Approach

This approach focuses on Black survival strategies within a racist and discriminatory macrosystem. As has been noted elsewhere in this chapter, the influence of the "melting pot" ideology has sometimes led social scientists to view Black adolescents through "color-blind" eyes, without sufficient regard for their ethnicity, socioeconomic status, and the social context in which they live. Yet Black adolescents live in environments where it becomes necessary to engage in coping behaviors because of problems uniquely associated with their skin color and society's reaction to it.

Ogbu (1985) described these coping behaviors as subsistence strategies on which Blacks judge competence. He presented an interesting list of hypothetical adult categories and activities exemplifying these strategies and competencies. The conventional worker, for example, holds a conventional job in the mainstream economy while the client (also called the "Uncle Tom") attaches himself or herself to a White patron in return for needed services or poor wages. Collective struggle (commonly associated with civil-rights activities) is used by Blacks to increase their pool of conventional resources in the inner city while entertainment exploits the social and economic resources within Black communities to satisfy people's needs for amusement and therapy in coping with problems. Mutual exchange relies on kin-based households and friendship networks in which members are expected to help each other with temporary shelter, food, clothing, childrearing, and other goods and services.

Hustling is a strategy used in the street economy to obtain money, goods, and services; pimping uses interpersonal relationships for monetary gain and is often an aspect of hustling activities. Finally, the "street man" uses physical strength to achieve desired ends—money, sex, services, and goods.

Membership in the above categories is not mutually exclusive. A person may belong to different categories at different points in time and/or in different situations. For example, the hustler or pimp may hold conventional employment at times or be involved in a mutual-exchange relationship. The importance of these categories or labels for our purposes is that they illustrate both traditional and alternative styles of coping.

Ogbu argued that an examination of the rearing and adjustment patterns shows that the majority of inner-city Blacks who acquire the knowledge, motivation, and skills to grow into confident adults have learned to adapt to two cultures simultaneously—the immediate environment and the wider world of the White middle-class. Assessments of behavior using criteria appropriate to a different milieu are thus likely to lead to diametrically opposed conclusions about an individual's capacity for adaptation.

Ogbu's adaptive cultural model, while intriguing and controversial, is without empirical support. More research is needed for a better understanding of Blacks' simultaneous and relatively successful adaptation to two cultures. The model does suggest, however, that some behaviors considered pathological in Black adolescents by White diagnosticians and therapists may, in fact, have adaptive value and that, as Ogbu argued, Black children and their families need to be seen in the context in which they live.

Major Relevant Health Issues

GENERAL HEALTH STATUS

Adolescents as a group are typically healthier than other age groups. Nevertheless, it is the only age group whose mortality rate has increased over the past three decades. Good health status is a function of many factors, including health education, nutrition, and access to health care; poverty and minority status affect each of these variables adversely. Low-income youth, for example, are much less likely to have public or private health insurance and, as a consequence, are 40%–50% less likely to receive physician and hospital care (Children's Defense Fund, 1985).

Disparities in mortality rates between Blacks and Whites begin at birth; Black infants are twice as likely to die as White infants. At the other end of the life cycle, the average life expectancy for Blacks is 69.6 years, as compared with 75.2 years for Whites (Gibbs et al., 1989). General health status differentials throughout life exhibit similar trends. Blacks, for example, have higher serum cholesterol levels and higher blood pressure levels than Whites. These general trends are apparent in adolescent age groups as well.

Black adolescents compared with their White counterparts have a higher incidence of mortality, chronic impairments, disabilities, physical handicaps, obesity, and elevated blood pressure (Brunswick, Merzel, & Messeri, 1985). Despite this greater vulnerability, they have had less access to needed services both in prevention and tertiary care. Blacks are twice as likely as Whites to have no regular access to health care and to rely more heavily on hospital emergency rooms and other outpatient facilities. This lack of services may contribute to their increased risk for health problems.

While technological advances have decreased mortality in general, there are many new environmental risk factors that are causing increased morbidity and mortality for adolescents. The three leading causes of death in adolescents are accidents, suicide, and homicide. One way of assessing these effects is by the years of potential life lost. Blacks of both sexes exhibit twice the number of potential years lost from these causes combined, but racial differences are not consistent across the categories. Whites show higher rates of suicide and death from automobile accidents, whereas Black adolescents have higher rates of other kinds of accidents and are five times more likely to die from homicides as are White youths. Mortality rates are also affected by gender. Males are much more likely to die during adolescence from most of these causes, particularly suicide (where White males show the highest rate) and homicide.

In addition to fatalities, a number of other societal conditions are related to increasingly significant physical- and mental-health problems in adolescents, including substance use and abuse (cigarettes, alcohol, and illicit drugs); physical abuse; careless sexual practices leading to teenage pregnancy and sexually transmitted diseases; and careless risk-taking behavior resulting in accidents and injuries.

Prenatal Care

Good health begins before birth. One of the most significant factors affecting the health of infants is the availability and quality of medical care during the mother's pregnancy. Women who do not receive such care are more likely to have birth complications, premature births, infants of lower birth weight, and increased infant mortality. Babies born to mothers receiving prenatal care are five times as likely to live and six times as likely not to be born prematurely as those not receiving care (U.S. Congress, Select Committee on Children, Youth, and Families, 1989). Low-birthweight infants

43

are associated with a variety of risk factors from birth on, including higher infant mortality, birth injury, poorer health, lower attention spans, and greater incidence of learning disorders.

The issue of appropriate prenatal care is particularly germane to Black adolescents in two ways: they themselves may be exhibiting the sequelae of nonexistent or poor quality care, and, if current trends continue, substantial numbers of Black females will be mothers before they reach the age of 20. While more than 75% of pregnant women in the U.S. do receive prenatal care in their first trimester, the 25% who do not are disproportionately represented in poor Black adolescents (Brown, 1988).

Although Medicaid was created in 1965 to increase the availability of medical and prenatal care for low-income individuals, substantial ethnic disparities continue to exist in the use of prenatal care. Black women are twice as likely as White women to receive late or no care. Those most at risk are low-income, unmarried, inner-city teenagers. Insufficient care is also more pronounced in some geographic areas than in others. A woman in New York State, for example, is three times as likely as one in Michigan or Connecticut to obtain late or no care. There are four major barriers to obtaining prenatal care: cost (inability to afford health insurance), fear of medical procedures, ambivalence about the pregnancy, and denial.

Lack of money or insurance appears to be the most significant factor obtained in almost all studies of this age group (Brown, 1988). Although employers are prohibited from discriminating against pregnant women with regard to medical insurance, most Black pregnant teenagers are not employed and their parents are not likely to have maternity coverage. Medicaid coverage is inadequate. An increasingly large portion of the poor is not enrolled in Medicaid programs because of eligibility requirements. In 1988 the average income eligibility ceiling for Medicaid was only 49% of the federal poverty level (Hill, 1988). Moreover, even those who are enrolled in Medicaid may not obtain early prenatal care because of cumbersome program enrollment requirements, reliance on overburdened clinics that may provide less adequate care, and a shrinking pool of obstetricians willing to work for low Medicaid rates as their malpractice insurance premiums soar. These issues exemplify problems at Bronfenbrenner's exosystem level.

A prestigious committee that studied prenatal care in the United States concluded that it had a maternity care system that is fundamentally flawed, fragmented, and overly complex with no direct, straightforward system for making maternity services easily accessible. Although well-insured, affluent women can be reasonably certain of receiving appropriate health care during pregnancy and childbirth, many other women cannot share this expectation (Brown, 1988, p.136). Poor Black teenagers have less access than most. In view of this glaring inequity and the proven cost-effectiveness of prenatal care across a wide variety of health problems, a macrosystem change is needed to ensure all pregnant women receive access to maternity health care.

Nutrition and Fitness

Over the past decade there has been increasing recognition that dietary and exercise practices play an important preventative role in a variety of illnesses. Poor nutrition is associated with poorer health during adolescence as well. Low-income Black children and adolescents are more likely than Whites to suffer from poor nutrition and its attendant health problems. It has been estimated (Children's Defense Fund, 1985) that 20%–30% of all low-income children suffer from health problems related to inadequate diet or chronic malnutrition, including iron deficiency anemia, fatigue, decreased attentiveness, impaired weight gain, stunted physical growth, and brain cell damage (Carter, 1983; Gibbs, 1988). High levels of anemia are found in low-income Black adolescents and may be associated with increased irritability, restlessness, and lowered attentiveness (Carter, 1983). Poor adolescent dietary habits are associated with increased later risk of illnesses such as cardiovascular problems, heart conditions, and diabetes.

The incidence of hunger and malnutrition and its sequelae has increased over the past decade, particularly for Black youth and their families (U.S. Congress, Select Committee on Hunger, 1985). Despite this trend, the Reagan and Bush administrations cut funds and restricted eligibility for food-stamp and nutrition programs. In the 1980s the federal government spent more to store the surplus products of farmers than it did to support food stamps and school-lunch programs.

Other Health Issues

A variety of syndromes are overrepresented in Black adolescents relative to other groups. One relatively rare genetically transmitted disease found primarily in Blacks is sickle-cell anemia. It is a chronic, disabling disease that affects one of every 600 Blacks. Symptoms during crises, which require hospitalization, include fevers, respiratory infections, eye problems, arthritic pain, extreme organ pains, and progressive damage. This illness, currently incurable, can result in premature death.

Tuberculosis (TB), a disease many believed was practically extinct, has recently exhibited an alarming increase among low-income Blacks. The tuberculosis rate in Blacks is five times that found in Whites. More than one third of recently recorded new cases are among Blacks, and Black males are four times as likely to contract TB as their White counterparts (Centers for Disease Control, 1987b). While there may be some genetic differences in predisposition to TB, it is also a disease generally associated with poverty, poor housing conditions, and poor health care. The increase may also be partially related to the increase in AIDS cases, for these individuals become vulnerable to this infection. The incidence seems to be on the increase in homeless families as well, where Blacks are again overrepresented.

Hypertension is a major chronic illness among adult Black males. This disease likely has its roots in the high proportion of Black male teenagers who show elevated blood pressure levels (Carter, 1983). In fact, cardiovascular disease is the fifth leading cause of death for Black adolescent males, and Black teenagers die from heart and congenital defects at twice the rate of White teenagers. Black teenage girls die from heart disease at three times the rate of their White counterparts. Little research attention has been directed to this problem.

It is interesting to note that prevalence rate for otitis media, which tends to be greater for ethnic groups than for Whites (see Fleming, Manson, & Bergeisen and Amaro, Messinger, & Cervantes, in this volume), is generally lower for Blacks than for Whites. For example, the Health Interview Survey of the National Center for Health Statistics (1975) showed the rate of otitis media for Black children to be only half (5.4%) the rate for White children (11.4%). These results were confirmed by other studies from various areas around the country (e.g., Robinson & Allen, 1984) and may be explained by anatomical differences.

A host of other health problems that are related to poor housing conditions are more common in Black youth. They include chronic respiratory problems, infestation from vermin, insect, and rat bites, and accidents due to poorly constructed buildings. Overcrowded households and lack of parental supervision also make Black youth particularly vulnerable to physical and sexual abuse (Hampton, 1986). These vulnerabilities are often attributable to both an exosystem and a macrosystem that devalue this group, assigning fewer resources to medical care for and research on particular health problems.

MENTAL HEALTH AND PSYCHOSOCIAL ISSUES

Precise estimates of the incidence of mental disorders in Black adolescents are difficult to arrive at. The major problem is the absence of large epidemiological surveys of mental-health problems in Blacks. Estimates that have been made are also often associated with bias in the diagnosis of Black patients, which may lead to either underestimates (e.g., with depression) or overestimates (e.g., psychoses or conduct disorders) of particular syndromes.

Despite these important concerns, a number of epidemiological and research studies give evidence of higher incidences of both behavioral disturbances and associated physical illnesses among Black urban youths than among their White counterparts. Childhood psychopathology has its highest rates among Black children in poor, urban communities. A study in Manhattan reported that proportionately twice as many Black as White children showed psychiatric impairment (Langer, Gersten, & Eisenberg, 1974). Studies of Black urban grade-school children report very high incidences of depression (see, e.g., Vincenzi, 1987). A number of recent investigators have further suggested that existing theories concerning mental illness may not be readily generalizable from the White population on which they are based. Additionally, there have been few people of color in fields such as psychiatry or clinical psychology, and, accordingly, training programs have paid little emphasis to subcultural differences in adaptation.

The omission in attention to subcultural differences is not limited to theories about mental illness; it is equally evident in our general developmental theories concerning adolescence. To take one example, Erikson's (1959) theory is widely cited as containing key concepts for understanding the psychological transitions of adolescence. Erikson postulated an eight-stage life-span theory, in which each stage contains a central crisis to be resolved. According to Erikson, the modal issue for adolescents is identity, and the characteristic crisis needing resolution is the establishment of a strong personal identity in various areas, including interpersonal, vocational, and philosophical spheres.

According to this theory, adolescents encounter various possible routes and pitfalls in this quest, and poor resolution of the crisis results in a diffuse or incomplete sense of one's adult roles. The path of adolescence begins with a period of identity diffusion in early adolescence, where no firm commitments are made, then continues to a period of identity moratorium, a period of active uncertainty in which different roles are tried out. The adolescent may proceed to (and presumably remain in) a phase of identity foreclosure, in which beliefs and life goals are chosen "prematurely" without weighing the many alternatives and options available. A mature identity is achieved by trying various alternatives, experiencing the associated anxiety, and emerging with more stable commitments associated with the phase of identity achievement in which adult roles are assumed. Research conducted within this framework (Marcia, 1980) suggests that many adolescents fail to reach the more mature stage of identity achievement.

Almost all the research dealing with adolescent identity development has been conducted with White middle-class samples. Some aspects of Eriksonian theory may be applicable to understanding some of the mental-health problems associated with Black adolescents as well. Undoubtedly, concern about identity cuts across all groups of adolescents. The theory, however, begins with the assumption that the developing youth has unlimited options. This assumption may not be tenable for less affluent groups who lack the time, the financial and psychological support, and the leisure to sample many roles.

Identity crises also do not emerge fully blown at adolescence. Rather, each stage is somewhat dependent on what has transpired in prior stages. According to Erikson, in the prior developmental stage of industry versus inferiority, children establish fundamental attitudes toward work. If they learn to master certain basic skills and are reinforced for doing so, they emerge with a positive sense of efficacy. If, on the other hand, they do not master societally valued skills and are negatively reinforced for the skills they do acquire, they are likely to develop feelings of lack of worth and negative self-esteem. Inadequate urban schools, then, may not only be failing these children in terms of basic education; they may also be contributing to their feelings of inadequacy by devaluing and rejecting them. This may, in turn, lead to the identity pathway that Erikson called negative identity, which is based on characteristics that oppose the dominant culture (i.e., becoming the rebel, the "meanest," or the most deviant).

A similar concept has been proposed by Steele and Nisbett (1989), namely, "protective identification." They argued that vulnerability to stigmatization causes individuals to "disidentify" with the mainstream orientation associated with the vulnerability and to turn to alternative types of identities. The results of both theories are similar but may indicate different modes of intervention.

Studies of child development have focused on White families and have erroneously assumed that cultural factors are the same for Blacks and Whites. Thus, our most widely accepted conceptualizations about adolescent development have tended to ignore subcultural differences about the very meaning of adolescence. What does preparation for an adult role mean to a teenager who has been alienated from and victimized by the very society that now expects conformity?

Gender is another variable associated with differing patterns of adaptation, dysfunctional behavior, and differential experiences of adolescence. Space limitations constrain discussions about the possible bases underlying gender differences, but these have been widely discussed elsewhere (see Kavanagh & Hops, 1994; Russo, 1990). Socialization practices associated with male and female development clearly differ in ways that influence adaptation and the development of coping strategies and symptoms (see Silvern & Katz, 1986; Katz, Boggiano, & Silvern, 1993). These patterns themselves vary within particular subcultural groups (see, e.g., Katz, 1987). Such interactions between race and gender are germane to a complete understanding of the data presented in this chapter, even though we are unable to consider them in detail. With these issues in mind, we now turn to the estimates of mental illness that have been made according to the traditional diagnostic categories.

Psychosis

Black youth have considerably higher (by about two to three times) rates of hospitalization than Whites. As previously noted, investigators (e.g., Gibbs, 1988) have questioned whether this finding reflects true sample differences or diagnostic bias. Blacks are often assigned more serious diagnoses than are Whites even though presenting symptoms are similar. This trend may well reflect institutional racism that uses White middle-class behavior patterns as normative.

Additional problems in assessing accurate rates of psychiatric disorder are that available statistics are based only on the minority of individuals who seek psychiatric treatment, and not the many who seek help from ministers, relatives, or the hospital emergency room. Despite these provisos, the level of stress experienced by inner-city Black youth clearly is often overwhelming and those who are unable to tolerate the continual microassaults of racism often develop a variety of mental disorders.

Gibbs (1988) is one of the many investigators who has eloquently described the kinds of stress Black youth are continuously and cumulatively exposed to: "a teacher calls him stupid; a White stranger gets up and walks away when he sits next to him on a crowded bus or subway; . . . a cab driver ignores him or refuses to take him to a 'Black' neighborhood; a police officer stops to question him in a White neighborhood . . . these daily interactions take an enormous toll on the mental health of Black youth in America, driving many of them to the depths of despair and the brink of madness" (p.242).

The incidence of schizophrenia in the general population (all age groups combined) is estimated at 1%. The incidence rate for adolescents is not essentially different than that for the general population, as most forms of schizophrenia begin during late adolescence and early adulthood. For Black males the rate is about twice as high. Schizophrenia is diagnosed in 25%–30% of all adolescents admitted to public mental hospitals, and Black adolescent males are six times as likely as White males to be so diagnosed. It is not clear why males should be more adversely affected than females.

The incidence of serious affective disorders (e.g., psychotic levels of depression or manic-depressive syndromes) is about 4% in adults, but this disorder tends to be less frequent in youth when hospital admissions are studied. Earlier studies suggested a lower prevalence of affective illness in Blacks than in the general population, but more recent studies have shown high rates of depression in low-income Black adolescents. Some have suggested the rates of serious depression may be between 5% and 15%. In White populations, much is made of greater incidence of female depression (see, e.g., Kavanagh & Hops, 1994); these gender differences are less pronounced in Blacks. Suicide rates for Black male adolescents have nearly tripled between 1960 and 1985 and have doubled for Black female teenagers in this time (Gibbs et al., 1989).

The ecological reality for most Black adolescents would seem to generate considerable depressive symptomatology, although it may not always be recognized as such. Investigators have suggested that depression is underestimated in this population because "depressive equivalents" may include high-risk behaviors and acting out. Additionally, typical depressive symptoms such as fatigue, loss of appetite, and difficulty in carrying out everyday activities may be interpreted by adolescents and their families as physical ailments rather than mental-health problems.

Black youth who are diagnosed as psychotic are more likely to be placed in state and county inpatient facilities and have lower rates of admission to private inpatient services. This trend has led some to suggest that a dual system of care exists concerning race (Thompson et al., 1986). Within the psychiatric facility itself, Black youth are also more likely to receive different kinds of treatment for the same diagnoses (Jones & Korchin, 1982). Mental-health workers often mistakenly believe that Black patients are unable to profit from psychotherapy (i.e., because of insufficient verbal skills, motivation, etc.); thus, they are more likely to receive supportive treatment and medication, which may be less effective. Some recent evidence suggests that this trend is true for physical ailments as well. Black patients, for example, are much less likely than Whites to receive kidney transplants (the more desirable treatment) and more likely to receive dialysis (the less effective treatment; Kutner & Brogan, 1991). Once again, the exosystem and macrosystem appear to interact to produce harmful outcomes.

A number of implications follow from these racial disparities in mental-illness diagnosis. First, there may be real problems in the accuracy of diagnoses as they are used for epidemiological purposes. It may be the case, for example, that health workers of different racial groups would interpret behavioral adaptations differently, leading to different diagnoses. Second, the diagnostic criteria themselves may be culturally or situationally inaccurate or biased. Third, whatever the underlying cause of the inaccuracy, intervention would be expected to be relatively ineffective if geared toward an inaccurate diagnosis (i.e., schizophrenia rather than depression). These issues point to dilemmas and conflicts in the recruitment and training of health-care professionals, where sensitivity to culturally formed adaptive behavior patterns is not adequately reinforced. They also illustrate a need for further research to help explicate whether the increased incidence in several mental disorders among Blacks is due to diagnostic bias or the increased stress that Blacks experience in a racist society.

Conduct Disorders, Juvenile Delinquency, and Criminal Behavior

Aggressive antisocial behavior patterns appear to be on the increase and have received a good deal of media attention. Such behavior is likely to first lead to difficulty in the school setting and later to delinquency. Black teenagers have a disproportionately high rate of conduct problems in school settings. They are suspended or expelled more often than Whites for truancy and aggressive behavior toward peers and teachers.

Aggressive, acting-out behavior outside school settings is likely to lead to trouble with law-enforcement agencies. While in absolute terms few adolescents are arrested (6.276 arrests per 100,000; U.S. Department of Justice, 1988), this age group accounts for proportionately more arrests for serious crimes than their numbers would suggest. The juvenile-justice system, as currently constituted, does little to modify acting-out behavior. Instead, boys convicted at an early age appear to become the most persistent offenders as adults. Self-reported offenders who are convicted between the ages of 14 and 18 are more likely to commit crimes at later ages than those who commit crimes as adolescents but are unconvicted (Farrington, 1977). Black adolescents are overrepresented in arrest statistics relative to their numbers, accounting for 54% of arrests of violent crimes by juveniles, 68% of arrests for aggravated assault, and 45% of arrests for robbery (U.S. Department of Justice, 1988). They are also twice as likely to be arrested for property crimes as Whites.

Black adolescents are also at greater risk of being victims of violent crimes. Homicide is currently the leading cause of death for Black male adolescents (Centers for Disease Control, 1986), and the homicide rate is nearly six times as great as for White males. These disparities, however, diminish considerably when socioeconomic levels are held constant (Dembo, 1988). Most homicides are perpetrated by peers and involve the use of guns. In addition, Black adolescents are more likely to be killed in confrontations with the police than are Whites (Pierce, 1986). Current estimates are that a young Black male has a 5% chance of being killed by violent means during his lifetime, a rate that is five times higher than for White males. This chilling rate has turned out to be an underestimate for the 1990s, and the seeming explosion of crimes of violence has received considerable attention.

Various interpretations have been given to these statistics. One is that criminal behavior may be used as a coping strategy where ecosystem alternatives are limited, as discussed earlier. Crime rates are strongly associated with low socioeconomic levels and urban location, which impinge profoundly on Black youth since poverty inhibits informal social control within families (Sampson & Laub, 1994). Statistics comparing racial groups do not typically control for such demographic factors. When only self-reports of offenses are examined (Krisberg et al., 1986), these disparities are much smaller than those typically reported in arrest statistics.

Arrest statistics themselves are not uniformly accepted as good indicators of levels of criminal behavior. Blacks are more likely to be arrested than Whites engaged in the same behavior (e.g., Huizinga & Elliot, 1986). Negative stereotypes about Blacks held by police may lead to more arrests if the behavior of Black youth is regarded as inherently suspicious. The initial acquittal of Los Angeles police officers in the beating of motorist Rodney King exemplifies the differences likely to be encountered by Blacks and Whites in the criminal-justice system. Antisocial behavior in many White adolescents is more likely to be interpreted and treated as an index of emotional disturbance, whereas the equivalent behavior in Black adolescents is more typically dealt with by the juvenile-justice system (Dembo, 1988).

Numerous theories have been proposed to explain juvenile delinquency, but few are associated with strong corroborative research. Two factors that have not been widely studied by criminologists merit further elaboration and investigation: television influences and father absence.

A recent report by the American Psychological Association (Huston et al., 1992) noted that, by early adolescence, "the young viewer will have witnessed approximately 8,000 murders and more than 22,000 assorted acts of violence—more than 30,000 violent acts before they hit the schools and streets of our nation as teenagers." Correlations are consistently obtained between amount of television violence viewed and degree of aggressive behavior displayed (Freedman, 1984), both in natural and experimental settings.

These findings may be particularly relevant for Black adolescents for several reasons. Television watching peaks in early adolescence (Huston et al., 1987), a period coinciding with initial delinquent forays. Low-income individuals watch more television (Greenberg, 1986). Blacks watch more than Whites, even when socioeconomic status is controlled, and rely on it for news and information more often (Staples & Jones, 1985). Additionally, research shows that adolescents as a group are underrepresented and devalued on television (Signorella, 1987), thereby providing few positive role models. Thus, the pernicious effects of television violence may be particularly pronounced on young, poor Black adolescents.

The issue of family composition is frequently mentioned in connection with Blacks because of the increasingly high incidence of single-parent, mother-headed families in this group. In 1960 single-parent families constituted 9% of all Black families. In 1980 this figure was 40%, and more recent census figures show a further increase to 44%. While the most deleterious effect associated with female-headed families is poverty, there may well be other negative effects of not having a resident father present, particularly on boys.

One of the hallmarks of adolescence is the differentiation of adult-oriented gender-role behavior within the context of physiological sexual maturity (Katz, 1986). According to some theorists (e.g., Hall, Lamb, & Perlmutter, 1982), early adolescence represents a time when behavioral gender stereotypes may become particularly pronounced; consequently, adolescents' behavior may appear to be caricatures of masculinity and femininity. In the absence of a consistently available, loving male model, adolescent boys may need to turn to others (including television characters) to learn how to behave in a masculine style.

Anthropological theories (e.g., Burton & Whiting, 1961) suggest that, in less industrialized societies, adolescent initiation rites are particularly stringent for boys who have lived their entire childhood in households with only adult women. Severe initiation rites to prove manhood are seen as counteracting earlier feminine identification in boys. It is not clear whether such a mechanism may be at work among Black adolescents from single-parent families, but this reasoning does suggest the need to parse out the effects of poverty from those of father absence.

In summary, we suggest that all adolescents have a need to define and enact gender-appropriate behavior, often in caricatured form. Boys who do not have access to consistently present, affectionate male models may be particularly vulnerable to the multiple television or street images that connect masculinity with violence.

Delinquent behavior typically begins in the early teen years; it is uncommon for crime to start in adulthood. The "typical" high-rate offender is a young male who begins crime in early adolescence, who comes from a troubled, low-income family, and whose parents are likely to have criminal records. He has a history of acting-out behavior in school, does poorly academically and often drops out, has difficulty finding a job, often becomes a frequent drug user, and commits crimes in the company of other young men (Farrington, Ohlin, & Wilson, 1986). It is apparent from this description that the same set of factors associated with delinquency underlies a wide variety of other adolescent problems.

The preceding discussion suggests a number of areas for preventative intervention. Societal concern with crime has led elected officials to stress apprehension and punishment rather than prevention. This emphasis may paradoxically have the opposite effect from that intended. Programs that attempt to frighten juveniles into stopping criminal activities by showing them the horrors of imprisonment often seem to backfire (see, e.g., Farrington et al., 1986; Lundman, 1984). Similarly, research on increasing the number of police shows that, while *fear* of crime decreases as more patroling officers are added to neighborhoods, crime *rates* do not seem to go down (Wilson & Kelling, 1982). Of the many different kinds of programs proposed for preventing delinquency, the most successful seem to be those that impart school-compatible skills to children (Dembo, 1988). Long-range solutions are more effective than short-term ones, but they are politically more difficult to enact.

While many theories have been proposed regarding the causes of delinquency, none of them have adequately addressed the most critical issue—individual differences. Most youth are not delinquent; a majority of crimes are committed by a relatively small proportion of chronic offenders (Wolfgang & Tracy, 1982). Some of the research attention currently devoted to why adolescents become delinquent should be redirected to ask why so many do not. Given the vast amount of social pathology, racism, and economic privation Black adolescents are often exposed to, how can we better understand the strengths and resiliencies of the many Black families whose teenagers do not get into trouble with the law? This question will be discussed later in the chapter.

Substance Abuse

Substance abuse represents a major health risk for adolescents. The statistics associated with substance abuse are staggering: half of the nation's hospital patients and most homeless people suffer from alcohol or drug abuse; the largest single cause of mental retardation is alcohol; one of every ten fetuses is exposed to illegal drugs; and three fourths of all homicides are drug or alcohol related, as are more than half the cases of rape, child abuse, and assault (Califono, 1989). Treatment is mostly unavailable (only 10% of those who need it get it) and unsuccessful (12% of those who enter drug programs are drug free after a year).

The most damaging substance is alcohol, despite its legality. It has been described as the number-one youth drug problem. It is also the most deadly since automobile accidents are the single largest cause of adolescent mortality, and almost half these are alcohol related. It is estimated that there are 3.3 million alcoholics under the age of 18 (Towers, 1987) and that alcoholism is on the increase for this age group. Although Black youth have somewhat lower rates of alcohol use than Whites, at least in early adolescence, rates of use are still substantial.

Another legal substance that is hazardous to health is nicotine. Despite the widely known adverse consequences of smoking, there are still 55 million smokers in the United States, and smoking habits usually start during adolescence. An earlier longitudinal study of inner-city Black youth in Harlem (Brunswick, 1979) found that 57% were smokers, a higher percentage than was reported for all high school seniors in 1988 (29%; National Institute on Drug Abuse, 1987).

Almost 60% of American teenagers try at least one illicit drug before they graduate from high school. White and Black adolescents have equal rates of marijuana use, which is the most widely used of the illicit drugs. Incidence of use among teenagers has been estimated at 13% in the National Survey on Drug Abuse. Heroin use appears to be on the decline, although it remains considerably more prevalent in Black communities than elsewhere. Cocaine use, including crack, is also higher among Black adolescents, whereas tranquilizers and stimulant pills are more frequently used by Whites. The earlier the onset of drug use, the longer and more heavily that substance will be used, but substances used are not independent. In the Brunswick study, for example, all heroin users also smoked marijuana, and 80% of them also used cocaine.

It is difficult to accurately determine rates of drug use in Black adolescents because most surveys have dealt with high school seniors who live with their families. Actual rates are probably higher for Black populations because school dropouts and those living away from their families are excluded from the analyses. Moreover, racial data typically aggregate Blacks from southern rural areas, who exhibit low drug usage, with those residing in inner-cities, who have high drug-use rates (Brunswick, 1988). These differences deserve more attention than they have received and demonstrate the significance of the social environment to drug usage, above and beyond race and economic level.

The health risks associated with high adolescent rates of drug use are considerable. Those Black adolescents who become addicted to heroin, for example, begin this usage at about age 15 and have a four times greater likelihood of dying before their midtwenties than those who do not use heroin. They are also more likely to be school dropouts, to have been incarcerated by their twenties (30% vs. 3% in the low drug-involved group), and have more skin problems, more accidents, a greater incidence of gonorrhea (45% vs. 3%), and a much greater likelihood of getting AIDS from intravenous drug use. The recent rise in the use of crack is equally problematical because of its extremely addictive properties and the monetary inducements for selling it, even among young children. As Gibbs (1988) noted, drug use in general is particularly problematic for many low-income Black youth because it is so often linked to a lifestyle that includes delinquency and selling drugs. Because of the competition associated with crack sales, violence is also increasing in ghetto communities. In large urban centers, such as Los Angeles, teenage gang activity related to drug sales has greatly increased, and this is generally attributed to both crack use and the ease with which guns are procured.

Like many of the other issues addressed in this chapter, society currently seems singularly unable to deal successfully with the increasing frequency of teenage drug abuse. A 40% *decrease* in support services occurred from 1980 to 1986 (U.S. Congress, Select Committee on Children, Youth, and Families, 1989). Many clinics have waiting lists for treatment from six to eighteen months, and the mental-health block grants funding some of these drug-treatment services have been cut 32% since 1981.

It is important to recall that Black adolescents exhibiting problem drug use represent a minority. Once again, research directed at understanding how so many adolescents manage to avoid the easy availability and economic lures of drug involvement could inform us about the strengths still available in disintegrating neighborhoods.

Educational Problems

It is important to note how frequently other psychosocial difficulties of Black youth are associated with school failure. While most of the research is correlational, making causality difficult to discern, academic problems appear to occur more often for those youth who become delinquent, drug abusers, and/or pregnant.

Much has been written about the lower scores obtained by Black youth on national achievement tests and the myriad problems associated with inner-city schools, and these are indeed causes for concern. Various theories have been propagated that focus on such factors as youth attitudes, bureaucratic rigidity, or lack of fit between school expectations and Black cultural values. In this latter vein Boykin (1980), for example, has argued that Black children and youth are less impersonal and more responsive and expressive than Whites and are, thus, turned off by an educational system that appears to them to be artificial and arbitrary. Since non-White students constitute more than 70% of the public-school populations in fifteen of the largest cities (e.g., 70.2% in Boston, 74% in Dallas, 92% in Atlanta, 78.2% in Los Angeles), the expectation for cultural sensitivity in public education is certainly a reasonable one.

Continued attention needs to be paid to why youth fail, but it is also necessary to recognize Black achievements. Fifteen percent of Black youth are below the national average in reading proficiency (Reed, 1988); we often ignore that the other 85% are at or above it. More Blacks receive low grades than Whites, but high percentages of Blacks who graduate from high school receive A's as well. The percentage of Black students completing high school rose dramatically from 12.9% in 1960 to 63% in 1990. While Black college enrollment has been declining since 1978, a cause for concern, the reasons for this decline appear to be based more on political and deteriorating economic conditions rather than academic factors. Most Black college students drop out for financial, not academic, reasons. An analysis of the family income levels of Black college students reveals that more than half of them were less than $20,000 a year, whereas only 15% of White students come from that income bracket (Reed, 1988). These statistics can be interpreted (although they are usually not) as indicative of the strength found in the Black family and a testimony to their belief in the positive value of education. In fact, parental school involvement is a major factor in success for Black youth (Connell, Spencer, & Aber, 1994).

Despite positive values associated with education, Black youth still can anticipate the economic consequences of a racist system that pays White high school dropouts more than Black high school graduates and in which high unemployment and discrimination further reduce the economic returns ordinarily associated with education and training.

Teenage Pregnancy

By the time Black females are 20 years old, 67% have been pregnant at least once (Joint Economic Committee, 1994). Birth rates for Black teenagers varied by state, ranging from 103.9 per 1,000 15–19-year-olds to 217.9 per 1,000 (as compared with a range of 46 per 1,000 to 105.6 per 1,000 for White teenagers; Centers for Disease Control, 1993). Of these pregnancies, an estimated 84% are unintended; Ladner (1987) estimated that 87% of births to Black teenagers were out-of-wedlock. Sixty percent of teenage mothers rely on Aid to Families with Dependent Children (AFDC) for economic support.

The problems associated with teen pregnancy have been widely discussed. From the teenagers' point of view, more medical problems, such as toxemia and premature or prolonged labor, are associated with early pregnancy (Moore & Burt, 1982). The psychological sequelae are even more far-reaching, often including dropping out of school and failing to develop the necessary vocational skills that would carry one beyond poverty levels of income. From the infants' point of view, there are many potential problems as well. Because teenage mothers are less likely to seek prenatal care, their infants are more likely to be born prematurely and/or be of low birthweight—both of which increase the likelihood of medical problems at birth and later in childhood. These children are also more likely to live in poverty.

Adolescent pregnancy rates in the United States are considerably higher than in other developed countries despite similar rates of adolescent sexual activity. Of the top ten industrialized countries, the United States has the highest fertility rate for 15–19-year-olds. Rates of out-of-wedlock births for Black women ages 15–19 have almost doubled between 1950 and 1980 (from 47% to 88%). The rate of increase is actually higher for White women of the same age (from 9% to 37%), but the absolute numbers are lower.

Early pregnancy is associated with urban poverty (Moore, Simms, & Betsey, 1986). It has been argued by some that AFDC money may encourage early pregnancy, but the data do not show this to be the case. It has also been suggested that female adolescents are particularly susceptible to peer influence and are, thus, more likely to "go along" with sexual activity. There are widely held erroneous beliefs among teenagers that pregnancy cannot occur if intercourse occurs infrequently or at young ages. Some other explanations given include the need to have somebody to love (Ladner, 1987), to prove their womanhood, or to identify with other women in their families who are mothers. Another possibility, not frequently discussed, is that having a baby may be one of the few positive events achievable for some of these teenagers and that, despite the negative financial aspects, birth and childrearing may be gratifying. While this possibility needs further research, statistics indicate that 80%–84% of all teenage births are unintended and unwanted. Finally, some cases of teenage pregnancy may be the result of poor sexual decision making on the part of young women who have been sexually abused or exploited as children. Victims of sexual abuse may have difficulty with refusal skills and may have higher rates of unwanted pregnancy and abortions than women who were not abused. Wyatt (1992) has also presented some evidence that Black women may report rape less often than White women, even though they are at equal (or greater) risk of actually being raped.

It is interesting to note that most theories of teenage pregnancy focus on the female, either forgetting that a male is also necessary for procreation or assuming that the responsibility for "saying no" or for using birth control should be the woman's. This focus omits several salient facts. First, many teenagers become pregnant as a result of rape or incest. Second, it is easier for males to obtain condoms than it is for females to obtain effective birth-control technology (e.g., pills, diaphragms) without medical services.

Lower-income males, however, often view contraceptive use as "unmanly." Only 43% of metropolitan males ages 17–21 in a national survey said they used some method of contraception, and only 17% used a condom during their first sexual experience (Pleck, Sonerstein, & Swain, 1988). As the males grew older, their female partners tended to use birth-control pills more, but withdrawal remained a frequently employed, albeit ineffective, technique. Older males were even less likely to use condoms, perhaps because females took more responsibility for contraception. Black males in this survey were somewhat more likely not to use any contraceptive method at either their first intercourse (66% vs. 55% for Black and non-Black groups, respectively) or their most recent intercourse (41% vs. 36%). Attendance in a sex-education course was not predictive of condom use at either first intercourse, which took place four years prior to the interview, or their most recent sexual experience.

The most effective pregnancy prevention program for females appears to be a combination of receiving information regarding sex, pregnancy, and contraception prior to the initiation of sexual activity. Despite these results, however, the Adolescent Family Life Act of 1981, which funds pregnancy-prevention efforts, specifically prohibited grantees from using funds to provide information about contraceptives. Abortion funding, counseling, and referral were also specifically prohibited. Programs that have provided both information and contraceptives, such as those in Saint Paul, Minnesota, have seen the teenage birth rate reduced by half from 1976 to 1984 (Rosauer, 1988). Even though surveys show 80% of adults favor providing sex education and contraceptives, institutions rarely seem able to muster the courage required to buck controversy. Thus, even while the effectiveness of providing contraceptives has been shown, eight states have recently forbidden school-based clinics to provide them (English & Tereszkiewicz, 1989).

Pleck et al. (1988) noted how little research attention has been devoted to adolescent male contraceptive behavior and beliefs. It is also of interest to note how frequently television presents sexual activity. No reference is ever made to contraception, and pregnancy rarely results. The message is that contraception is unnecessary or irrelevant. Our institutions are clearly doing youth a disservice by not providing more realistic information. In their perhaps misguided zeal not to offend adults who oppose birth-control techniques, schools and the media have forgotten that more than 80% of the public favor sex-education programs that teach adolescents about contraception. It is difficult to understand why youth should be repeatedly shown messages about how much fun it is to drink beer and commit violence, while the depiction of sexually responsible behavior should be off-limits. As noted in the APA report previously cited, the young adolescent will have witnessed 8,000 murders on television by the age of 13 but not one instance of contraceptive use.

Sexually Transmitted Diseases and AIDS

Societal failure to provide youth with easily accessible contraception, combined with negative attitudes about its use, continues to have dire health consequences beyond pregnancy for teenagers. The rate of sexually transmitted diseases has been dramatically increasing among adolescents. As noted earlier, high percentages (45%) of heroin users have gonorrhea (Brunswick, 1988). Eighty percent of all new cases of syphilis are among Blacks (Centers for Disease Control, 1987a). Young Black males have somewhat higher rates of other sexually transmitted diseases than are found in the general population, which may be because of earlier initiation of sexual activity or negative attitudes about condom use (Gibbs, 1988). The increase in syphilis was associated with higher rates of HIV infection. Intravenous–drug users are also at considerably higher risk for AIDS, now becoming a leading cause of death for young adults. In late 1987, 35% of Blacks in whom AIDS was diagnosed had contracted it through intravenous drug use.

In 1988, Black adolescents represented 50% of 1,212 persons under age 20 diagnosed as having AIDS, 289 cases of AIDS among 13–19-year-olds (Centers for Disease Control, 1988), but more than 14,000 cases reported for the age 20–29 group. The individuals who developed the symptoms in their twenties probably became infected as teenagers (Hein, 1988) because of the long incubation period for this disease.

According to Gibbs (1988), AIDS occurs 2.6 times more often among Black men than among Whites. Among this group homosexual and bisexual men represented 46% of the cases, and heterosexual intravenous-drug users constituted 35%. Black youth account for 50% of identified AIDS cases under the age of 20. Of the AIDS cases reported in 1992, 34.9% were Blacks, 32% of AIDS deaths were Blacks, and Black males will be an increasing proportion of this population (Mays & Cockran, 1987). Because of less access to medical services, Black AIDS patients have a much lower average survival rate of eight months, compared with 18–24 months for Whites (Houstin-Hamilton, 1986). Despite the extent of this problem, services available for counseling these youth, their families, and their sexual partners are extremely inadequate (Honey, 1988).

Service Delivery Issues

AVAILABILITY OF MEDICAL CARE FOR ADOLESCENT HEALTH PROBLEMS
As noted earlier, Black teenagers are less likely than Whites to receive either preventative health care or appropriate medical services. In a medical study of Black Job Corps volunteers, for example, only half of those who needed corrective lenses had them. Dental services are also less likely to be available.

Various reasons underlie the lower accessibility of health-care services for low-income Black adolescents. As stated earlier, the primary causes appear to be financial inability to purchase private health-insurance and the changed eligibility requirements for Medicaid for the working poor. An analysis of the health insurance status of adolescents (U.S. Congress, Office of Technology Assessment, 1989) revealed that 15% of those between 10 and 18 years of age lacked public or private coverage. The corresponding figure for poor adolescents was 30%. The proportion of uninsured adolescents increased by 25% in the 1980s because of limitations on Medicaid eligibility. The most important determinant of coverage was family income.

In the absence of insurance coverage or funds to pay fees of private physicians, inner-city youth are most likely to turn to public clinics and hospitals. Although many of these services are adequate, many more are understaffed, have less well-trained, foreign doctors, are underfinanced, and have outmoded equipment. The emergency services of public hospitals are often scarcely able to cope with the quantity of presenting problems.

MENTAL-HEALTH SYSTEM DELIVERY

It has generally been recognized that there is an acute need for attention to adolescents' mental-health and psychosocial problems, both at the treatment and prevention levels. This need, however, does not reflect more severe emotional disturbances in adolescents than in other groups. Epidemiological studies have estimated adolescent emotional disturbances at 10%–20%, a figure comparable to the adult population (Powers, Hauser, & Kilner, 1989). Rather, this need is due to the absence of research, trained professionals, and programs aimed at the unique requirements of this age group, which health professionals have only recently begun to recognize and document.

Additional issues, such as cultural match between patients and therapists and problems of access, are particularly germane to Black youth. Most White mental-health professionals lack intercultural training. White therapists are often ignorant of the dynamics and interpretations of Black behavior in therapy and may, therefore, reach erroneous conclusions or pursue ineffective strategies. Additionally, insufficient numbers of Blacks are entering the mental-health field. Blacks, for example, constituted only 1.8% of the psychiatrists belonging to the American Psychiatric Association in 1984 (Liu & Yu, 1985).

Inpatient treatment often required by diagnosis of psychosis is met in this population by state and county mental hospitals. In 1984 there were 280 such hospitals, with an occupancy rate of almost 90%. Black patients constituted 18% of these admissions. As previously noted, even within mental-health settings, Black adolescents often obtain less optimal care than Whites. The conduct behaviors of Black adolescent males are also much more likely to result in their commitment to a correctional institution. In 1980 for every thousand Black males ages 15–24, 2.02 were inmates of mental hospitals, whereas 26.65 were in correctional institutions. In 1990, 30.8% of all juvenile court cases were Black adolescents; 42% of the inmates in public juvenile facilities were Black.

As noted earlier, services for the treatment of some psychosocial problems, such as substance abuse, are particularly sparse. The bulk of federal funds in the drug areas have gone into law enforcement rather than treatment. Little work has been done on development of substance-abuse treatment programs specifically for adolescents. Only 5% of the 3,000 facilities organized to treat drug and alcohol abuse served predominantly adolescent groups. Most teen referrals (typically made by the juvenile-justice system) are made to drug-free programs, which include drop-in centers, clinics, and challenge experiences (such as Outward Bound). Many are also sent to residential programs or alternative schools that provide counseling, education, and social activities. Residential programs appear to be more effective than drug-free programs. The most successful programs are those that obtain family involvement.

Prevention programs for substance abuse have received more attention. While the general strategy of prevention seems more promising, most of the commonly used approaches do not seem to work very well. These include moral exhortation, fear-provoking programs, increased information (which sometimes arouses interest in trying the drug), and programs aimed at developing values and interpersonal skills in a general context. Media efforts in the form of antidrug public service announcements have also not been particularly effective, perhaps because of the redundancy of advertisements proclaiming the value of taking legal drugs for so many ailments. The most successful programs are those that focus on factors involved in the initiation of drug use and that train adolescents how to withstand peer pressure. This psychosocial approach has been effective in smoking-prevention efforts directed at middle-class White early adolescents but has not yet been as widely used with alcohol, marijuana, or cocaine use prevention. One recent longitudinal program, Project Alert, is currently being undertaken in California, starting with seventh graders (Ellickson et al., 1988), but more such studies are needed.

ALTERNATIVE HEALTH-CARE SYSTEMS FOR BLACK ADOLESCENTS
For all ethnic groups, the hallmark of the adolescent years is change. Adolescence is often characterized by upheavals and conflicts associated with making the transition into adulthood. An interesting model by Jessor (1984) suggested that a number of factors inherent in adolescence affect behavioral health, including the attainment of reproductive maturity and sexual interest and the exaggerated influence of peers. The challenge to practitioners and researchers is to understand the specific ecosystems of Black adolescents so that more effective health services can be designed. Traditional helping professionals are likely to hold values and attitudes that are at variance with this subculture (Jones & Korchin, 1982). Health caretakers need to discard deficit models of Black culture and expend more effort to examine and understand these differences in order to raise the probability of a successful treatment outcome. This section will briefly describe several less traditional approaches that capitalize on subcultural differences to increase treatment efficacy.

Family Community Networks
Black families often serve the pivotal function as recipients and "circuit breakers" for stress, conflict, and confusion, despite their own greater vulnerability within society. For Black urban adolescents, problems of stress and conflict are compounded by problems of poverty, illiteracy, unemployment, and racism. The consequences of these bleak circumstances for many Black youths and their families are revealed in the previously noted high rates of institutionalization (psychiatric and correctional) and academic failure. Thus, management of adolescent health problems can be especially difficult. Many key strengths in Black family life have been identified that assist in this process, including strong kinship bonds, adaptability of family roles, strong religious orientation, and strong educational and work orientations. Sociologists have paid a great deal of attention to strengths in Black families (McAdoo, 1981; White, 1980). The models described below have been useful in explicating the strengths found in Black culture and family life. They afford avenues to uncovering alternative coping mechanisms, specifically for Black adolescents.

Informal Adoption. Informal adoption has a long tradition as an effective strategy used in stabilizing Black families. Hill (1972) described the tradition of "doubling up," in which Black families have taken in children and elderly people from other families. This practice, dating back to the time of slavery, has been a source of social, psychosocial, and economic support for many Blacks. The process of "child keeping" is a valuable resource for Black adolescents who do not have a strong family.

Additionally, informal adoption is important because Black children are notoriously more difficult to place through formal adoption practices than White children. The Black family becomes a vehicle through which a number of uncles, aunts, and others may participate in the rearing of any one Black child (White, 1980).

Genograms or Kinship Ties. Genograms are used in family therapy to help track and utilize the totality of family patterns and broaden the focus of nuclear family therapy. "Network" therapists recognize that the basic social unit for the Black adolescent may not be the nuclear family, or even a family kinship, but a collage of persons united through a psychosocial kinship. These observations have led to the establishment of therapy groups that include not only the nuclear family but also persons related by blood, marriage, friendship, neighboring residence, or work association. The genogram is based on the concept of this extended family tree (genealogy). The concept, borrowed from the field of anthropology, allows the therapist to organize and structure important information about the roles of family members and other significant individuals, their interrelationships, and their conflicts.

Boyd (1983) described how the genogram has been an essential part of her treatment process with Black families. She argued that caution must be used because the genogram requires the gathering of important "family secrets" that are not readily shared with strangers or even with clinicians prior to the establishment of a relationship of trust. To date little research has been conducted on the genogram, but its potential usefulness with Black adolescents lies in the ways in which intricate kinship patterns that seldom completely conform to bloodlines can be organized. Similarly, Brisbane and Womble (1985) noted that many Black teenagers have social or blood relatives (other than parents) whom they take into their confidence. They advocated utilizing this informal support system in treating Black adolescents for alcoholism. Research on such use should be encouraged.

The Church

The Black church is more than a religious institution; it is a viable mental-health resource. Hill (1972) elaborated the ways Blacks use religion to provide emotional release of tensions accumulated through experiences in an oppressive society. Singing, preaching, and social exchange all help to promote solidarity and a sense of attachment and identity. Additionally, many parishioners use pastors to discuss their problems. Religious social networks in which the minister and other congregates take on aspects of an extended family constitute important social services provided by Black churches. For example, counselors at the Harlem Interfaith Counseling Service, a Black agency in New York City, noted that many of their clients also receive mental-health and other forms of assistance from churches—especially during times of crisis (Boyd, 1983).

Ministers and other parishioners serve as a community-support system. Many Black adolescents are able to take advantage of pastoral counseling during troubled times, and in some instances ministers have agreed to serve as "cotherapists" in family-therapy settings. Religion has also been used as a vehicle for explaining and manipulating "reality" among some Black patients, especially adolescents (Allen, 1988). Black alcoholics can be helped in greater numbers through Alcoholics Anonymous if emphasis is placed on the spirituality that exists in the Alcoholics Anonymous program. In treating the Black teen alcoholic many authors cite the importance of the church, in addition to employee assistance programs and other social action and community organizations (Brisbane & Womble, 1985). Yet, few clinicians utilize the information on clients' religion as an aspect of the treatment process.

Alternative Religious Beliefs and Health Practices

Blacks have brought beliefs and practices regarding health and illness from diverse areas of the world. In addition to organized churches, Blacks who experience unendurable stress often have access to a folk medical system as an alternative health system. For many Blacks, health beliefs and practices have their roots in a composite of African culture, early European folklore, and traditional religion. They may use herbal medicines from Africa, the voodoo religions of the Caribbean, fundamental Christianity, and magic.

In some communities, spiritual advisers heal the sick. The range of treatments may include herbs, roots, religious rituals, and faith healing. Treatment sometimes includes items worn on the body to ward off danger (e.g., amulets) and items used in the home to keep away evil spirits or to bring good luck, such as candles, incense, voodoo dolls, and ritual kits (Snow, 1979). There are many types of folk healers, including herbal shop operators, faith healers, and neighborhood prophets.

Other religious sects also provide emotional and social support. Rastafarianism has figured prominently in explanations of mental health, especially among West Indians. The cult identifies strongly with African blackness, rejects Western culture as decadent, and views Christianity as a system of Black oppression and exploitation. Although Rastafarianism is mostly a religious system, it is also a form of political protest—and more important, a self-help economic movement (similar to the Black Muslims). Members wear their uncut hair in "locks," live in communes detached from society, and commonly use marijuana to aid meditation (Allen, 1988). Rastafarianism has been described as a logical form of indigenous self-understanding and meaning especially for the rural underclass and the urban ghetto poor at the bottom of a color-class system.

Middle class and socially mobile adolescents, in rebelling against authority, sometimes assume Rastafarianism as a negative or alternate identity and a repudiation of their parents and society. Many schizophrenic and some manic-depressive patients use Rastafarianism as a means of compensating for identity loss and the search for meaning (Allen, 1988). Rastafarians, however, are usually productive and as well integrated as the average population. Some clinicians believe that the Rastafarian lifestyle and belief systems may have a protective function in an alienating society. Islamic religious movements have also attracted many followers, in part because they provide self-help and other compensatory approaches to handling problems.

Community-Based Paraprofessionals

Black low-income families often do not, or cannot, make use of office-based or hospital facilities, and other alternatives are sometimes available. Epstein and Shainline (1974) conducted an experimental program to provide in-home paraprofessional parental-aide guidance and counseling to low-income Black families. Parent aides supervised by mental-health practitioners provided the sole therapeutic intervention. Results indicated that in-home interventions often led to effective outcomes, in part because of greater frequency of counselor-client interactions than is possible in a traditional office setting. Differences were less likely to be labeled as pathological, barriers between counselor and client were easier to surmount, and telephone communications occurred more often than in traditional settings. This approach suggests possibilities for reaching greater numbers of Black adolescents who are shut out from traditional services.

Parent aides should not be used simply to cut cost but should rather be integrated with traditional approaches. Black families could well benefit from mental-health teams that combine the parent-aide approach with in-office services. Paraprofessionals may also serve a facilitating role in helping Black families and their adolescents feel more comfortable with traditional systems.

The School

Schools represent an important community resource that provides adolescents with a variety of peers and other socialization agents. In some instances, such influences may override the family in importance. Although we have not found any special programs that represent alternatives to traditional health-giving services, we do note that the need for special-education services is an important aspect of health-care management. Practitioners must be sensitive to circumstances that indicate a need to intervene in the health process. Evidence of emotional, behavioral, or developmental problems provides useful insight into reasons for poor school performance.

The federal mandate of PL94–142, enacted in 1975, and the related Rehabilitation Act of 1973 makes it possible to design individualized programs of instruction for individuals with handicaps. These laws, recently updated, prohibit discrimination against any handicapped person in programs receiving federal funds. Further, they provide for program accessibility and availability of nonacademic services. Thus, the educational system also provides a variety of services to Black adolescents who suffer from various learning disabilities.

School-Based Clinics

As noted earlier, two major barriers to appropriate health care for Black adolescents are geographic and financial accessibility. Additionally, adolescents often mistrust adults and would, therefore, not be likely to return to places that seem insensitive to their concerns.

One of the most promising approaches to health services for Black adolescents is the school-based health clinic, which appears to overcome some of these barriers (Donovan & Waszak, 1989). As Millstein (1988) noted, the problem behaviors of adolescents are complex, interrelated, and unresponsive to simple interventions. Thus, a comprehensive approach appears to be needed, which is often provided in school-based health programs.

While these programs currently serve less than 1% of the adolescent population, they are aimed at minority youth (50% of all such clinic users are Black). They offer a wide array of important services, including physicals (21% of services, including those for sports), treatment of acute illnesses (25%), mental-health counseling (11%), reproductive services (10%), treatment of acne (4%), chronic illnesses (4%), and other conditions including hearing and vision problems (20%) (Carnegie Corporation, 1989). Services are offered at low or no cost, are easily accessible in the school, and are comprehensive in their offerings as well as in their referral networks. Judging from the high (71%) average enrollment rate and the relatively low cost of $50 to $150 per student per year (Millstein, 1988), one can infer that they are being well received, are sensitive to adolescents, and are cost-effective.

Conclusions

Although psychologists no longer think of adolescence as a time of invariable storm and stress, it clearly can be for some. Adolescence is a developmental period that represents the congruence of physiological sexual maturity, enhanced abstract cognitive capacity (Piaget, 1972), and the formation of adult identity (Erikson, 1959; Marcia, 1966). For many adolescents this confluence of factors increases their levels of stress. The advent of adolescence also has an impact on families. As Powers and colleagues noted, "Not only do families affect adolescent development, but aspects of adolescent development (e.g., puberty and cognitive change) affect the life of the family" (1989, p. 203).

Dealing with adolescents often reinvokes in parents adult memories of their own adolescent conflicts. Parents seem to expect to have difficulty with their adolescents. Thus, many adults have negative attitudes toward adolescents. Such negative attitudes toward adolescents in general combined with increasing racism (Katz & Taylor, 1989) may make Black teenagers particularly vulnerable to societal discrimination.

The nature of adolescents' social and physical environment clearly influences their goals, values, and behavior. The authors have reviewed the particular vulnerabilities of Black adolescents and have noted that they are more at risk for a variety of physical and mental-health problems than their White counterparts. Persistent and rising poverty, mounting social disruption, epidemic teen pregnancy, alcoholism, and divorce all pose risks to Black adolescents' physical and mental health. These factors rarely occur in isolation. Their interaction with each other and with other aspects of the social ecology, such as racism and discrimination, unfulfilled expectations, poor quality of life in the inner city, and limited opportunities may produce both maladjustment in Black adolescents and greater risk for later problems.

At present, there are limited programs for treatment or reduction of substance abuse, alcoholism, and unwanted pregnancies. There are many positive aspects of the Black community, however, that do provide adequate support for Black adolescents. Family and community networks play prominent roles in the Black community by providing a strong sense of work ethics, high achievement, strong kinship bonds, strong religious beliefs, and flexibility in roles. The church is also a strong and viable resource for support and emotional release.

Several nontraditional approaches to treatment, including the use of genograms in family therapy and the use of paraprofessionals to augment traditional office-based treatment, appear promising. Schools may also help in identifying adolescents with emotional, behavioral, and developmental problems needing attention.

Despite the alternative approaches described in this chapter, there is a continuing need for local, state, and federal programs to bring parity in health care for all Americans—especially Black Americans. To accomplish this task, major initiatives will be required. These include but are not limited to drug-abuse programs emphasizing treatment and education regarding AIDs in the Black community, clinical programs for the detection of sickle-cell disease in newborns, teen pregnancy counseling, and improved prenatal care facilities. School-based clinics have provided an effective avenue for providing health-care services. There is a dire need, however, for more Black trained professionals in the health fields to pursue other effective strategies.

Many of the behaviors that are problematical during the teenage years would be less so in adulthood. Many activities that are detrimental to good health, such as drinking and smoking, are age graded and are, therefore, symbolic of growing up. Within this context, however, there are clearly those that engage in a variety of abusive behaviors that go way beyond trying out "forbidden" adult behaviors. In studying adolescent transitions to nonhealthy behavior, Jessor and Jessor (1977) found that proneness to problem behavior was associated with particular personality patterns, including a high concern for personal autonomy, a lack of interest in conventional goals, a jaundiced view of society at large, and more tolerant attitudes about transgressions.

Although this longitudinal study primarily assessed White adolescents, many of these factors appear to also be characteristic of Black adolescents, particularly those who are poor and live in inner cities. Continued exposure to racist incidents elicits jaundiced views of society. A poor educational system and a deteriorating economy make conventional goals particularly problematic for this group. Finally, the relative absence of successful conventional role models and alternative avenues to financial success may well make inner-city youth more tolerant of illegal behavior.

It appears from this review that neither medical nor psychological practitioners have been successful in designing programs that adequately deal with the interrelated and complex psychosocial issues of Black adolescents. A better understanding of the developmental and social issues involved in adolescent acting-out behavior might improve our prevention and treatment programs.

One of the implicit social expectations for adolescents is that they will find a path to enter adult roles successfully. They must be able to attain their full intellectual, emotional, and behavioral potentials, both for their own mental health and for their future contributions to societal productivity. Attainment of these goals has been labeled "self-actualization" by Maslow (1970). Maslow's concept of a hierarchy of needs may be particularly applicable to understanding Black adolescent development. Within this theoretical system, the more basic needs must be satisfied before the higher-level ones. Thus, before adolescents are capable of self-actualization, they must have had their physiological needs, needs for safety, needs for belonging, needs for love, and needs for self-esteem satisfied, in that order. As we have demonstrated, inner-city Black youth are often hungry, live in unsafe environments, do not feel as if they belong, and are subjected to other ecological realities that would appear to make it difficult to establish positive self-esteem. Because so many of the factors underlying these trends can be changed, the lack of health in this group reflects the lack of health in our society. While we certainly would endorse the provision of additional physical and mental-health services to this subpopulation, we suggest that the problems are best dealt with in a proactive spirit. The symptoms have to be treated, but the underlying systemic issues need to be addressed.

The information provided in this chapter should be helpful in expanding treatment modalities for distressed Black adolescents. The synthesis of novel and traditional strategies is clearly needed to ameliorate the multiple problems among Black adolescents. This challenge must be met by all institutions dealing with this population so that they develop to their fullest potential.

References

Allen, E. A. (1988). West Indians. In L. Comas-Diaz & E. E. H. Griffith (Eds.), *Clinical guidelines on cross-cultural mental health* (pp. 303–332). New York: Wiley.

Boyd, N. (1983). Family therapy with black families. In E. E. Hones & S. J. Korchin (Eds.), *Minority mental health* (pp. 227–249). New York: Praeger.

Boykin, A. W. (1980, November). *Reading achievement and the social cultural frame of reference of Afro American children.* Paper presented at NIE Roundtable Discussion on Issues in Urban Reading, Washington DC.

Brisbane, F. L., & Womble, M. (1985). *Treatment of black alcoholics.* New York: Haworth.

Bronfenbrenner, U. (1979). *The ecology of human development: Experiments by nature and design.* Cambridge: Harvard University Press.

Brown, S. S. (1988). *Prenatal care, reaching mothers, reaching infants.* Washington DC: National Academy Press.

Brunswick, A. F. (1979). Black youths and drug-use behavior. In G. Beschner & A. Friedman (Eds.), *Youth drug abuse: Problems, issues and treatment* (pp. 443–492). Lexington MA: Lexington.

Brunswick, A. F. (1988). Young black males and substance use. In J. T. Gibbs (Ed.), *Young, black, and male in America: An endangered species* (pp. 166–187). Dover MA: Auburn House.

Brunswick, A. F., Merzel, C., & Messeri, P. (1985). Drug use initiation among urban black youth: A seven-year follow-up of developmental and secular influences. *Youth and Society, 17*, 189–216.

Burton, R. V. & Whiting, J. W. M. (1961). The absent father and cross-sex identity. *Merrill-Palmer Quarterly, 7*, 85–95.

Califano, J. A., Jr. (1989, December 8). Drug war: Fool's errand no.3. *New York Times,* p. A19.

Carnegie Corporation (1989 June). *Turning points, preparing American youth for the 21st century.* New York: Carnegie Corporation of New York.

Carter, J. H. (1983). Vision or sight: Health concerns for Afro-American children. In G. Powell, J. Yamamoto, A. Romero, & A. Morales (Eds.), *The psychosocial development of minority group children* (pp. 13–25). New York: Brunner/Mazel.

Centers for Disease Control. (1986). Premature mortality in the United States: Public health issues in the use of years of potential life lost. *Morbidity and Mortality Weekly Report, 35,* 11–115.

Centers for Disease Control. (1987a, July 3). Increases in primary and secondary syphilis—United States. *Morbidity and Mortality Weekly Report, 36,* 393–397.

Centers for Disease Control. (1987b, April 17). Tuberculosis in Blacks—United States. *Morbidity and Mortality Weekly Report, 36,* 212–220.

Centers for Disease Control. (1993). Teenage pregnancy and birth rates—United States 1990. *Morbidity and Mortality Weekly Report, 42,* 236–238.

Children's Defense Fund. (1985). *Black and White children in America.* Washington DC: Author.

Comer, J. P., & Hill, H. (1985). Social policy and the mental health of black children. *Journal of the American Academy of Child Psychiatry, 24,* 175–181.

Connell, J. P., Spencer, M. B., & Aber, J. L. (1994). Education risk and resilience in African-American youth: Context, self, action, and outcomes in school. *Child Development, 65,* 493–506.

Dembo, R. (1988). Delinquency among black youth. In J. T. Gibbs (Ed.), *Young, black, and male in America: An endangered species* (pp. 129–165). Dover MA: Auburn House.

Donovan, P., & Waszak, C. D. (1989). *School-based clinics enter the '90's: Update, evaluation and future challenges.* Washington DC: Center for Population Options.

Ellickson, P. L., Bell, R. M., Thomas, M. A., Robyn, A. E., & Zellman, G. L. (1988). *Designing and implementing Project ALERT: A smoking and drug prevention experiment.* Santa Monica CA: Rand.

English, A., & Tereszkiewicz, L. (1989). *School-based health clinics: Legal issues.* Washington DC: Adolescent Health Care Project, National Center for Youth Law. Support Center for School-Based Clinics, The Center for Population Options. National Center for Youth Law.

Epstein, N., & Shainline, A. (1974). Paraprofessional parent-aides and disadvantaged families. *Social Casework, 55,* 230–236.

74

Erikson, E. H. (1959). Identity and the life cycle. *Psychological issues, Monographs 1*, (pp. 1–171). New York: International Universities Press.

Farrington, D. P. (1977). The efforts of public labeling. *British Journals of Criminology*, *17*, 112–125.

Farrington, D. P., Ohlin, L. E., & Wilson, J. Q. (1986). *Understanding and controlling crime toward a new research strategy*. New York: Springer.

Freedman, J. L. (1984). Effect of television violence on aggressiveness. *Psychological Bulletin*, *100*, 372–378.

Gibbs, J. T. (1988). *Young, black, and male in America: An endangered species*. Dover MA: Auburn House.

Gibbs, J. T., Huang, L. N., and Associates (Eds.) (1989). *Children of color: Psychological interventions with minority youth*. San Francisco: Jossey-Bass.

Greenberg, B. S. (1986). Minorities and the mass media. In J. Bryant & D. Zillman (Eds.), *Perspectives on media effects* (pp. 165–188). Hillsdale NJ: Erlbaum.

Hall, E., Lamb, M. E., & Perlmutter, M. (1982). The development of sex roles. *Child psychology today* (2nd ed.). New York: Random House.

Hampton, R. L. (1986). Family violence and homicide in the black community: Are they linked? In *Report of the secretary's task force on black and minority health* (Vol. 5, pp. 69–73). Washington DC: Department of Health and Human Services.

Hein, K. (1988, March). AIDS *in adolescents: Exploring the challenge*, 20–21. Paper presented at the National Invitational Conference, New York.

Hill, I. (1988). *Reaching women who need prenatal care: Strategies for improving state prenatal programs* (Vol. 8). Washington DC: National Governors' Association, Center for Policy Research.

Hill, R. (1972). *The strengths of black families*. New York: Emerson Hall.

Honey, E. (1988). AIDS and the inner city: Critical issues. *Social Casework*, *69*, 365–370.

Houstin-Hamilton, A. (1986). A constant increase: AIDS in ethnic communities. *Focus*, *1*, 1–2.

Huizinga, D., & Elliot, D. S. (1986). *Juvenile offenders: Prevalence, offender incidence and arrest rates by race*. Paper presented at the meeting on Race and the Incarceration of Juveniles, Racine WI.

Huston, A. C., Donnerstein, E., Fairchild, H., Feshbach, N. D., Katz, P. A., Murray, J. P., Rubinstein, E. A., Wilcox, B. L., & Zuckerman, D. (1992). *Big world, small screen: The world of television in American society*. Lincoln: University of Nebraska Press.

Huston, A. C., Wright, J. C., Rice, M. L., Kerkman, D., & St. Peters, M. (1987, April). *The development of television viewing patterns in early childhood: A longitudinal investigation*. Paper presented at the meeting of the Society for Research in Child Development, Baltimore.

Jessor, R. (1984, November). *Adolescent problem drinking: Psychological aspects and developmental outcomes*. Paper presented at the meeting of the Carnegie Conference on Unhealthful Risk-Taking Behavior Among Adolescents, Stanford CA.

Jessor, R., & Jessor, S. L. (1977). *Problem behavior and psychosocial development: A longitudinal study of youth*. New York: Academic Press.

Jones, E. E., & Korchin, S. J. (1982). *Minority mental health*. New York: Praeger.

Katz, P. A. (1986). Gender identity: Development and consequences. In R. D. Ashmore & F. K. Del Boca (Eds.), *The social psychology of female-male relations: A critical analysis of central concepts* (pp. 21–67). Orlando FL: Academic Press.

Katz, P. A. (1987). Family constellation: Effects on gender schemata. In L. S. Liben & M. Signorella (Eds.), *Children's gender concepts: New directions in child development* (pp. 39–56). San Francisco: Jossey-Bass.

Katz, P. A., Boggiano, A. K., & Silvern, L. (1993). Theories of female personality. In F. Denmark & M. Paludi (Eds.), *Handbook of the psychology of women* (pp. 237–280). Westport CT: Greenwood.

Katz, P. A., & Taylor, D. A. (1989). *Eliminating racism: Profiles in controversy*. New York: Plenum.

Kavanagh, K., & Hops, H. (1994). Good girls? Bad boys? Gender and development as contexts for diagnosis and treatment. In T. H. Ollendick & R. J. Prinz (Eds.), *Advances in clinical child psychology* (Vol. 16, pp. 45–79). New York: Plenum.

Krisberg, B., Schwartz, I., Fishman, G., Eiskovits, Z., & Guttman, E. (1986). *The incarceration of minority youth*. Minneapolis: Hubert H. Humphrey Institute of Public Affairs, Center for the Study of Youth Policy.

Kutner, N. G., & Brogan, D. (1991). Sex stereotypes and health care: The case of treatment for kidney failure. *Sex Roles: A Journal of Research, 24* (5/6), 279–290.

Ladner, J. A. (1987). Black teenage pregnancy: A challenge for educators. *Journal of Negro Education, 56,* 53–63.

Langer, T., Gersten, J., & Eisenberg, J. (1974). Approaches to measurement and definition of the epidemiology of behavior disorders. *International Journal of Health Services, 4,* 483–501.

Liu, W. T., & Yu, E. S. H. (1985). Ethnicity, mental health, and the urban delivery system. In J. W. Moore & L. W. Moldonado (Eds.), *Urban ethnicity in the United States: New immigrants and old minorities* (pp. 211–247). Beverly Hills: CA Sage.

Lundman, R. J. (1984). *Prevention and control of juvenile delinquency*. New York: Oxford University Press.

Marcia, J. E. (1966). Development and validation of ego identity status. *Journal of Personality and Social Psychology*, *3*, 551–558.

Marcia, J. E. (1980). Identity in adolescence. In J. Adelson (Ed.), *Handbook of adolescent psychology* (pp. 159–187). New York: Wiley.

Maslow, A. H. (1970). *Motivation and personality* (2nd ed.). New York: Harper & Row.

Mays, V. & Cochran, S. (1987). Acquired immunodeficiency syndrome and black Americans: Special psychosocial issues. *Public Health Reports*, *102*, 221–231.

McAdoo, H. P. (1981). *Black families*. Beverly Hills CA: Sage.

Millstein, S. G. (1988). *The potential of school-linked centers to promote adolescent health & development*. Carnegie Council on Adolescent Development, Working Papers. Washington DC

Moore, K., & Burt, M. (1982). *Private crisis, public costs: Policy perspectives on teenage childbearing*. Washington DC: Urban Institute.

Moore, K. A., Simms, M. C., & Betsey, C. L. (1986). *Choice and circumstances: Racial differences in adolescent sexuality and fertility*. New Brunswick NJ: Transaction.

National Center for Health Statistics. (1975). *Persons with impaired hearing, United States–1971*. Series No. 10, No. 101. Rockville MD: Health Researchers Administration, U.S. Public Health Service.

National Institute on Drug Abuse. (1987). *National trends in drug use and related factors among American high school students and young adults, 1975–1986*. Washington DC: U.S. Department of Health and Human Services.

Ogbu, J. U. (1985). A cultural ecology of competence among inner-city blacks. In M. B. Spencer, G. K. Brookins, & W. R. Allen (Eds.), *Beginnings: The social and affective development of black children* (pp. 45–66). Hillsdale NJ: Erlbaum.

Panem, Sandra (1988). *The AIDS bureaucracy*. Cambridge: Harvard University Press.

Piaget, J. (1972). Intellectual evolution from adolescence to adulthood. *Human Development*, *15*, 1–12.

Pierce, H. B. (1986). Blacks and law enforcement: Towards police brutality reduction. *The Black Scholar*, *17*, 49–54.

Pleck, J. H., Sonerstein, F. L., & Swain, S. O. (1988). Adolescent male's sexual behavior and contraceptive use: Implications for male responsibility. *Journal of Adolescent Research*, *3*, 275–284.

Powers, S., Hauser, S., & Kilner, L. (1989). Adolescent mental health. *American Psychologist, 44*, 200–208.

Reed, R. J. (1988). Education and achievement of young black males. In J. T. Gibbs (Ed.), *Young, Black, and male in America: An endangered species* (pp. 37–96). Dover MA: Auburn House.

Robinson, D. O., & Allen, D. V. (1984). Racial differences in tympanometric results. *Journal of Speech and Hearing Disorders, 49*, 140–144.

Rosauer, R. (1988). *Teen pregnancy.* ECS survey of state initiatives for youth at risk. ECS Publication No. AR-87-55. Denver: Education Commission of the States.

Russo, N. (1990). Overview: Forging research priorities for women's mental health. *American Psychologist, 45*, 368–373.

Sampson, R. J., & Laub, J. H. (1994). Urban poverty and the family context of delinquency: A new look at structure and process in a classic study. *Child Development, 65*, 523–540.

Signorella, N. (1987). Children and adolescents on television: A consistent pattern of devaluation. *Journal of Early Adolescence, 7*, 255–268.

Silvern, L. E., & Katz, P. A. (1986). Gender roles and adjustment in elementary school children: A multidimensional approach. *Sex Roles, 14*, 181–202.

Snow, L. F. (1979). Folk medical beliefs and their implications for care of patients: A review based on a study of Black Americans. *Annals of Internal Medicine, 81* (1), 82–96.

Staples, R., & Jones, T. (1985, May/June). Culture, ideology and Black television images. *Black Scholar, 16*, 10–20.

Steele, C. M., & Nisbett, R. E. (1989). *Protective disidentification as mediation of academic outcomes among Black college students.* Unpublished manuscript, University of Michigan.

Thompson, J., Rosenstein, M., Milazzo-Sayre, L., & MacAskill, R. (1986). Psychiatric services to adolescents: 1970–1980. *Hospital and Community Psychiatry, 37*, 584–590.

Towers, R. L. (1987). *How schools can help combat student drug and alcohol abuse.* Washington DC: National Education Association.

U.S. Bureau of the Census. (1993). *We, the American Blacks.* Washington, DC: U.S. Department of Commerce, Bureau of the Census.

Joint Economic Committee. (1994). *Teenage pregnancy: The economic and social costs.* Hearing before the Subcommittee on Education and Health of the Joint Economic Committee, One Hundred and Second Congress, Second Session. Washington DC: U.S. Government Printing Office.

U.S. Congress. Office of Technological Assessment. (1989). *Adolescent health insurance status: Analyses—Background paper*. Washington DC: U.S. Office Government Printing.

U.S. Congress. Select Committee on Children, Youth, and Families. (1989). *Children and families: Key trends in the 1980s*. Washington DC: U.S. Government Printing Office.

U.S. Congress. Select Committee on Hunger. (1985). *Hearings on poverty and hunger in the black family*. Washington DC: U.S. Government Printing Office.

U.S. Department of Justice. Bureau of Justice Statistics. (1988, March). *Report to the nation on crime and justice* (2nd. ed.) (NCS-105506). Washington DC: Author.

Vincenzi, H. (1987). Depression and reading ability in sixth-grade children. *Journal of School Psychology, 25*, 155–160.

White, J. L. (1980). Toward a black psychology. In R. Jones (Ed.), *Black Psychology* (pp. 5–7). New York: Harper & Row.

Wilson, J. (1988, April). *The American underclass: Inner-city ghettos and the norms of citizenship*. The Godkin Lecture, John F. Kennedy School of Government, Harvard University.

Wilson, J. Q. & Kelling, G. L. (1982, March). Broken windows. *Atlantic Monthly*, pp. 29–38.

Wolfgang, M. E. & Tracy, P. E. (1982). *The 1945 and 1985 birth cohorts: A comparison of the prevalence, incidence, and severity of delinquent behavior*. Paper presented at Conference on Public Danger, Dangerous Offenders, and the Criminal Justice System, Cambridge MA.

Wyatt, G. E. (1992). The sociocultural context of African American and White American women's rape. *Journal of Social Issues, 48* (1), 77–91.

3

The Health of Latino Youth:
Challenges for Disease Prevention

Hortensia Amaro, Miriam Messinger, and Richard Cervantes

Latino is the term used to refer to persons living in the United States who are of Spanish-speaking background and ancestry from Latin America. It is used in a manner equivalent to the term *Hispanic* as found in most government documents.

Latinos represent a rich mosaic of groups with distinct racial, class, and age characteristics. In addition, these groups differ in national origin, immigration history, settlement patterns, legal status (Portes & Rumbaut, 1990), and social and cultural adaptation (Bean & Tienda, 1987). These historical, demographic, and sociocultural features shape the health and disease experience of individual Latinos. As a result, Latinos have multiple and distinct health-care and prevention needs; this fact has distinct implications for prevention efforts.

In addition, there is a controversial assertion that Latinos as a group are a superhealthy population (Hayes-Bautista, 1992). Some researchers and Latino health advocates have concluded that Latinos have a more favorable health profile than would be expected from their general socioeconomic and minority status. They attribute this to sociocultural characteristics that operate as protective factors or to selective immigration patterns (Hayes-Bautista, 1992). Thus, the unexpected "good" health of Latinos has been viewed by some as a paradox in public health. Unfortunately, variations in health status among Latinos are often lost because data are aggregated, thus easily leading to erroneous conclusions and misguided public-health approaches.

For the purpose of this chapter, we define youth as representing the age range from 10–18 years. Unfortunately, specific data are not always available for the 10–18-year-old age range. Furthermore, the years immediately preceding adolescence (before age 10) are critical to the initiation of risk behaviors and the presence of risk factors for youth. At the higher end of the age spectrum, young adulthood is often the time when risk behaviors and risk factors become manifest through clinical health problems. Therefore, we provide data for the available age range, which at times extends to age 25.

Demographic Profile of Latinos

According to the U.S. Census Bureau (U.S. Bureau of the Census, 1991), there were 22.3 million Latinos residing in the mainland United States in 1990, with an additional 3.5 million living in Puerto Rico. These numbers represented an increase of approximately 50% from the period between 1980 and 1990. In 1990, Latinos accounted for 9% of the total population of the United States.

Chapa and Valencia (1993) provided an excellent overview of demographic trends for the U.S. Latino population. The population of Mexican origin is the largest of all Latino groups: Mexican Americans make up approximately 60.4%, Puerto Ricans 12.2%, and Cuban Americans 4.7% of the total Latino population. Other Latinos, primarily from Central and South America, represented 22.8% of the mainland Latino population.

In 1990, California had approximately one third of the nation's Latinos, and California, Texas, and New York had approximately two thirds of the entire mainland Latino population. Latinos are typically highly urbanized: about 67% of Latinos resided in sixteen metropolitan areas (Chapa & Valencia, 1993). The highly urbanized areas of Southern California, New York, New Jersey, and Miami contained the largest concentration of Latinos, with just under 8 million persons. In general, Latinos of Mexican origin are the predominant group in the southwestern states, with Puerto Ricans concentrated in the Northeast and Cubans mostly in the Southeast, primarily in Florida. The Midwest has substantial populations of Latinos from nearly all groups.

In the 1990 census, one of most striking demographic characteristic of the overall Latino population was its youthfulness. Compared with White non-Latinos, Latinos had the greatest proportion of their population under age 18 (25.7% vs. 36.5%) and had a median age of 26 compared with 33.5 for all other ethnic groups. Among Latinos, those of Mexican origin were the youngest (with median age 24.1), while those of Cuban origin were the oldest (with median age 39.1) (Chapa & Valencia, 1993). Population projections indicate a steady growth of the general Latino population, particularly among the young. The Latino population under 18 years of age may well triple by the year 2020 and comprise 25% of the nation's total youth population (Pallas, Natriello, & McDill, 1989).

As the Latino population grows, there is reason to believe that the economic and educational status of Latinos may remain somewhat bleak. While Latino educational attainment levels seem to be increasing, they continued to be much lower than for White non-Latinos at every school level (Chapa & Valencia, 1993). According to the 1990 census, only one in two Latinos completed high school, compared with four of five White non-Latinos. Within the Latino population, Mexican-origin youth had the lowest high school completion rate (44%). Fewer Latinos (9%) than White non-Latinos (22%) completed a four-year college. Among Latinos, however, Mexican-origin youth only had a 5% college completion rate, compared with 20% for Cuban-origin Latinos. These trends cannot be attributed solely to the influx of immigrant students because American-born Latinos have considerably lower levels of education than American-born White non-Latino youth (American Council on Education, 1990).

Several factors probably contribute to the poor educational attainment of Latinos: the lack of access to equal educational resources, including bilingual education resources, low levels of funding for educational facilities in predominantly minority communities, shrinking public funding for education in general, low performance expectations on the part of schools for Latino students, and lack of effective ways to involve Latino parents, including the absence of bilingual support services for them.

According to the U.S. Census, about one in four Latinos were reported to be living in poverty (Chapa & Valencia, 1993). Puerto Ricans had the highest percentage of individuals living below the federally established poverty level, compared with about one in eight non-Latinos (Chapa & Valencia, 1993). The high proportion of female-headed households also contributed to their high poverty rate (Chapa & Valencia, 1993). Puerto Ricans had a higher proportion of female-headed households (39.0%) than Mexican Americans (20.0%) and Cubans (19.0%). In analyzing the 1990 Census, Chapa and Valencia (1993) reported the annual average family income for White non-Latinos was $29,400 per year, compared with $15,800 for Latino families. Given the larger average family size for most Latino groups when compared to White non-Latinos (3.8 vs. 3.1), per capita income for Latinos was considerably lower than per capita income for White non-Latinos (Chapa & Valencia, 1993). Consequently, 37.6% of all Latino children were living below the federally established poverty level, as compared with 17.3% of white non-Latino children (Chapa & Valencia, 1993). Thus, Latino children may be at higher risk for a variety of health-related problems.

Limitations of Data on Latino Youth

Historically, conceptualization and measurement problems in research have resulted in grouping of Latinos into the larger category of minorities (General Accounting Office, 1992). Many researchers assumed that generalizations derived from such health profiles covered Latinos because they were exposed to similar social conditions as other minorities. However, recent research has demonstrated that minority populations differ in important ways from each other, with significant subgroup differences as well (Williams, Lavizzo-Mourey, & Warren, 1993; Vega & Amaro, 1994; National Center for Health Statistics, 1992a). The conceptualization that often grouped all minorities into one category and sometimes grouped Latinos with White non-Latinos has resulted in a profound lack of information on the specific health profiles of Latinos, including Latino youth (Vega & Amaro, 1994; Williams et al., 1993).

The effect of the lack of precise information on Latino youth has been especially noticeable in documents that describe the health of Americans and identify strategies for addressing health problems and service needs. The 1986 Secretary's Task Force on Black and Minority Health report (U.S. Department of Health and Human Services, 1986) contained many apologies for the lack of health data on Latinos. In 1990, the Healthy People 2000 Report (U.S. Department of Health and Human Services, 1991) had no specific Latino initiatives for the majority of measurable objectives because of lack of data. This failure of the U.S. health data system to provide information on mortality and morbidity trends for Latino populations was noted in a recent report by the General Accounting Office (1992).

In 1978, the Office of Management and Budget set standards for assessment of race and ethnicity information in national datasets (Office of Management and Budget, 1978). In addition, the Disadvantaged Minority Health Improvement Act of 1990 (H.R. 5702, 1990) created clear directives to the federal agencies that collect health information under the Department of Health and Human Services to employ ethnicity identifiers for the major racial and ethnic populations. The legislation also directed agencies to ensure that study samples included sufficiently large numbers of persons from the major groups and subgroups in order to provide adequate information on the health status of the major categories of race and ethnicity.

To date, however, most national health–data systems do not provide adequate data on the health of Latino youth because they do not collect appropriate and accurate data on ethnicity, they do not sample sufficiently large numbers of Latino youth, or they fail to tabulate and report data separately for Latinos (Amaro, 1993; Vega & Amaro, 1994). Moreover, Latino mortality data have serious limitations due to the inadequacy of ethnicity identifiers in death certificates, as well as the lack of available updated census information. For example, accurate estimates of Latino death rates are impossible to determine because, until 1988, the national model for death certificates did not contain Latino identifiers. Although some states have incorporated Latino origin into their death certificates, such reporting is not uniform and lacks demographic precision (Council on Scientific Affairs, 1991).

Another problem is in the national health data, a major source for information on the health status of youth. The age breakdowns used are ill suited to reveal the specific health problems of adolescents. In the mortality data reports, for example, the most common age categories used are 1–14 years and 15–24 years, or the data are not systematically available at all.

Much of the national data on adolescent health behavior originates from the Youth Risk Behavior Survey (YRBS), which samples grades 9–12. While the YRBS reports on a large sample, there are several problems in generalizing from this survey to Latino youth. First, all Latinos, both those living in Puerto Rico and on the mainland, are grouped under "Latino." Second, school-based samples underestimate health problems because of the high rate of out-of-school Latino youth and the differences between the two groups (in school and out) on many factors of research interest.

Mortality and Morbidity among Latino Youth
MORTALITY
Unless noted, the data presented here represent only the three major Latino groups: Mexican American, Puerto Rican, and Cuban American. At the

present, indicators of health for those of Central or South American origin are generally unavailable. Three commonly used indicators are used to compare mortality between Latinos and White non-Latino youth: leading causes of death, years of potential life lost, and death rates for selected causes of death. For each of these, data are first presented for Latinos overall; whenever data are available on specific Latino groups, such data are presented.

Leading Causes of Death

There are important differences between Latino youth and White non-Latino youth in the leading causes of death and their rankings. Data from death certificates in 1989 indicate that diabetes mellitus was one of the ten leading causes of death among Latinos 15–24 years of age, but not for White non-Latino youth (National Center for Health Statistics, 1992b). Homicide and legal intervention and HIV infection/AIDS ranked somewhat higher among Latino youth (second and fifth, respectively) than among White non-Latino youth (third and seventh, respectively) (National Center for Health Statistics, 1992b). One year later, 1990 data indicated that HIV/AIDS was the sixth leading cause of death among Latino youth ages 15–24 (National Center for Health Statistics, 1993b). However, this change from fifth to sixth leading cause of death in 1990 may be an artifact due to exclusion of data on deaths from New York City. This could easily have resulted in an underestimation of specific causes of death disproportionately found in New York City Puerto Ricans, such as HIV/AIDS, infant mortality, tuberculosis (TB), and sexually transmitted diseases (STDs).

Moreover, currently available death statistics are further limited in that they only provide the absolute number of Latino deaths and the ranking of the causes of death. Because of inadequate denominator data from the 1990 census, death rates have not been calculated for the major Latino groups since 1979–1981, except for 1987–1989.

Years of Potential Life Lost (YPLL)

The measurement of YPLL was generated to investigate premature death because crude mortality rates are weighted toward deaths among the elderly. The measurement weights causes of death that disproportionately affect younger age groups, and it is calculated by multiplying deaths for each age group under 65 by the numbers of years lost before age 65. Age-specific YPLLs are summed by specific cause of death and for all causes (Desenclos &

Hahn, 1992). Data from 1986–1988 on YPLL have been published for Latinos less than 65 years of age (Desenclos & Hahn, 1992) but without a break-down of YPLL for Latino youth. Latino men (YPLL 74.3) have higher YPLL rates than White non–Latino men (68.3), while YPLL rates for Latinas (32.9) were slightly lower (35.7) than those of White non–Latinas (Desenclos & Hahn, 1992). The YPLL rates differed significantly across Latino groups: Puerto Ricans had the highest rates compared with Mexican Americans and Cuban Americans (Desenclos & Hahn, 1992). It is evident that YPLL rates for the overall Latino population were significantly affected by the high mortality rates among youth (ages 15–24) due to suicide, homicide, and legal intervention (YPLL 43.4) and accidents and adverse effects (51.3), especially when compared with White non–Latino rates for the same cause of death (22.3 and 48.1, respectively) (Desenclos & Hahn, 1992).

Death Rates for Latinos

The most recently available general death rates for Latinos use an overall ethnicity category (Latino) without Latino group breakdowns (National Center for Health Statistics, 1993a, 1933b). The most relevant age category is 15–24 years of age. Interpretation of the data on youth is further limited because rates are provided for only two causes of death, homicide and legal intervention and accidents and adverse effects. Overall death rates for La-tino youth (103.3) exceeded those of White non–Latinos (89.3) (National Center for Health Statistics, 1993a). The 1990 death rate for homicide and legal intervention among Latino youth (43.4) greatly exceeded those of White non–Latinos (22.3) (National Center for Health Statistics, 1992b). Deaths due to accidents and adverse effects for this period also reflect slightly higher rates for Latino youth (51.3) compared with White non–Latinos (48.1) (National Center for Health Statistics, 1992a).

General data from 1979–1981, although less recent and with less cover-age of the Latino population, have some advantages over more recent data because they provide death rates by sex and age (Maurer, Rosenberg, & Keemer, 1990). These data represented deaths from fifteen reporting states and included 45% of the Latino population; their accuracy may vary across Latino groups (Maurer et al., 1990). These data showed that the higher Latino mortality rate for those under age 45 was attributable to the re-ported state death rates for males in the 15–24 year and 25–34 year age cate-gories.

Death Rates for Specific Latino Groups

As previously stated, mortality statistics grouping Latinos mask important differences in health conditions within specific groups. Available data on overall death rates by Latino groups (1979–1981) showed that death rates for Puerto Ricans of all ages (512.4) were higher than for other Latino groups (Mexican Americans, 489.4, Cuban Americans, 345.2; other Latinos, 341.3) (Maurer et al., 1990). It is reasonable to speculate that, among youth, similar differences in overall death rates would also occur. Where data were specifically calculated for deaths due to homicide and legal intervention, the rate was more than eight times greater among Puerto Ricans, almost six times greater for Mexican Americans, and more than three times greater for Cuban Americans than for White non-Latinos.

MORBIDITY

Indicators of health status, such as the incidence of chronic conditions and infectious diseases, bed disability days, and specific health behaviors, also vary across Latino groups and reflect different patterns of disease and prevention needs among these groups (Vega & Amaro, 1994). Several Latino health experts have argued that such morbidity indicators provide better measures of the health status of the overall population than do mortality indicators (Hayes-Bautista, 1992; Novello, Wise, & Kleinman, 1991).

Because of the youthfulness of the Latino population, morbidity among its youth will almost certainly have a significant impact on the level and type of demands for health-care resources for Latinos overall.

Unintentional Injury

Accidents and their adverse effects are the leading cause of death for Latino adolescents and so it would be expected that injuries also contribute significantly to morbidity among Latino adolescents. Among high school youth sampled in a national survey in 1990–1991, motor-vehicle crashes accounted for the largest portion of hospital and emergency-room costs associated with injuries (Centers for Disease Control, 1993a). A major limitation of the morbidity reports on unintentional injuries is that they fail to provide for subgroups of Latino youth. Of those students who ride motorcycles, significantly more White non-Latinos (59.8%) than Latinos (39.3%) wore helmets, which can prevent serious head trauma (Centers for Disease Control, 1993a). Only 47.3% of the sample reported wearing seat belts all or most of the time, and there was no significant difference by race or ethnicity.

Violence

Interpersonal violence caused 20,000 deaths and 2.2 million injuries in the United States in 1986 (Centers for Disease Control, 1992c). National data from high school students (Centers for Disease Control, 1992c) indicated that Latino boys (16.2%) and girls (4.4%) more often reported being in a fight in which at least one person required medical attention during the thirty days preceding the survey than did White non–Latino adolescents (boys, 10.1%; girls, 2.4%). Latino high school students (22 per 100,000) had a thirty-day incidence rate of physical fighting higher than did White non–Latinos (13) but lower than that for Blacks (31) (Centers for Disease Control, 1992c).

The YRBS also documented weapon carrying among high school students. Twenty percent of all students sampled (31.5% of males and 8.1% of females) had carried a weapon to school during the previous month (Centers for Disease Control, 1993b). Latino males had the highest percentage of students who had carried a weapon (41.1%) as well as the highest thirty-day incidence of weapon carrying. Knives and razors were the most common weapons involved (Centers for Disease Control, 1993b).

Prevalence estimates for violence-related behaviors are invariably confounded by socioeconomic status and geographic location. The data do not consider the context in which youth live; therefore, the data fail to discern the contributions of environment and ethnicity or the possible synergistic effect of these two factors. Most Latino youth live and attend school in poor urban areas, which are more likely to foster interpersonal violence, gangs, drug dealings, and the subsequent use of weapons. Research is needed on the role of social and environmental factors in violent behavior among Latino youth in order to inform prevention and intervention efforts.

ENVIRONMENTAL RISKS

Children who live in housing with peeling lead paint or in neighborhoods with lead-contaminated soil are at high risk for lead contamination. Data have shown that, among Latinos, Puerto Rican children had both the highest mean blood levels and the highest percentage with elevated blood levels of lead. One in nine Puerto Rican children, one in twenty Mexican American children, and one in twenty-nine White non-Latino children had elevated blood levels. The highest levels were found in 4- and 5-year-old children (Carter-Pokras et al., 1990). High blood levels of lead often create significant chronic health problems such as decreased stature (Frisancho & Ryan, 1991), hearing impairments (Schwartz & Otto, 1991), mental retardation, and peripheral neuropathies.

Other health issues related to the enviromental conditions of poverty include malnutrition, exposure to unsanitary conditions, and violence. Mexican American youth who assist their parents in fieldwork are often exposed to dangerious pesticides.

Chronic Medical Conditions

Past studies have not sufficiently examined the prevalence, incidence, and severity of chronic illnesses among Latino youth. Limited data exist on some illnesses and conditions for some segments of the Latino population. These data are often flawed because they do not control for socioeconomic status; they tend to rely on parental reports of medical conditions and may underestimate true rates because of unrecognized, undiagnosed, or untreated conditions such as diabetes.

The 1988 National Health Interview Survey lists musculosketal impairments, deafness and hearing loss, blindness and vision impairments, speech defects, cerebral palsy, diabetes, sickle cell anemia, asthma, and respiratory allergies as the eleven most prevalent chronic conditions among children younger than 18 years of age (Newacheck, Stoddard, & McManus, 1993). The survey found that parents of White non-Latino youth (younger than 18) were more likely to report chronic conditions for their children: (336/1,000) compared with Blacks (246/1,000) and Latinos (242/1,000) (with Latino group not specified) (Newacheck et al., 1993). However, it appears that Latino children may have a higher rate of severe chronic conditions. For example, while data from the earlier 1978–1980 National Health Survey also indicated lower rates of chronic conditions among Latino youth (younger than 17) it documented that Latino children had significantly higher rates of conditions severe enough to interfere with school attendance (Trevino & Moss, 1984).

What data are available indicate that Mexican American and Cuban American children have a prevalence of chronic medical conditions similar to those of White non-Latino children. Mainland Puerto Rican children, however, showed a higher prevalence (6.2%) than did Mexican Americans

(3.9%), Cuban Americans (2.5%), and children overall (Mendoza et al., 1992). The small sample of Cuban American children made those data unreliable as a population estimate and therefore only reflected attributes of the subjects examined.

The methods for collecting data on chronic conditions in children may be affected by reporting differences across ethnic groups. It is not clear whether the ethnic differences that emerge are due to differences in parental knowledge of chronic conditions in their children (related to lower access to health care) or to actual differences in health status. There is a need for better and more complete data on chronic conditions among Latino children and youth.

Asthma. Greater attention has been paid recently to the emergence of asthma as a significant contributor to childhood mortality and morbidity for Latino youth, particularly Puerto Ricans (Colp et al., 1993; Guarnaccia, 1992). Active asthma is two to four times higher among Puerto Rican children (11.2%) than any other U.S. group, including White (3.3%) and Black (5.9%) non-Latinos, Mexican Americans (2.7%), and Cuban Americans (5.2%; Carter-Pokras & Gergen, 1993). There are also gender and age variations in asthma prevalence across Latino groups. Puerto Rican and Mexican American boys are more likely to develop asthma than girls of the same groups (Guarnaccia, 1992). All Puerto Rican children, regardless of socioeconomic status, have higher active asthma rates than Mexican American children living in poverty and they develop asthma at a younger age than Mexican Americans (Carter-Pokras & Gergen, 1993).

A Texas study of asthmatic Mexican American youth 6 to 16 years of age identified several morbidity factors including at least occasional limitations in their daily activities (74%) and approximately one day of impairment per week. Other effects of the asthma were school absences (mean of thirteen days), acute-care medical visits (three per year), and hospitalizations (about one per year) (Wood et al., 1993). Morbidity associated with asthma, however, seems to be more severe among Puerto Rican children than all other Latino children (Carter-Pokras & Gergen, 1993).

Another study of Mexican American youth with asthma found that 44% were exposed to cigarette smoke in the home (Wood et al., 1993). Exposure to passive smoke may exacerbate asthma symptoms among these Latino youth; smoking has been associated with a twofold increase in bronchitis among other Latinos (Bang, Gergen, & Carroll, 1990).

Smoking among parents of Latino children with asthma may reflect a lack of knowledge regarding the nature of the disease and its treatment. There is evidence that Latino parents of asthmatic children lack thorough knowledge about the effects of smoking on asthma (Wood et al., 1993). Lack of insurance and access to consistent and ongoing medical care because of poverty also complicates the management of childhood and adolescent asthma, resulting in greater morbidity (Guarnaccia, 1992; Wood et al., 1993).

Diabetes Mellitus. Diabetes is a significant contributor to morbidity among Latino adults (Flegal et al., 1991; Stern & Haffner, 1992). Populations with Southwest Indian genetic contribution and Puerto Ricans tend to have a higher incidence of obesity and diabetes (Flegal et al., 1991; Webber et al., 1991). There is a paucity of information on the epidemiology of childhood and adolescent diabetes among Latinos.

Latino youth, however, demonstrate risk factors for diabetes. For example, higher levels of triglycerides and truncal obesity have been reported among Mexican American children and adolescents in Texas when compared with levels in White and Black non-Latino peers (Webber et al., 1991). Both factors are associated with higher rates of obesity and diabetes among adults.

Cardiovascular Risk. Researchers have begun examining predictors of cardiovascular disease (e.g., blood pressure, cholesterol, and lipoprotein levels) among young people. High blood pressure, high levels of low-density lipoprotein and total cholesterol (TC), and high TC/high-density lipoprotein (HDL) ratios are often indicative of increased risk for cardiovascular disease. Low HDL levels are related to obesity and hyperinsulinemia, particularly in individuals with a family history of diabetes.

Latino youth, especially boys, have shown evidence of increased risk for cardiovascular disease. For example, Latino youth exhibited an earlier rise to adult cholesterol levels than did other ethnic groups (Webber et al., 1991). Another study of high school seniors in Texas found significantly lower HDL cholesterol levels and higher TC/HDL ratios in Mexican American adolescents than in White non-Latinos (Troxler et al., 1991). Overall, boys in that study had significantly lower levels of HDL and higher TC/HDL ratios compared with girls (Troxler et al., 1991). While research is needed to document the prevalence of these risk factors among other groups of Latino youth, existing data clearly suggest the need for prevention efforts especially targeted to Latino boys.

Infectious Disease (Other than STDs). Infectious diseases are increasing in Latino communities, and diseases such as hepatitis A, measles, TB, and typhoid fever are causing excessive morbidity for Latinos (Sumaya, 1991). High rates of poverty, poor living conditions with inadequate hygiene (e.g., contaminated drinking water), barriers to health care, low rates of immunization, and infections brought by immigrants from their countries of origin all contribute to infection rates for Latinos.

For example, while TB declined 4.8% among non-Latino Whites between 1985 and 1987, it increased 12.7% among Latinos (Snider, Salinas, & Kelly, 1989). The Centers for Disease Control findings for 1993 report 5,194 cases of TB among the Latino population, with a median age of 33: 65% of patients were male and 454 cases were reported in the 15–24-year age group (Centers for Disease Control, 1994). While rates among adolescents appeared to be much lower, the significantly higher rates of TB among foreign-born persons raise concerns that TB may become a much larger problem among Latino adolescents since its incidence in the general U.S. population is rising (Centers for Disease Control, 1994).

SEXUALITY AND HEALTH

Data on sexuality and sexual behavior among Latinos are lacking (Amaro, 1992). Many studies on sexual behavior among Latino adolescents and young adults are of limited value because of their use of nonrepresentative school or community samples and the narrow scope of questions asked about sexuality. Although the available studies provide little insight into how Latino youth learn about sexuality and how their cultural norms affect sexual behavior, the studies do provide some useful information about sexual and contraceptive practices and their health implications.

Sexual Behavior

Latino boys seem to have rates of sexual activity between those of White and Black non-Latinos. For example, a 1990 national study (Centers for Disease Control, 1992d, 1992e) of high school students found that Latino boys (45%) reported having sexual intercourse during the three months preceding the survey more often than White non-Latinos (39%) but less often than Black non–Latinos (68%). Latino boys, however, had slightly more sexual partners than non–Latino Black boys (Centers for Disease Control, 1992d, 1992e). In contrast, Latina girls reported less overall sexual activity and a lower percentage who had four or more sexual partners in their lifetime than girls of other ethnic groups (Brindis, 1992; Centers for Disease Control, 1992d, 1992e). An older study using data from the 1982 National Survey of Family Growth reported that 42% of Latina adolescents (15–19 years) were sexually active, with no significant differences across Latino groups (Durant, Pendergrast, & Seymore, 1990a).

Contraceptive Use

Latino youth are generally less likely to use contraception than other groups, placing them at greater risk for both pregnancy and STDs. Latina high school students who were sexually active reported less contraceptive use (47%) than either White (88.1%) or Black (75%) non–Latinas (Centers for Disease Control, 1992e). Young Latino males were also less likely than White or Black non–Latino peers to report any contraceptive use (69.1%, 80.1%, and 76.3%, respectively) or condom use at most recent sexual intercourse (46.8%, 50%, and 54.5%, respectively) (Centers for Disease Control, 1992e). Intention to use condoms has also been noted to be lower among White or Black non–Latina adolescent girls (Norris & Ford, 1992).

Mexican American and Central or South American youth seem more likely to use effective birth control than Cuban American, Puerto Rican, or other Latinos. A major predictor of ineffective contraceptive use was the failure to use birth control at first coitus (Durant et al., 1990b).

In general, Latinas ages 15–19 seem less likely to have initiated sexual activity, less likely to use contraception, and more likely to become pregnant and to deliver a child than White non–Latina adolescents (Brindis, 1992). These differences may not be explained by socioeconomic status alone since sexually experienced Mexican American girls were twice as likely as White non–Latinas to have been pregnant even after socioeconomic status and social stability were taken into account (Aneshensel, Fielder, & Becerra, 1989). The high pregnancy rate among Latinas has both health and social implications because Latina adolescent mothers are more likely than White and Black non–Latina adolescent mothers to demonstrate poor school performance, be grade delayed, or to have dropped out of high school (Brindis, 1992; Linares et al., 1991).

Religious beliefs and cultural norms regarding women's roles, sexuality, and contraception may be important factors in contraceptive use and pregnancy among some Latina youth, as has been found with Mexican American women (Amaro, 1988).

Sexually Transmitted Diseases

Sexually transmitted diseases are on the rise among adolescents and young adults, and Latino youth are no exception (Brindis, 1992; Holmes, 1991). Latino boys have gonorrhea rates nearly three times higher and syphilis rates approximately twenty times greater than their White non-Latino peers (Brindis, 1992). In contrast, the prevalence for both gonorrhea and syphilis among Latinas was similar to that of White non-Latinas (Brindis, 1992), although rates varied significantly by geographic location. For example, in Massachusetts, a study found Latina adolescents had thirty-eight times the rate of syphilis as White non-Latina adolescents (Holmes, 1991).

HIV/AIDS. Rates of HIV infection show a disproportionate number of Latino adolescents infected with HIV. Although Latinos represented approximately 9 percent of the U.S. population in 1990, they constituted nearly 20% of adolescents diagnosed with AIDS (Centers for Disease Control, 1992a). Latinos represented 27.9% of all adolescent boys diagnosed with AIDS, and Latinas represented 16.8% of adolescent girls with AIDS. Latino adult military recruits (17–24-years-old) were 2.5 times more likely to be HIV positive than were White non-Latinos (Centers for Disease Control, 1987; Holmes, 1991). Among Job Corps entrants (ages 16–21) Latinos had twice the sero-prevalence HIV rate of White non-Latinos and half the rate of Black non-Latinos (St. Louis et al., 1991).

Infection rates also differed by geographic location. Among women younger than age 20 delivering babies in New York State, the infection rate was 5.8 per 1,000 in New York City and 1.3 per 1,000 elsewhere in the state, while the rates for the Latinas in the same samples were 5.7 per 1,000 and 5.1 per 1,000, respectively (Bowler et al., 1992). Among adolescents with AIDS, the ratio of male to female (3:1) was much smaller than that among adults (10:1), highlighting the growing importance of heterosexual transmission among girls and women in the United States (Centers for Disease Control, 1991). Given the approximately ten-year incubation period from infection to AIDS, HIV infection rates among teenagers would be a much better indicator of morbidity and mortality related to AIDS than rates of AIDS cases.

Out-of-school youth, who are generally not included in national surveys, seem to be at especially high risk for HIV infection. In a New York City study, 32% of gay or bisexual adolescent boys and 71% of runaway adolescent boys reported never or rarely using a condom during genital or anal sex (Rotheram-Borus et al., 1992). Puerto Rican gay and bisexual adolescent boys in that sample reported sexual behaviors that fitted a high-risk pattern (Rotheram-Borus, Rosario, & Koopman, 1991).

Risky sexual behaviors of adolescents of all ethnicities, as well as Latino adolescents, have changed little since the early 1980s, despite increasing knowledge about HIV infection (Centers for Disease Control, 1992b; Goodman & Cohall, 1989). Use of condoms at most recent intercourse did not increase significantly between 1990 and 1991, although use by sexually active teens younger than age 15 did increase slightly (Centers for Disease Control, 1992b).

Latino youth appear to lack both knowledge about HIV infection and AIDS and risk behaviors such as unprotected intercourse (Amaro & Gornemann, 1992; Smith et al., 1991). Many Latino youth seemed to talk to others about HIV/AIDS, but the information obtained was often limited and superficial (Amaro & Gornemann, 1992; Ford & Norris, 1991).

Lack of knowledge may be a significant contributing factor to the lower use of contraception among Latino youth. Research on sexuality has indicated that Latino adolescents and young adults were less knowledgeable about physiology, reproduction, pregnancy, contraception, and HIV/AIDS (Amaro, 1992; Amaro & Gornemann, 1992; Davis & Harris, 1982; DiClemente, Boyer, & Morales, 1988; Moore & Erickson, 1985; Norris & Ford, 1991; Padilla & O'Grady, 1987; Scott et al., 1988). Latina adolescents appeared to be especially uninformed about sexuality and contraception (Norris & Ford, 1991; Scott et al., 1988) and to hold more conservative attitudes than both Latino boys and girls of other ethnic groups (Moore & Erickson, 1985; Padilla & O'Grady, 1987). There is a need for research that investigates the contributions of factors such as knowledge and religious or cultural beliefs to rates of sexual activity and pregnancy.

MENTAL HEALTH

No national study has been conducted to examine the mental health of Latino youth. However, studies that investigated psychosocial issues among Latino adolescents using local or regional samples provide some useful information. Mexican American adolescents score lower on measures of self-esteem and self-concept (Grossman, Wirt, & Davids, 1985) and higher on measures of depression (Centers for Disease Control, 1993e; Roberts & Sobhan, 1992; Swanson et al., 1992) than do White non-Latinos.

Suicidal ideation and suicide attempts, which are often associated with depression, seem to be more common among Latino youth, especially for girls (Razin et al., 1991). The 1990 YRBS found that more Latino students than White or Black non-Latino students had experienced suicidal ideation, made a plan to commit suicide, attempted suicide, or received medical attention for a suicide attempt (Centers for Disease Control, 1993e). Girls reported higher percentages for each of the categories than did boys, and Latinas had the highest percentage of attempted suicide (14.9% compared with 12% for Latino boys and 10.7% for White non-Latina girls) (Centers for Disease Control, 1993e).

Both depression and anxiety related to trauma among Latino adolescents may have increased with the growth of the population of Latino refugee youth from Central and South America (Tyler et al., 1992). A study of thirty Latin Americans 8–12 years old in Montréal found that a history of more frequent and intense trauma was significantly correlated with anxiodepressive symptoms and introversion (Rousseau, Corin, & Renaud, 1989).

In addition, research is just emerging on the results of trauma sustained by poor urban youth in the United States as a result of exposure to domestic and social violence (Groves et al., 1993), which we have already noted to be high among Latinos. Finally, suicidal ideation and depression are strongly related to substance use, both as predictors and as possible consequences of use (Centers for Disease Control, 1993e; Razin et al., 1991). Some evidence has suggested that increased exposure to mainstream U.S. culture may also be associated with these problems (Swanson et al., 1992).

SUBSTANCE USE

Although there is probably more published research on substance use than on any other health issue affecting Latinos, much is yet to be understood. One important limitation of the current research is that most of the national school-based studies aggregate Latino groups, making findings difficult to interpret given the probable differences in drug use among these groups.

Data from the 1992–1993 Monitoring the Future Study (Johnston,

O'Malley, & Bachman, 1994) highlight several important patterns regarding substance use among Latino youth. First, among eighth-grade students, Latinos have the highest prevalence for the use of marijuana, hallucinogens, LSD, cocaine, and tranquilizers. For example, by the eighth grade, more Latino than White non-Latino or Black students have used marijuana (20.3%, 11.0%, and 9.3%, respectively). Thus, it appears that illicit drug use is initiated earlier among Latino youth.

The second pattern is that, for the more dangerous drugs, such as cocaine, crack, and heroin, Latino youth continue to show higher rates of use through the senior year of high school, even though Latino youth "have a considerably higher school drop out rate . . . than whites or blacks, which would tend to diminish any such differences by senior year" (Johnston et al., 1994).

Third, alcohol use among Latino and White non-Latino students shows similar prevalence rates that are higher than those of Blacks. For example, among eighth graders, the thirty-day prevalence of alcohol use has increased to 50.5% among Latinos, 55.6% among White non-Latinos, and 32.4% among Blacks. Similarly a significantly larger proportion of Latino (24.8%) and White non-Latino (33.6%) seniors than Black (12.5%) seniors report having gotten drunk in the last thirty days. A similar patten is also evident for binge drinking, where 21.4% of eighth-grade Latino students report drinking five or more drinks in a row in the past two weeks, compared with 12.6% of White non-Latinos and 10.7% of Blacks.

Another important finding in the Monitoring the Future Study is that Latino youth start out in the eighth grade with similar rates of daily cigarette use as White non-Latino youth (7.2% vs. 8.8%). A greater percentage of Puerto Rican male adolescents smoke cigarettes (21.7%) than do their Mexican American (12.9%) or Cuban American (7.9%) counterparts (Gregory & Clark, 1992). The same trend existed for Latina adolescents (Puerto Ricans 19.1%; Mexican Americans 7.9%; Cuban Americans 8.1%). By the twelfth grade, however, daily cigarette use among Latinos is significantly lower (11.8%) than that of White non-Latino youth (21.4%).

Overall, initiation of substance use among Latino youth, as with other groups, occurs earlier in boys, among whom the onset of cigarette and alcohol use has been found to start as early as the fifth and sixth grades (Vega, Zimmerman, Warheit, Apssori, & Gil 1993).

Two important confounding factors must be kept in mind. First, these comparisons do not control for socioeconomic status. Second, the differential dropout rates across ethnic groups may also account for the relatively lower reported rates of smoking among twelfth-grade Latino youth and may also underestimate the overall use of substances among Latino youth since it is students who drop out who have the highest rates of substance use (Chavez, Edwards, & Oetting, 1989).

Because substance use among dropouts is generally much higher than for in-school youth and there are high rates of noncompletion of high school for Latinos, the surveys of high school youth are likely to grossly underestimate the prevalence of drug use among Latino adolescents. One study in the Southwest reported that dropouts had the highest prevalence of alcohol and drug use, followed by "at risk" students. While White non-Latino dropouts reported higher usage rates than did the Mexican American dropouts, the prevalence was high for both groups: more than 50% overall had tried cocaine and more than 75% had tried marijuana (Chavez et al., 1989). Another study of Central American youth in Washington DC who lived apart from their families also revealed greater prevalence and frequency of drug use (particularly marijuana and cocaine) than for Latino adolescents reported through household surveys (Tommasello et al., 1993).

Other studies reported higher prevalence and earlier initiation for some substances and highlighted intergroup differences among Latinos. In a separate study of New York City seventh graders, Dominicans had a higher rate of drinking than did Puerto Ricans or White or Black non-Latinos (Bettes et al., 1990). In a national survey, White non-Latino eighth graders reported a higher prevalence of usage of pills, alcohol, and smokeless tobacco, whereas Mexican Americans reported higher rates of marijuana, crack, cocaine, heroin, and cigarette use (Chavez & Swaim, 1992). By the twelfth grade, the White non-Latinos in the same study reported a higher lifetime prevalence for nearly every substance (Chavez & Swaim, 1992). There is also some evidence that urban Latino males have elevated rates of cocaine use (Marzuk et al., 1992).

One study reported that risk factors and predictors of substance use were similar across ethnic groups, with peer influence the major predictor of use (Dusenberry et al., 1992). Factors found to be significantly related to these differential rates among groups include geography and community (urban or rural) (Rebach, 1992); gender (Centers for Disease Control, 1992d, 1993d; Chavez et al., 1989); family structure (Sokol-Katz & Ulbrich, 1992); and acculturation (Brook et al., 1992; Vega et al., 1993). Acculturation was examined in a study of Mexican American teenagers. Those with two U.S.-born parents had higher rates of illicit drug use than those for which one or both parents were foreign born, and the Mexican Americans had nearly four times the rate of drug use as the comparison group living in Mexico (Swanson et al., 1992). A study comparing Puerto Rican adolescents living in New York City with those in San Juan, Puerto Rico, with and without histories of cross-migration found that rates of drug use paralleled an individual's exposure to the host society of New York City, with the greatest impact found for Latinas (Velez & Ungemack, 1989). Studies on drug use among Latino adults have also documented a positive relation between acculturation and use of marijuana and cocaine (Amaro et al., 1990).

Gender Norms and Their Impact on Health Status

The process of acculturation, as well as differences within the subgroups of the Latino population, makes it difficult to rely on global definitions of norms related to gender role. Few empirical studies exist to guide a precise understanding of Latino gender roles, a problem even more profound when one reviews the scant literature on developmental issues specific to Latino youth (Arroyo & Cervantes, in press).

Numerous misconceptions and stereotypes of Latino families were promoted in early social- and behavioral-science literature, and many still persist. For example, Mexican American children have been described as being raised in families with a rigid patriarchal structure, rural family values, and culture of poverty traits (Diaz-Guerrero, 1975; Madsen, 1964). The idea of male superiority and dominance has probably received more attention than any other single characteristic of Latino families. Some authors have challenged the sparse empirical support for such negative and simplistic stereotypes about Latinos (Andrade, 1982; Cromwell & Cromwell, 1978; Vasquez & Gonzalez, 1981; Zapata & Jaramillo, 1981).

As in other ethnic groups, gender-role socialization among Latinos is influenced by many factors, including socioeconomic status and acculturation. A more dynamic view of the Latino family's gender roles may be more accurate and useful than the stereotypic notions of rigid and static gender roles (Vasquez, 1994; Zapata & Jaramillo, 1981).

There is clearly a great need for research on how Latino families socialize children with respect to gender roles and sexuality. Such information is needed to inform prevention efforts related to reduction of HIV infection and sexually transmitted diseases among Latino youth. For example, there is very little research on Latino gay and lesbian youth or on their health problems. Latino gay youth may fear and/or experience considerable alienation from family because of the stigma among Latinos associated with a gay identity and relationships (Rotheram-Borus et al., 1991, 1994). In addition, many of these youth are at high risk for problem behaviors including sexual and drug-use behaviors (Rotheram-Borus et al., 1994). Latino gays and lesbians appear to experience difficulties in coming out for fear of rejection from family members and the Latino community at large (Espin, 1984, 1987; Gutierez, 1992; Morales, 1989, 1992). This fear becomes a barrier particularly among Latino men who are HIV seropositive and may want to share their serostatus with family and friends. Fear that such disclosure would bring rejection because they are gay leaves them isolated emotionally and socially (Mason et al., 1994).

Research on gender-role socialization and sexuality could also prove useful for understanding the high rates of adolescent pregnancy among Latina girls and its impact on the sexual behavior of young Latino men. For example, Pleck and colleagues (1993) found that the degree of young men's traditional masculinity ideology was associated with attitudes (e.g., belief that pregnancy is a way to validate their masculinity) and behaviors (e.g., having a greater number of sexual partners and not using condoms) that placed their sexual partners at risk for pragnancy and sexually transmitted diseases. Studies are needed to document better the beliefs and behaviors of Latino youth related to gender role and how these affect sexual behavior.

There is some evidence that acculturation affects other health behaviors differently for Latino women and men. For example, alcohol and cigarette use has appeared to increase with acculturation among women while it has had little or the opposite effect among men (Caetano, 1986; Marin, Perez-Stable, and Marin, 1989). Some authors have reported that, for alcohol use, this effect appears to be especially important among young women (Markides et al., 1990). Changes in gender roles brought about by acculturation may differentially affect the health of young Latino women and men.

Health-Care Utilization
PHYSICAL-HEALTH SYSTEM
Latinos appear to be poorly served by our medical, dental, and mental-health systems. National data were first collected on Latino health utilization in the National Health Interview Survey during 1976 and 1977. The re-

sults indicated that only 69% of Latinos reported seeing a physician in the year prior to being interviewed, compared with 76% of White non-Latinos and 74% of Black non-Latinos (Health Resources Administration, 1980). Latinos also averaged the fewest visits to a physician per year.

Trevino and Moss (1984) developed nationwide estimates for Latinos by national origin based on data from the National Health Interview Survey conducted between 1978 and 1980. Their findings revealed that the aggregate Latino population experienced an approximately equal number of physician visits per year when compared with White and Black non-Latinos, even after controlling for age; significant differences existed among Latino groups. Mexican Americans, for example, averaged fewer visits to a physician (3.7) than did non-Latino Whites (4.8) and Blacks (4.6), while Puerto Ricans and Cuban Americans averaged more visits (6.0 and 6.2 visits, respectively) (Trevino & Moss, 1984).

In their analysis, Trevino and Moss (1984) also found that 20% of Mexican Americans over the age of 4 years had never been to a dentist, compared with 2.5% of White non-Latinos, 9.2% of Black non-Latinos, 6.9% of Puerto Ricans, and 3.1% of Cuban Americans. Additionally, Mexican Americans were the least likely to be admitted to a hospital and demonstrated fewer days per hospital stay than any other ethnic group. In contrast, Puerto Ricans and Cuban Americans were likely to be hospitalized for a longer period of time, compared with Mexican Americans, White non-Latinos, and Blacks.

Aday, Flemming, and Andersen (1984) suggested that having a regular source of medical care contributes to continuity and quality of health services and is a good predictor of health-services utilization. From the 1976 National Health Interview Survey, Latinos, especially those living in the Southwest, were less likely to have a regular source of medical care than White and Black non-Latinos. Kasper and Barrish (1982) reported similar findings: 19% of those sampled reported not having a regular source of health care, compared with 13% of the total U.S. population.

Very few utilization studies focus on specific health care for Latino youth. In a study by the Centers for Disease Control (1992b), Latino children were reported to be the least likely to see a physician for a number of childhood illnesses compared with White and Black non-Latinos. In 1988, the National Survey of Family Growth showed that Latino adolescents were the least likely to use family planning services (Mosher & Bachrach, 1986).

MENTAL-HEALTH SYSTEM

Karno and Edgerton (1969) describe an epidemiological paradox to characterize the contrast between mental-health needs of Mexicans Americans and their low levels of utilization of services. Multiple studies have indicated gross underutilization of mental-health services by Latinos in general and Mexican Americans in particular.

In local, regional, and national surveys, Latino adults were consistently found to underutilize mental-health services (Hough et al., 1987; Yamamoto & Silva, 1987). Mexican Americans who suffered from diagnosable psychiatric disorder are half as likely as others to have used a specialty mental-health service in the year prior to their interview (Hough et al., 1987).

In general, health-service utilization is significantly related to factors of accessibility and affordability of services. Trevino and Moss (1983) examined a variety of cost factors related to utilization of health services by Latinos. They found that, for all groups, regardless of ethnicity, those without third-party health insurance were 50% less likely to have visited a physician in the past year. Such benefits are not available to undocumented Latinos. It is unknown how health-care reforms will affect unemployed Latinos and undocumented immigrants.

For Latinos, accessibility issues also include language, transportation, location of health services, available child care, and availability of bilingual or bicultural health-care staff. For mental-health services, there is consensus that the presence of bilingual or bicultural clinicians improves utilization of services, as well as the appropriateness of such services for non-English-speaking clients and their families.

Health-service research for Latino youth is sorely needed. As seen from this review, few data are available, and it is difficult to ascertain the actual level of need, availability, or use of services, but it appears that many Latino children and adolescents may not be receiving the level of care necessary to ensure both physical and emotional health.

Implications for Prevention

The role of sociocultural variables in illness and health among Latinos is largely unexplored, and this is even more true for Latino youth (see Cervantes & Castro, 1985). The review provided in the previous sections of this chapter suggests that at least five sociocultural factors are critical to consider in understanding the health status of Latino youth: poverty, the process of immigration and cultural adaptation, cultural beliefs (e.g., regarding health, gender roles, and adolescence), structural barriers to healthy development and access to health and other resources, and heterogeneity of the Latino population.

The review provided in this chapter also makes it clear that the health status of Latino youth from different groups is inextricably linked to the specific historical, geographic, sociological, and economic context of each group.

Morbidity and mortality data demonstrate that, while some Latino groups appear to be healthier than others, there is little support for the general assertion that Latinos are a superhealthy population. A prime example is the overall mortality rate among Latino youth, which exceeds that of White non-Latinos (National Center for Health Statistics, 1992b; L. Fingerhut, personal communication, 1994).

Studies that rely on parental reports indicate that Latino youth seem to be less severely affected by traditional major chronic health conditions in comparison with White non-Latinos, although there are some exceptions (e.g., asthma and infectious diseases). The data on chronic conditions affecting Latino youth, however, are too sparse. They do not allow for analyses by separate Latino groups and often do not account for rates of undiagnosed conditions, which are higher among Latino youth and which are likely to affect the accuracy of data that rely on parental reports.

Latino youth are disproportionately affected by environmental and infectious health problems. In addition, some evidence suggests that they manifest increased risk factors for diabetes and cardiovascular disease. Compounding the problems for the development of intervention programs is the lack of epidemiological data on Latino youth.

Peer influence is a major factor in substance use for Latinos, as with other youth, which suggests that interventions should be community based and affect entire networks of youth rather than focus on individual behavior.

Sexuality and sexual behavior are central to several health problems facing Latino youth (e.g., sexually transmitted diseases and pregnancy). The rates of unprotected intercourse and adolescent pregnancy among Latino youth present major challenges to the health and development of this population. These patterns are not explained by individuals' socioeconomic status alone. Social *structural* barriers to resources, such as jobs, education, and positive role models may exacerbate the health risks of Latino youth.

For example, Latino children and youth who observe and experience the lack of opportunity and inequity in resources between themselves and mainstream America may become discouraged or even cynical toward the social and politidal system. Adjustment to these conditions often includes becoming part of a gang for a sense of belonging or even for mere survival, which further fosters unhealthy behaviors.

A substantial proportion of Latino youth live in poverty; this must be considered when developing public-policy strategies for improving health and well-being in this population. Medical approaches that take a disease-specific focus rather than a community-encompassing approach will be ineffective in the long run in addressing the poverty-related major public-health problems confronting Latino youth. A broad public-health approach in conjunction with economic development is needed to address the conditions of poverty that jeopardize the health and development of Latino children and youth.

Approaches that actively engage Latino youth and their parents in the identification of problems and the design of prevention and intervention programs promise to be the most useful and cost-effective strategies to reduce behavioral and environmental health risks to Latino youth. This approach may not be easy for those of us trained to think of ourselves as experts, with the professional perspective that we have the necessary knowledge that community members lack to change such conditions.

Prevention efforts that engage parents in efforts to decrease sexual risk behaviors are examples of a community-based approach. The Strengthening Families Project, developed by the National Coalition of Latino Health and Human Service Organizations (COSSMHO), works closely with parents to improve communication with youth regarding a variety of issues including sexuality, HIV and AIDS, and sexually transmitted diseases (Szapocznik & COSSMHO, 1994). This model prevention program was developed with the input of Latino parents and communities in three geographic locations representing major Latino groups. Rather than employ methods that ignore culturally tied gender-role socialization and sexual norms, the program engages parents to improve their effectiveness in communicating with youth and facilitating a discussion of these issues within the family.

Participatory education is another model that has been effectively applied in communities worldwide (Amaro & Aguiar, 1994; Freire, 1970, 1990; Freire & Faundez, 1989; Magaña, 1992; Wallerstein, 1992; Werner & Bower, 1982). This approach uses the concept of dialogue and collective learning (Balance et al., 1986; Clinchy & Zimmerman, 1985) or relational empowerment (Surrey, 1991) as the primary means to help community members identify the problems faced by their community and make desired changes.

Programs that seek to address risk factors among Latino youth must be built on the understanding that the life conditions among poor Latino youth and families and the compounded effects of discrimination leave many Latino families fearful of contacting health-care and government agencies. They also feel marginalized and isolated, with low self-esteem and low self-worth. Public-health methods that focus solely on changing individual characteristics such as attitudes and behaviors to an imposed norm have a further disempowering effect because people are acted on by the system and the world that surrounds them. In contrast, public health efforts that address individual and contextual social factors and that work for social change are more empowering because they stress people's ability to act on the system and the world (Werner & Bower, 1982).

To meaningfully improve the health of Latino youth, we need to refocus our efforts from an emphasis on individual factors and behaviors to approaches that address the contextual factors such as poverty, racism, and disempowerment that so forcefully affect health and development.

References

Aday, L. A., Flemming, G. V., & Andersen, R. M. (1984). *Access to medical care in the United States: Who has it, who doesn't?* Chicago: Pluribus.

Amaro, H. (1988). Women in the Mexican-American community: Religion, culture, and reproductive attitudes and experiences. *Journal of Community Psychology, 16,* 6–20.

Amaro, H. (1992). *Hispanic sexual behavior: Implications for research and HIV prevention.* Washington DC: National Coalition of Hispanic Health and Human Services Organizations.

Amaro, H. (1993, July). *Health data on Hispanic women: Methodological limitations.* Paper presented at the 1993 Public Health Conference on Records and Statistics, Washington DC.

Amaro, H., & Aguiar, M. (1994). Programa Mama/Mom's Project: A community-based outreach model for addicted women. In J. Szapocznick & H. Munoz (Eds.), *A Hispanic family approach to substance abuse prevention* (pp. 125–154). Washington DC: Department of Health and Human Services.

Amaro, H., & Gornemann, I. (1992). *HIV/AIDS related knowledge, attitudes, beliefs and behaviors among Hispanics in the Northeast and Puerto Rico: Report of findings and recommendations.* Boston: Northeast Hispanic AIDS Consortium.

Amaro, H., Whitaker, R., Coffman, G., & Heeren, T. (1990). Acculturation and marijuana and cocaine use: Findings from the Hispanic HANES. *American Journal of Public Health, 80,* 54–60.

American Council on Education. (1990). *Minorities in higher education: Ninth annual status report.* Washington DC: Author.

Andrade, S. J. (1982). Social science stereotypes of the Mexican-American woman: Policy implications for research. *Hispanic Journal of Behavioral Sciences, 4,* 223–244.

Aneshensel, C. S., Fielder, E. P., & Becerra, R. M. (1989). Fertility and fertility-related behavior among Mexican American and non-Hispanic white female adolescents. *Journal of Health and Social Behavior, 30* (1), 56–76.

Arroyo, W., & Cervantes, R. C. (In press). The Mexican American child. In J. D. Nopshitz (Ed.), *Handbook of child and adolescent psychology.* New York: Basic Books.

Balance, M. F., Clinchy, B. M., Goldberger, N. R., & Tarule, J. M. (1986). *Women's ways of knowing: The development of self, voice and mind.* New York: Basic Books.

Bang, K. M., Gergen, P. J., & Carroll, M. (1990). Prevalence of chronic bronchitis among U.S. Hispanics from the Hispanic Health and Nutrition Examination Survey, 1982–84. *American Journal of Public Health, 80,* 1495–1497.

Bean, F. D., & Tienda, M. (1987). *The Hispanic population of the United States.* New York: Sage.

Bettes, B. A., Dusenbury, L., Kerner, J., James-Ortiz, S., & Botvin, G. J. (1990). Ethnicity and psychosocial factors in alcohol and tobacco use in adolescence. *Child Development, 61,* 557–565.

Bowler, S., Sheon, A. R., D'Angelo, L. J., & Vermund, S. H. (1992). HIV and AIDS among adolescents in the United States: Increasing risk in the 1990s. *Journal of Adolescence, 15,* 345–371.

Brindis, C. (1992). Adolescent pregnancy prevention for Hispanic youth: The role of schools, families, and communities. *Journal of School Health, 62* (7), 345–351.

Brook, J. S., Whiteman, M., Balka, E. B., & Hamburg, B. A. (1992). African-American and Puerto Rican drug use: Personality, familial, and other environmental risk factors. *Genetic, Social, and General Psychology Monographs, 118*, 417–438.

Bureau of the Census. (1991). *Census Bureau releases 1990 census counts on Hispanic population groups.* U.S. Department of Commerce News (Press Release CB91-216), Washington DC.

Caetano, R. (1986). Patterns and problems of drinking among U.S. Hispanics. In *Report of the secretary's task force on black and minority health* (pp. 142–186). Washington DC: U.S. Department of Health and Human Services.

Carter-Pokras, O. D., & Gergen, P. J. (1993). Reported asthma among Puerto Rican, Mexican-American, and Cuban children, 1982 through 1984. *American Journal of Public Health, 83*, 580–582.

Carter-Pokras, O., Pirkle, J., Chavez, G., & Gunter, E. (1990). Blood lead levels of 4–11-year-old Mexican American, Puerto Rican, and Cuban children. *Public Health Reports, 105*, 388–393.

Centers for Disease Control. (1987). Trends in immunodeficiency virus infection among civilian applicants for military service—United States. October 1985–December 1986. *Morbidity and Morality Weekly Report, 36*, 273–276.

Centers for Disease Control. (1991). *HIV/AIDS surveillance: Year-end edition.* Atlanta: Author.

Centers for Disease Control. (1992a). *HIV/AIDS surveillance: Third quarter edition.* Atlanta: Author.

Centers for Disease Control. (1992b). HIV instruction and selected HIV-risk behaviors among high school students—United States, 1989–91. *Morbidity and Mortality Weekly Report, 41* (46), 866–868.

Centers for Disease Control. (1992c). Physical fighting among high school students—United States, 1990. *Morbidity and Mortality Weekly Report, 41* (6), 91–94.

Centers for Disease Control. (1992d). Selected behaviors that increase risk for HIV infection among high school students—United States, 1990. *Morbidity and Mortality Weekly Report, 41* (14), 231, 237–240.

Centers for Disease Control. (1992e). Sexual behavior among high school students—United States, 1990. *Morbidity and Mortality Weekly Report, 40* (51 & 52), 885–888.

Centers for Disease Control. (1993a). Safety-belt and helmet use among high school students—United States, 1990. In *Chronic disease and health promotion: Reprints from the MMWR. 1990–1991 Youth Risk Behavior Surveillance System* (pp. 41–44). Atlanta: Author.

Centers for Disease Control. (1993b). Weapon-carrying among high school students—United States, 1990. In *Chronic disease and health promotion: Reprints from the MMWR. 1990–1991 Youth Risk Behavior Surveillance System* (pp. 17–19). Atlanta: Author.

Centers for Disease Control. (1993c). Tobacco use among high school students—United States, 1990. In *Chronic disease and health promotion: Reprints from the MMWR. 1990–1991 Youth Risk Behavior Surveillance System* (pp. 5–7). Atlanta: Author.

Centers for Disease Control. (1993d). Current tobacco, alcohol, marijuana, and cocaine use among high school students—United States, 1990. In *Chronic disease and health promotion: Reprints from the MMWR. 1990–1991 Youth Risk Behavior Surveillance System* (pp. 13–16). Atlanta: Author.

Centers for Disease Control. (1993e). Attempted suicide among high school students—United States, 1990. In *Chronic disease and health promotion: Reprints from the MMWR. 1990–1991 Youth Risk Behavior Surveillance System* (pp. 9–11). Atlanta: Author.

Centers for Disease Control. (1994). *Reported TB cases in the United States, 1993*. Atlanta: Author.

Cervantes R. C., & Castro, F. G. (1985). Stress, coping and Mexican American mental health: A systematic review. *Hispanic Journal of Behavioral Science, 7*, 1–73.

Chapa, J., & Valencia, R. R. (1993). Latino population growth, demographic characteristics, and educational stagnation: An examination of recent trends. *Hispanic Journal of Behavioral Sciences, 15*, 165–187.

Chavez, E. L., Edwards, R., & Oetting, E. R. (1989). Mexican American and white American school dropouts' drug use, health status, and involvement in violence. *Public Health Reports, 104*, 594–604.

Chavez, E. L., & Swaim, R. C. (1992). An epidemiological comparison of Mexican-American and white non-Hispanic 8th- and 12th-grade students' substance use. *American Journal of Public Health, 82*, 445–447.

Clinchy, B., & Zimmerman, C. (1985). *Growing up intellectually: Issues for college women*. Wellesley MA: Stone Center, Wellesley College.

Colp, C., Pappas, J., Moran, D., & Lieberman, J. (1993). Variants of antitrypsin in Puerto Rican children with asthma. *Chest, 103*, 812–815.

Council on Scientific Affairs. (1991). Hispanic health in the United States. *Journal of the American Medical Association, 265*, 248–252.

Cromwell, V. L., & Cromwell, R. E. (1978). Perceived dominance in decision making and conflict resolution among Anglo, Black and Chicano couples. *Journal of Marriage and the Family, 40*, 749–759.

Davis, S. M., & Harris, M. B. (1982). Sexual knowledge, sexual interests, and sources of sexual information of rural and urban adolescents from three cultures. *Adolescence*, *17*, 471–492.

Desenclos, J. C. S., & Hahn, R. A. (1992). Years of potential life lost, before age 65, by race, Hispanic origin, and sex—United States, 1986–88. *Morbidity and Mortality Weekly Report*, *41* (SS 6), 13–23.

Diaz-Guerrero, R. (1975). *Psychology of the Mexican.* Austin: University of Texas Press.

DiClemente, R., Boyer, C., & Morales, E. (1988). Minorities and AIDS: Knowledge, attitudes, and misconceptions among Blacks and Latino adolescents. *American Journal of Public Health*, *78*, 55–57.

Durant, R. H., Pendergrast, R., & Seymore, C. (1990a). Sexual behavior among Hispanic female adolescents in the United States. *Pediatrics*, *85*, 1051–1058.

Durant, R. H., Seymore, C., Pendergrast, R., & Beckman, R. (1990b). Contraceptive behavior among sexually active Hispanic adolescents. *Journal of Adolescent Health Care*, *11*, 490–496.

Dusenbury, L., Kerner, J. F., Baker, E., Botvin G., James-Ortiz, S., & Zauber, A. (1992). Predictors of smoking prevalence among New York Latino youth. *Americal Journal of Public Health*, *82*, 55–58.

Espin, O. (1984). Cultural and historical influences on sexuality in Hispanic/Latina women: Implications for psychotherapy. In C. Vance (Ed.), *Pleasure and danger: Exploring female sexuality* (pp. 149–163). London: Routledge & Kegan Paul.

Espin, O. (1987). Issues of identity in the psychology of Latina lesbians. In Boston Lesbian Psychologies Collective (Ed.), *Lesbian psychologies: Explorations and challenges* (pp. 35–51). Champaign: University of Illinois Press.

Flegal, M. K., Ezzatti, T. M., Harris, M. I., Haynes, S. G., Juarez, R. Z., Knowler, W. C., Perez-Stable, E. J., & Stern, M. P. (1991). Prevalence of diabetes in Mexican Americans, Cubans, and Puerto Ricans from the Hispanic Health and Nutrition Examination Survey, 1982–1984. *Diabetes Care*, *14* (7, Suppl. 3), 628–638.

Ford, K., & Norris, A. (1991). Urban African-American and Hispanic adolescents and young adults: Who do they talk to about AIDS and condoms? What are they learning? *AIDS Education and Prevention*, *3*, 197–206.

Freire, P. (1970). *Pedagogy of the oppressed.* New York: Continuum.

Freire, P. (1990). *Education for critical consciousness.* New York: Continuum.

Freire, P., & Faundez, A. (1989). *Learning to question: A pedagogy of liberation.* New York: Continuum.

Frisancho, A. R, and Ryan, A. S. (1991). Decreased stature associated with moderate lead concentrations in Mexican-American children. *American Journal of Clinical Nutrition, 54*, 516–519.

General Accounting Office. (1992). *Hispanic access to health care: Significant gaps exist.* Washington DC: U.S. Government Printing Office.

Goodman, E., & Cohall, A. T. (1989). Acquired immunodeficiency syndrome and adolescents: Knowledge, attitudes, beliefs, and behaviors in a New York City adolescent minority population. *Pediatrics, 84*, 36–42.

Gregory, S. J., & Clark, P. I. (1992). The "big three" cardiovascular risk factors among American Blacks and Hispanics. *Journal of Holistic Nursing, 10* (1), 76–88.

Grossman, B., Wirt, R., & Davids, A. (1985). Self-esteem, ethnic identity, and behavioral adjustment among Anglo and Chicano adolescents in west Texas. *Journal of Adolescence, 8*, 57–68.

Groves, B. M, Zuckerman, B., Maran, S., & Cohen, D. (1993). Silent victims: Children who witness violence. *Journal of the American Medical Association, 269*, 262–264.

Guarnaccia, P. J. (1992). Asthma, the Puerto Rican child, and the school. In A. N. Ambert & M. D. Alvarez (Eds.), *Puerto Rican children on the mainland: Interdisciplinary perspectives* (Vol. 10, pp. 237–272). New York: Garland.

Gutierrez, E. (1992). Latino issues: Gay and lesbian Latinos claiming La Raza. In B. Berzon (Ed.), *Positively gay* (pp. 240–246). Berkeley CA: Celestial Arts.

Hayes-Bautista, D. E. (1992). Latino health indicators and the underclass model: From paradox to new policy models. In A. Furino (Ed.), *Health policy and the Hispanic* (Vol. 4, pp. 32–47). Boulder CO: Westview.

Health Resources Administration. (1980). *Health of the disadvantaged. Chart book II* (DHHS Publication No. 890-633). Washington DC: U.S. Government Printing Office.

Holmes, M. D. (1991). Editorial: AIDS in communities of color. *American Journal of Preventive Medicine, 7*, 461–462.

Hough, R. L., Landsverk, J. A., Karno, M., Burnam, M. A., Timbers, D., Escobar, J., & Regier, D. (1987). Utilization of health and mental health services by Los Angeles Mexican Americans and non-Hispanic whites. *Archives of General Psychiatry, 44*, 702–709.

Johnston, L., O'Malley, P., & Bachman, J. (1994). *National survey results on drug use from the Monitoring Future Study, 1975–1993.* U.S. Department of Health and Human Services. PHS Vol. 1. Ann Arbor: University of Michigan, Institute for Social Research.

Karno, M., & Edgerton, R. B. (1969). Perceptions of mental illness in a Mexican American community. *Archives of General Psychiatry, 20*, 233–238.

Kasper, J. A., & Barrish, C. (1982). *Usual sources of medical care and their characteristics Data preview 12.* (DHHS Publication No. 82-3324). Washington DC: U.S. Government Printing Office.

Linares, L. O., Leadbeater, B. J., Kato, P. M., & Jaffe, L. (1991). Predicting school outcomes for minority group adolescent mothers: Can subgroups be identified? *Journal of Research on Adolescence, 1*, 379–400.

Madsen, W. (1964). *The Mexican Americans of South Texas.* New York: Holt, Rinehart & Winston.

Magaña, J. R. (1992). Una pedagogia de concientización para la prevención del VIH/SIDA. *Revista Latinoamericana de Psicología, 24* (1–2), 97–108.

Marin, G., Perez-Stable, E. J., & Marin, B. (1989). Cigarette smoking among San Francisco Hispanics: The role of acculturation and gender. *American Journal of Public Health, 79*, 196–199.

Markides, K. S., Ray, L. A., Stroup-Benham, C. A. & Trevino, F. (1990). Acculturation and alcohol consumption in the Mexican American population of the Southwestern United States: Findings from HHANES 1982–84. *American Journal of Public Health, 80* (Suppl.), 42–46.

Marzuk, P. M., Tardiff, K., Leon, A. C, Stajic, M., Morgan, E. B., & Mann, J. J. (1992). Prevalence of cocaine use among residents of New York City who committed suicide during a one-year period. *American Journal of Psychiatry, 149*, 371–375.

Mason, H. R. C., Marks, Q., Simoni, J., Ruiz, M. S., & Richardson, J. L. (1994). Culturally sanctioned secrets? Latino men's nondisclosure of HIV infection to family, friends, and lovers. *Health Psychology, 14*, 6–12.

Maurer, J. D., Rosenberg, H. M., & Keemer, J. B. (1990). Deaths of Hispanic origin, 15 reporting states, 1979–1981. *Vital and Health Statistics, 20* (18), 1–47.

Mendoza, F. S., Ventura, S. J., Saldivar, L., Baisden, K., & Martorell, R. (1992). The health status of U.S. Hispanic children. In A. Furino (Ed.), *Health policy and the Hispanic* (Vol. 8, pp. 97–115). Boulder CO: Westview.

Moore, D. S., & Erickson, P. I. (1985). Age, gender, and ethnic differences in sexual and contraceptive knowledge, attitudes and behaviors. *Family and Community Health, 8*, 38–51.

Morales, E. (1989). Ethnic minority families and minority gays and lesbians. *Marriage and Family Review, 14*, 217–239.

Morales, E. (1992). Latino gays and Latina lesbians. In S. Dworkin & F. Gutierrez (Eds.), *Counseling gay men and lesbians: Journey to the end of the rainbow*
(pp. 125–139). Alexandria VA: American Association for Counseling and Development.

Mosher, W. D., & Bachrach, C. A. (1986). Contraceptive use: United States, 1982.
Vital and Health Statistics, 23 (12), 1–51.

National Center for Health Statistics. (1992a). *Health, United States, 1991.* Hyatts-
ville MD: Public Health Service.

National Center for Health Statistics. (1992b). Advance report of final mortality
statistics, 1989. *Monthly Vital Statistics Report,* 40 (8, Supplement 2).

National Center for Health Statistics. (1993a). Advance report of final mortality statistics, 1990. *Monthly Vital Statistics Report,* 41 (7, Supplement).

National Center for Health Statistics. (1993b). *Health, United States, 1993.* Hyatts-
ville MD: Public Health Service.

Newacheck P. W., Stoddard, J. J., & McManus, M. (1993). Ethnocultural variations in the prevalence and impact of childhood chronic conditions. *Pediatrics, 91,*
1031–1039.

Norris, A. E., & Ford, K. (1991). AIDS risk behaviors of minority youth living in
Detroit. *American Journal of Preventive Medicine, 7,* 416–421.

Norris, A. E., & Ford, K. (1992). Beliefs about condoms and accessibility of condom intentions in Hispanic and African American youth. *Hispanic Journal of Behavioral Science, 14,* 373–382.

Novello, A. C., Wise, P. H., & Kleinman, D. V. (1991). Hispanic health: Time for
data, time for action [Editorial]. *Journal of the American Medical Association, 265,*
253–255.

Office of Management and Budget. (1978). Directive No. 15: Race and ethnic standards for federal statistics and administrative reporting. In *Statistical policy handbook* (pp. 37–38). Washington DC.: Office of Federal Statistical Policy and Standards, U.S. Department of Commerce.

Padilla, E. R., & O'Grady, K. E. (1987). Sexuality among Mexican-Americans: A
case of sexual stereotyping. *Journal of Personality and Social Psychology, 52,* 5–10.

Pallas, A. M., Natriello, G., & McDill, E. L. (1989). The changing nature of the
disadvantaged population: Current dimensions and future trends. *Educational
Researcher, 18,* 16–22.

Pleck, J. H., Sonenstein, F. L. & Leighton, C. K. (1993). Masculinity ideology: Its
impact on adolescent males' heterosexual relationships. *Journal of Social Issues,
4993,* 11–29.

Portes, A., & Rumbaut, R. G. (1990). *Immigrant America: A portrait.* Berkeley and Los Angeles: University of California Press.

Razin, A. M., O'Dowd, M. A., Nathan, A., Rodriguez, I., Goldfield, A., Martin, C., Goulet, L., Sceftel, S., Mezan, P., & Mosca, J. (1991). Suicidal behavior among inner-city Hispanic adolescent females. *General Hospital Psychiatry, 13,* 45–58.

Rebach, H. (1992). Alcohol and drug use among American minorities. *Drugs and Society, 6* (1/2), 23–57.

Roberts, R. E., & Sobhan, M. (1992). Symptoms of depression in adolescence: A comparison of Anglo, African, and Hispanic Americans. *Journal of Youth and Adolescence, 21,* 639–651.

Rotheram-Borus, M. J., Meyer-Bahlburg, H. F. L., Rosario, M., Koopman, C., Haignere, C. S., Exner, T. M., Matthieu, M., Henderson, R., & Gruen, R. S. (1992). Lifetime sexual behaviors among predominantly minority male runaways and gay/bisexual adolescents in New York City. *AIDS Education and Prevention, Supplement,* 34–42.

Rotheram-Borus, M. J., Rosario, M., & Koopman, C. (1991). Minority youths at high risk: Gay males and runaways. In M. E. Colten & S. Gore (Eds.), *Adolescent stress: Causes and consequences* (pp. 181–200). New York: de Gruyter.

Rotheram-Borus, M. J., Rosario, M., Meyer-Bahlburg, H. F. L., Koopman, C., Dopkins, S. C., & Davies, M. (1994). Sexual and substance use acts of gay and bisexual male adolescents in New York City. *Journal of Sex Research, 31,* 47–57.

Rousseau, C., Corin, E., & Renaud, C. (1989). Armed conflict and trauma: A clinical study of Latin-American refugee children. *Canadian Journal of Psychiatry, 34,* 376–385.

Schwartz, J., & Otto, D. (1991). Lead and minor hearing impairment. *Archives of Environmental Health, 46,* 300–305.

Scott, C. S., Shifman, L., Orr, L., Owen, R. G., & Fawcett, N. (1988). Hispanic and Black American adolescents' beliefs relating to sexuality and contraception. *Adolescence, 23,* 667–688.

Smith, K. W., McGraw, S. A., Crawford, S. L., Costa, L. A., & McKinlay, J. B. (1991). *Estimates of human immunodeficiency virus infection risk among Latino adolescents in two New England cities.* Report of the New England Research Institute, Watertown MA.

Snider, D. E., Salinas, L., & Kelly, G. D. (1989). Tuberculosis: An increasing problem among minorities in the United States. *Public Health Reports, 104,* 646–653.

Sokol-Katz, J. S., & Ulbrich, P. M. (1992). Family structure and adolescent risk-taking behavior: A comparison of Mexican, Cuban, and Puerto Rican Americans. *International Journal of the Addictions, 27,* 1197–1209.

St. Louis, M. E., Conway, G. A., Hayman, C. R., Miller, C., Petersen, L. R., & Dondero, T. J. (1991). Human immunodeficiency virus infection in disadvantaged adolescents: Findings from the U.S. Job Corps. *Journal of the American Medical Association, 266,* 2387–2391.

Stern, M. P., & Haffner, S. M. (1992). Type II diabetes in Mexican Americans: A public health challenge. In A. Furino (Ed.), *Health policy and the Hispanic* (Vol.6, pp.55–75). Boulder CO: Westview.

Sumaya, C. V. (1991). Major infectious diseases causing excess morbidity in the Hispanic population. *Archives of Internal Medicine, 151,* 1513–1520.

Surrey, J. L. (1991). The "self-in-relation": A theory of women's development. In J. D. Jordan, A. G. Kaplan, J. B. Miller, I. P. Stiver, & J. L. Surrey (Eds.), *Women's growth in connection: writings from the stone center* (pp.162–180). New York: Guilford.

Swanson, J. W, Linskey, A. O., Quintero-Salinas, R., Pumariega, A. J., & Holzer, C. E. (1992). Binational school survey of depressive symptoms, drug use, and suicidal ideation. *Journal of the American Academy of Child and Adolescent Psychiatry, 31,* 669–678.

Szapocznik, J., & COSSMHO (1994). Structural family therapy. In J. Szapocznik & COSSMHO (Eds.), *Hispanic-Latino family approaches to substance abuse prevention* (pp.41–74). Rockville MD: Center for Substance Abuse Prevention.

Tommasello, A., Tyler, F. B., Tyler, S. L., & Zhang, Y. (1993). Psychosocial correlates of drug use among Latino youth leading autonomous lives. *International Journal of the Addictions, 28,* 435–450.

Trevino, F. M., & Moss, A. J. (1983). Health insurance coverage and physician visits among Hispanic and non-Hispanic people. *Health, United States, 1983* (DHHS Pub. No.84-1232). Washington DC: U.S. Government Printing Office.

Trevino, F. M., & Moss, A. J. (1984). Health indicators for Hispanic, Black and White Americans. *Vital and Health Statistics, 10* (148), 1–88.

Troxler, R. G., Park, M. K., Miller, M. A., Karnavas, B. A., & Lee, D. H. (1991). Predictive value of family history in detecting hypercholesterolemia in predominantly Hispanic adolescents. *Texas Medicine, 87* (11), 75–79.

Tyler, F. B, Tyler, S. L., Tommasello, A., & Zhang, Y. (1992). Psychosocial characteristics of marginal immigrant Latino youth. *Youth and Society, 24,* 92–115.

U.S. Department of Health and Human Services. (1986). *Report of the Secretary's Task Force on Black and Minority Health. Volume 8: Hispanic health issues.* Washington DC: U.S. Government Printing Office.

U.S. Department of Health and Human Services. (1991). *Healthy People 2000: National health promotion and disease prevention objectives.* Washington DC: Public Health Service.

Vasquez, M. T. J. (1994). Latinas. In L. Comas-Diaz & B. Greene (Eds.), *Women of color: Integrating ethnic and gender entities in psychotherapy* (pp. 114–138). New York: Guilford.

Vasquez, M. T. J., & Gonzalez, A. M. (1981). Sex roles among Chicanos: Stereotypes, challenges, and changes. In A. Baron, Jr. (Ed.), *Explorations in Chicano psychology* (pp. 50–70). New York: Praeger.

Vega, W. A., & Amaro, H. (1994). Latino outlook: Good health, uncertain prognosis. *Annual Review of Public Health, 15,* 39–67.

Vega, W. A., Zimmerman, R. S., Warheit, G. J., Apssori, E., & Gil, A. G. (1993). Risk factors for early adolescent drug use in four ethnic and racial groups. *American Journal of Public Health, 83* (2), 185–189.

Velez, C. N., & Ungemack, J. A. (1989). Drug use among Puerto Rican youth: An exploration of generational status differences. *Social Science and Medicine, 29,* 779–789.

Wallerstein, N. (1992). Powerlessness, empowerment, and health: Implications for health promotion programs. *American Journal of Health Promotions, 6,* 197–205.

Webber, L. S., Harsha, D. W., Phillips, G. T., Srinivasan, S. R., Simpson, J. W., & Berenson, G. S. (1991). Cardiovascular risk factors in Hispanic, White, and Black children: The Brooks County and Bogalusa heart studies. *American Journal of Epidemiology, 133,* 704–714.

Werner, D., & Bower, B. (1982). *Helping health workers learn.* Palo Alto CA: Hesperian Foundation.

Williams, D. R., Lavizzo-Mourey, R., & Warren, R. C. (1993, March). *Race in the health of America: Problems, issues, and directions.* Paper presented at the workshop on the Use of Race and Ethnicity in Public Health Surveillance, sponsored by the Centers for Disease Control and Prevention and Agency for Toxic Substances and Disease Registry, Atlanta.

Wood, P. R., Hidalgo, H. A., Prihoda, T. J., & Kromer, M. E. (1993). Hispanic children with asthma: Morbidity. *Pediatrics, 91,* 62–69.

Yamamoto, J., & Silva, A. (1987). *Do Hispanics underutilize mental health services?* Paper presented at the Conference on Health and Behavior: Research Agenda for Hispanics, Chicago.

Zapata, J. T. & Jaramillo, P. T. (1981). The Mexican American family: An Adlerian perspective. *Hispanic Journal of Behavioral Sciences, 3,* 275–290.

4

American Indian Adolescent Health

Candace M. Fleming, Spero M. Manson, and Lois Bergeisen

Indian and Native Population Characteristics

According to the 1990 census (Bureau of the Census, 1992), the American Indian and Alaska Native population numbers 1,959,234. The population is quite young compared with the overall U.S. population (median ages of 26.2 years and 31.7 years, respectively); almost 19% of the Indians and Alaska Natives fell within the 10–19 age group, compared with 14% for all races. In fiscal year 1992, the service population of the Indian Health Service (IHS) (count of those American Indians and Alaska Natives who are eligible for IHS services) was approximately 1.16 million and is increasing at a rate of about 2.6% per year.

Socioeconomic status in Indian and Native population lags all other races (U.S. Department of Health and Human Services, Public Health Service, Indian Health Service, 1991). However, the Indian and Native population is diverse; there are more than 300 federally recognized tribes, each with its own culture, history, geography, and demography. Social and economic characteristics vary considerably from reservation to reservation. For example, unemployment rates for the Choctaw Reservation in Mississippi are below those of the state, while unemployment on the Pine Ridge Reservation in South Dakota is approximately 70%, the highest in the country.

In the thirty years since the inception of the IHS, major advances have

---

Portions of the analysis in this chapter are based on Spero M. Manson's research for *Indian Adolescent Mental Health* (U.S. Congress, Office of Technology Assessment, OTA-H-446, 1986).

been accomplished in improving the health status of Indians living in reservation states. For example, from 1957 to 1986–1988, the maternal mortality rate has decreased 91% and is now only slightly higher than that of the U.S. average (U.S. Department of Health and Human Services, Public Health Service, Indian Health Service, 1991), infant mortality has decreased 85%, and life expectancy at birth for Indians residing in reservation states increased to 71.1.

Yet, despite some gains, the age-adjusted mortality rates for all reservation states in 1988 were considerably higher than for the U.S. population for tuberculosis (400% greater), alcoholism (438% greater), accidents (131% greater), diabetes mellitus (155% greater), homicide (57% greater), and suicide (27% greater) (U.S. Department of Health and Human Services, Public Health Service, Indian Health Service, 1991).

Indian and Native Adolescent Physical Health Concerns

The health-related issues and personal concerns facing Indian adolescents, such as peer pressure, alcohol and drug use, violence, and premature sexual activity, are not unlike those facing adolescents throughout the United States. But specific additional concerns to Indian and Native adolescents spring from their strong traditional background. The complex relation between Indian tribes and the federal government further complicates the delivery of health and social services.

MORTALITY

The death rate for Indian youth 15–24 years of age was 1.6 times higher than that for the U.S. general populations. The two leading causes of deaths of Indian youth were accidents (89.1 deaths per 100,000) and suicide (23.5 deaths per 100,000), as compared with accidents and homicide for U.S. youth. Indian males ages 15–24 were more at risk for early death than females of this same age group (9.5% and 4.2%, respectively; U.S. Department of Health and Human Services, Public Health Service, Indian Health Service, 1991).

ADOLESCENT PREGNANCY AND SEXUALITY

Despite extensive data on adolescent pregnancy in the United States, scant attention has been paid in the published literature to Indian adolescents. There does, however, appear to be much concern within the Indian communities about teen pregnancy. Adolescent pregnancy appears to be a major reason for dropping out of school for Indian females. While there appears to be little stigma attached to adolescent births in Indian communities, the social and economic consequences of teen births are not unlike those for other teenagers.

In 1986–1988, just over 19% of births in IHS service areas were to women under the age of 20 (U.S. Department of Human Services, Public Health Service, Indian Health Service, 1991), compared with 12% for the 1987 general U.S. rate. While the proportion of births to adolescents has been declining for the general U.S. population, it has remained relatively stable for Indian adolescents younger than 15 while increasing slightly for those in older age cohorts (Centers for Disease Control, 1988). Little is known about the abortion patterns for Indian women, and pregnancy rates of any age cohort cannot be calculated using existing IHS data.

Indian females under 15 years of age were twice as likely to seek early prenatal care in 1986 than in 1980 (33% vs. 17%). Indian women under age 19 are only somewhat less likely to receive first trimester prenatal care than the U.S. general population (Centers for Disease Control, 1988).

Indian women, including adolescents, are much less likely to give birth to low-birthweight infants (5% of Indians compared with 14% for all adolescents). This statistic may appear to be a positive indicator but is most likely due to the influence of the high rates of diabetes in Indian populations.

Adolescent Sexual Behavior

Few data were available on the sexual behavior of Indian adolescents until the recent completion of the Indian Adolescent Health Survey (IAHS) (Blum et al., 1992), administered in the schools of several reservation communities served by the IHS. Some 13,454 Indian youth from seventh to twelfth grades were surveyed; 49.2% were male and 50.7% were female. A subsample of 6,184 rural non-Native youth was also compiled, referred to as the Minnesota Adolescent Health Survey (MAHS) sample for comparison.

The proportion of males in the IAHS subsample who reported ever having sexual intercourse was higher than that of rural White Minnesota males (35% vs. 28%), while females showed comparable numbers (27% vs. 24%). The data indicated that, for twelfth-grade Indian females, the average age at first intercourse was 14, while it was 13.6 for twelfth-grade males. About 7% of females indicated they had been pregnant at some time; about 5% of males said they had fathered a child.

The IAHS showed that Indian adolescents are aware of AIDS as a health threat. Of those youth who are not sexually active, more than one quarter indicated fear of disease as a reason for not having sex. However, only 49% of sexually active males and 24% of sexually active females reported they or their partners use condoms.

OTITIS MEDIA

Otitis media (middle-ear infection) is widely regarded as the most frequently identified disease of Indian children. It is most prevalent from birth to approximately 7 years of age (Howie, Ploussard, & Stoyer, 1975). Its special significance for adolescents lies in its contribution to hearing loss (Paradise, 1980), delays in cognitive and psycholinguistic development (Zinkus & Gottleib, 1980), lowered educational achievement (DiSarno & Barringer, 1987), and reading problems and emotional difficulties (Bennet, Ruuska, & Sherman, 1980). The potential scope of these problems is reflected in estimates that as many as 75% of all Indian children experience otitis media, that 13,000 Indians are in need of hearing aids, and that as many as 22,000 may require otologic surgery (Stewart, 1975).

INJURIES

As stated previously, injuries, primarily as a result of motor vehicle accidents, account for the largest proportion of deaths to Indian youth. Some 45% and 34% respectively, of those males and females in grades 10–12 who drink indicated they drink and drive (Blum et al., 1992). Nearly 22% of all Indian adolescents indicated they sometimes or often ride with someone who has been drinking. Seat belts have proved to significantly reduce the risk of severe and fatal injury in automobile crashes, yet well over 40% of Indian adolescents indicated they rarely or never wear a seat belt.

More than 40% of Indian males and 28% of females indicated riding a motorcycle or similar vehicle at least once a month (Blum et al., 1992). However, of those, 40% of males and nearly half of females rarely or never wear a helmet when riding such vehicles, and 40% of Indian adolescents also place themselves at risk for injury at least occasionally when riding in the back of pickup trucks (a common vehicle on reservations), which are rarely equipped with occupant safety devices.

Additionally, according to the IAHS, fighting appears to be common for Indian adolescents. Almost one quarter of Indian adolescents participated in a group fight within the last year, and more than 30% of Indian adolescents, compared with 5% of Minnesota non-Indian youths, were worried about the violence in their neighborhood.

TOBACCO USAGE

Smokeless tobacco use is increasing among children and adolescents. Prevalence rates for Indian adolescents are higher than those of any other ethnic group. Data from the IAHS support the findings of previous research. Comparing data from the IAHS and the MAHS, smokeless tobacco use is higher across all grades among not only Indian males, but also Indian females (Blum et al., 1992). Twenty percent of twelfth-grade Indian males use smokeless tobacco on a daily basis; 10% of ninth-grade Indian females do so. For every grade level after the seventh, Indian females were more likely to be daily cigarette smokers than males.

Indian Adolescent Emotional and Mental-Health Concerns

Most psychiatric disorders documented in the *Diagnostic and Statistical Manual* (American Psychiatric Association, 1987) are represented at least as frequently among American Indian and Alaska Native adolescents as in the adolescent population at large (Bechtold, Manson, & Shore, 1994). Several disorders may be found more frequently among Indian adolescents, including mental retardation, specific developmental disorders, identity disorder, substance-use disorder, depression disorders, posttraumatic stress disorder, and adjustment disorders. More valid estimates of the extent of diagnosable mental disorders among Indian adolescents (and non-Indian adolescents) await systematic epidemiologic study. Much of the data for this section is drawn from *Indian Adolescent Mental Health* (U.S. Congress, Office of Technology Assessment, 1986a). Readers are encouraged to review that report for detailed information and tables.

DEVELOPMENTAL DISORDERS

Mental retardation and other developmental disabilities may occur with greater frequency among Indian adolescents, although prevalence is not well established (O'Connell, 1987). The Native American Rehabilitation and Training Center concluded that neurosensory disorders and certain developmental disabilities appear to be from four to thirteen times greater for American Indians than for the U.S. population in general (Native American Rehabilitation and Training Center, 1979). A more recent analysis of national data from 1984 observed that almost 10% of American Indian students in public schools had some form of developmental disability (O'Connell, 1987). These data suggest that developmental disabilities are a serious problem among Indian adolescents and may be related to the high prevalence of otitis media and fetal alcohol syndrome (FAS) among Indian children.

FETAL ALCOHOL SYNDROME

The pioneering work on FAS and fetal alcohol effects (FAE) was conducted by May and his colleagues (May et al., 1983). They found that one group of Indians had a higher incidence of FAS than any that had been reported previously, while two other Indian groups had lower rates but the incidence appeared to be growing. Of all the fetal alcohol children, 73% had been adopted or placed in foster homes because of abandonment or neglect by their natural mothers. Twenty-three percent of biological mothers had died, almost always from an accident, cirrhosis of the liver, or other alcohol-related trauma or illness. May and his colleagues noted that a relatively small number of mothers were responsible for the prevalence of FAS and FAE, which suggests that prevention can be targeted to high-risk mothers.

DEPRESSION

Depression has long been a concern with respect to Indian adolescents. Numerous clinicians and investigators have argued, for example, that behavioral difficulties such as conduct disorder, learning problems, or substance abuse may reflect underlying depression. Unfortunately, the systematic study of depression among adolescents in general, much less their Indian counterparts, has advanced more slowly than among adults, as theories about childhood depression are still evolving (U.S. Congress, Office of Technology Assessment, 1986c).

Nonetheless, depression is frequently cited among the troubles experienced by Indian youth. Of the studies comparing the level of depression among Indian adolescents with a sample of non-Indians (Ackerson et al., 1990; University of Minnesota, 1989b), most reported more depression among Indian adolescents. When self-report screening methods are used, at least half of Indian adolescents have reported serious depressive symptoms (Manson et al., 1990; National Center for American Indian and Alaska Native Mental Health Research, 1989a, 1989b). It is no surprise that, when the more restrictive diagnostic criteria for clinical depression are used, the proportion of Indian adolescents found to be depressed is smaller (Ackerson et al., 1990; Beiser & Attneave, 1982; May, 1983).

SUICIDE

While suicide is the second leading cause of death for Indian and Alaska Native adolescents, the actual number of deaths is relatively low (e.g., thirty deaths among 10–19-year-old Indians in 1986; U.S. Congress, Office of Technology Assessment, 1989). Bechtold's (1988) analysis suggests that serial suicides by Indian adolescents are fueled by the same interpersonal and social dynamics as in the population at large.

In 1986, the age-specific mortality rate for suicide for 15–19-year-old Indians was an estimated 26.3 deaths per 100,000 population, compared with 10.0 per 100,000 in the general population. For 15–19-year-olds, death rates from suicide have decreased somewhat, but rates for 10–14-year-olds are approximately four times higher than that for the general U.S. population and have increased steadily (U.S. Congress, Office of Technology Assessment, 1989).

SUICIDE ATTEMPTS

In 1988, there were 424 hospitalizations for Indian adolescents ages 10–19 that involved a suicide attempt. Seventy percent (298) were females, with the majority (55%) in the 15–17 range. Nearly half (47%) of male suicide discharges were also in this age range (U.S. Department of Health and Human Services, Public Health Service, Indian Health Service, 1989b).

Nearly 12% of Indian males and 20% of Indian females in a subset of IAHS data collected from approximately 2,700 students in some Plains, Southeast, and Southwest tribes indicated they had ever attempted suicide, compared with 7% of males and 14% of females in the MAHS (American Alliance for Health, 1988). The IAHS noted that 75% of adolescents who had attempted suicide reported they received no mental-health care.

ANXIETY

Beiser and Attneave (1982) reported that anxiety was the fourth most common mental-health problem for youth (8% of males and females ages 15–

19) seen in IHS mental-health programs in 1974, nearly equal to the frequency of depression. May's (1983) survey revealed that, in 1981 and 1982, about 18% of all males and nearly 10% of all females seen for anxiety in the IHS Albuquerque area office mental-health program were between 10 and 19 years of age. Studies of boarding school and college students suggested remarkably high levels of different forms of anxiety among Indian adolescents and suggest that anxiety may be an important factor contributing to social and academic problems in school (National Center for American Indian and Alaska Native Mental Health Research, 1989a, 1989b).

SUBSTANCE ABUSE AND DEPENDENCE

Given the high rate of deaths among young Indians due to causes related to substance use, particularly alcohol (U.S. Congress, Office of Technology Assessment, 1986b), there is considerable interest in this problem among Indian tribes and health providers. Several recent surveys point to different conclusions about the extent of substance use among Indian adolescents.

Surveys by Beauvais and Oetting have found high rates of alcohol and drug experimentation among Indian adolescents relative to non–Indian adolescents (Beauvais et al., 1989). Preliminary data from the more recent IAHS found a much lower use of drugs among Indian adolescents than did the Beauvais and Oetting surveys. Alcohol and cocaine use were comparable between Indian and non–Indian students, while marijuana use was higher among Indians than among the mostly non–Indian Minnesota sample.

The number of adolescents dependent on or otherwise abusing drugs as opposed to experimenting with them a single time is unclear from existing data. In a survey of attitudes toward drugs on the Wind River Reservation in Wyoming, Indian adolescents were found to have a more favorable attitude toward the use of marijuana and other drugs and to be more likely to try using them, but they were no more likely to continue using such drugs after trying them than were White adolescents from the same geographic area (Cockerham, Forslund, & Raboin, 1976).

Nonetheless, persistently high drug use is still the norm across most categories for young Indian people, especially in regard to marijuana, inhalants, and stimulants (Beauvais et al., 1989). In addition, American Indians begin abusing various substances at a younger age than their White counterparts (Weibel, 1984). Indian adolescents also seem particularly prone to using alcohol and other drugs in combination. Inhalant use appears to decline, however, as other substances such as marijuana and alcohol become more accessible.

IDENTITY DISORDER, ALIENATION, AND SELF-ESTEEM

Indian adolescent identity disorder has yet to appear in the published literature as a formal focus for discussion, although it is relevant to the life experiences of many Indian adolescents. The literature does address self-esteem and alienation, which are central to identity disorder. The missing dimension is the associated degree of functional impairment, and thus this topic marks an area of transition from the mental disorders to serious but less diagnostically specifiable problems.

For the most part, studies on self-esteem and alienation suggest that Indian adolescents have negative views of themselves. They may characterize themselves as being friendly, helpful, easygoing, and more interested in happiness than in success, but not as being particularly smart, strong, good-looking, or at ease in front of groups. Attendance at a segregated Bureau of Indian Affairs (BIA) school or an integrated public school does not appear to affect self-esteem or sense of alienation (Development Associates, 1983). A review by Development Associates (1983) concluded that, while Indian students test at lower than normative levels with respect to their personal self-concept, they hold their own cultural group in high regard.

CONDUCT DISORDER AND DELINQUENCY

The literature does not allow an analysis of the incidence and prevalence of diagnosable conduct disorder among Indian adolescents. However, studies exist concerning several of the symptoms characteristic of conduct disorder. These studies provide some information about the possibility of conduct disorder among Indian adolescents but, because they are only single behaviors, do not necessarily mean that the adolescents involved have a diagnosable mental disorder. Running away, dropping out of school, and behaving delinquently may indicate that an adolescent is experiencing emotional stress and/or may be responding relatively rationally to environmental problems.

Delinquency is thought to be a large and growing problem among Indian adolescents. There is, however, relatively little information to substantiate this assumption. Forslund and Meyers (1974) summarized early studies indicating that delinquency among Indian youth was characterized by a preponderance of petty offenses and misdemeanors. In 1982, the most frequent causes for arrest were disorderly conduct (25.9%), liquor law violations (11.2%), curfew violations (9.8%), drunkenness (9.6%), and running away from home (6.6%; May, 1983).

Youth from both Indian and non-Indian communities reported having frequently engaged in delinquent acts, but there were significant differences between Indian and non-Indian males on only seven offenses and between Indian and non-Indian females on only sixteen offenses (Forslund & Cranston, 1975). Jensen, Straus, and Harris (1977) demonstrated that, when alcohol-related offenses (to which Indian youth, in their data, were three times more prone than Anglo or Hispanic children) were eliminated, delinquency rates were comparable. Fifty-eight percent of juvenile arrests were for alcohol use: 63% for males and 37% for females (May, 1983).

SCHOOL DROPOUT RATES

Indian students drop out of school at rates substantially higher than the general population. Estimates range between 15% and 60%, whereas the frequency of dropout in the general population ranges from 5% to 30% (Development Associates, 1983). Regional studies confirmed these findings, although the differences between Indian and non-Indian students appeared negligible in two surveys of New Mexico schools (Corwin, 1978; Horton & Annalora, 1974; Squires, 1978; Young, 1981).

Culture-specific factors help to account for Indian students dropping out of school. Szasz (1974), for example, argued that lack of participation and failure within the educational system—coupled with its historic failure to address Indian cultural values and ideals—have led Indian people to perceive schools as irrelevant. In addition, many Indian families function on the basis of family needs assuming priority over personal desires and larger societal demands. Indian dropouts have frequently cited being needed at home to care for younger siblings and older family members as a reason for leaving school (Hanks, 1973).

Other family-related factors like mobility and instability also contribute to Indian student dropout rates. Wax and Wax (1974) found a strong relation between dropping out and irregular employment of fathers among Indian high school students. The families of many Indian school dropouts are characterized by marital conflict, divorce, unstable residence patterns, and parental alcoholism (Brown, 1973).

RUNNING AWAY

Runaway Indian youth are reportedly a growing problem and have captured recent interest. Data are relatively sparse, however, reflecting the difficulty in identifying and reaching this population. According to one study, runaway Indian youth are comparable to runaway youth in general (Indian Center, 1986). Half of the adolescents in this study had run away from two to five times; 9% had run away more frequently. Age was strongly and positively related to the frequency, duration, and distance of running away as well as to the likelihood of using public services.

Conflict with parents including parental alcohol and drug abuse and home-related problems was the predominant cause of running away, but school difficulties, problems with siblings, and other problems were also cited. On returning home, few runaways (17%) reported using services that might help them cope more effectively with these stresses.

CHILD AND ADOLESCENT ABUSE AND NEGLECT

Child and adolescent abuse and neglect are of increasing concern in Indian communities (U.S. Congress, Senate, Select Committee on Indian Affairs, 1989). It is unclear whether the variation in estimates of prevalence is due to widely divergent definitions of the phenomena, to differential reporting methods, or to true epidemiologic differences that reflect the particular stresses and strains of local communities (Wichlacz & Wechsler, 1983). Moreover, there is no mechanism for systematic reporting of child abuse and neglect cases to the BIA or tribal contract social-service agencies, and these data do not include urban Indians. Data from the BIA (U.S. Department of the Interior, Bureau of Indian Affairs, 1989) and self-reports by adolescents reflect that a minimum of 1% of Indian children in BIA service areas may have been abused or neglected in a single year. In the IAHS survey, 8.3% of male and 24% of female seventh to twelfth graders reported they had been abused physically, sexually, or both at some time in their lives (University of Minnesota, 1989a). Non-Indians were much less likely to report either physical or sexual abuse but more likely to indicate that they had ever discussed the abuse with a friend, family member, or helping professional (University of Minnesota, 1989a).

The dynamics of abused and neglected Indian children probably mirror those of abusive families in general (Helfer & Kempe, 1987). Interpersonal conflict, marital disruption, single parenting, chaotic family situation, parental alcoholism, inadequate caregiver-child bonding, severe educational deficits, chronic physical illness, unemployment, and violent death are common (Fischler, 1985; Piasecki et al., 1989). Variables that are more specific to Indian communities include stresses resulting from rapid sociocultural change, gender role changes, failed parenting skills, the changing nature of the extended family, and special risks attached to boarding schools.

More Indian children residing with foster or adoptive families had had histories of abuse or neglect than their counterparts who lived either with parents or in such institutional settings as boarding schools (Piasecki et al., 1989). The troublesome aspect of these findings is that, at the time of the survey, 61% of the children with histories of abuse or neglect resided within the familial households that likely gave rise to these conditions. Several recent, highly publicized cases of sexual abuse in BIA schools indicate, however, that the home is not the only arena in which Indian children are at risk for abuse (U.S. Congress, Senate, Select Committee on Indian Affairs, 1989).

PARENTAL ALCOHOLISM

The extent of alcohol abuse in Indian communities is of long-standing concern (U.S. Congress, Office of Technology Assessment, 1986b) and is implicated in many of the major causes of morbidity and mortality for Indians. Recently, a total of 22.5% of Indian adolescents surveyed perceived that their parents had a drinking problem (University of Minnesota, 1989a), compared with 14% of Minnesota non-Indian adolescents (University of Minnesota, 1987).

FAMILY DISRUPTION

Compared with Minnesota students, Indian students reported their biological parents were much less likely to be living together (84% vs. 44%) (National Center for American Indian and Alaska Native Mental Health Research, 1989a; University of Minnesota, 1987). Perhaps most disturbing, 12% of Indian adolescents reported that one or both parents were dead, compared with approximately 3% of Minnesota students. As a consequence, Indian adolescents were more than twice as likely to report living in a single-parent household, and almost ten times as likely to report living without a parent as the Minnesota students.

SCHOOL ENVIRONMENT

In school, alcohol consumption was seen as the most frequently occurring behavior for all students, although rural Minnesota youth saw more drinking behavior than either metropolitan Minnesota or Indian students. On the other hand, Indian students were much more likely to indicate that students were using drugs, destroying property, getting into fights, and stealing.

Plains adolescents are more likely to see drinking, fighting, and drugs as more common in their environment than do Indian teenagers from other parts of the United States. Perceptions of somewhat lower alcohol usage by Southeast Indian adolescents is probably reflective of restrictive liquor laws in the area. Southeast students were much more likely to perceive that students were sniffing substances (glue, paint, Liquid Paper, etc.) than students elsewhere but less likely to perceive the use of other drugs.

School pressures were a substantial source of stress for students (National Center for American Indian and Alaska Native Mental Health Research, 1989a). Indian adolescents in high school were more likely to identify concerns about families and friends. Many more Indians than Whites report having had stressful experiences related to school academically and economically and found them of equal or greater concern (Dise-Lewis, 1988).

HEALTH–SERVICE DELIVERY SYSTEMS

The IHS is the agency most directly responsible for providing health services to Indian adolescents living on or near Indian communities or reservations. In fiscal year 1992, the number of American Indians and Alaska Natives eligible for IHS services was estimated to be approximately 1.16 million. Eligibility is determined by residence on or near the twelve geographic area offices of the IHS. Other important health- and human-service systems that address Indian adolescents' needs are tribal health programs, urban health programs, BIA, and state and local service agencies.

Indian Health Service Primary Health Care Services

Most of IHS's budget is devoted to the provision of primary acute health care services. In every IHS service area, medical providers are scarce (Dougherty, 1989; U.S. Congress, Office of Technology Assessment, 1986c; U.S. Congress, Office of Technology Assessment, Health Program, 1987) and the ratio of providers to population is well below accepted standards (Dougherty, 1989; U.S. Congress, Office of Technology Assessment, Health Program, 1987). This overextension is due to a combination of widespread needs among Indians for physical health care, the fact that the financial resources of the IHS have not increased relative to inflation since 1978, and difficulties in recruiting clinical personnel to IHS service areas.

Indian Health Service Maternal and Child Health (MCH) Program

The MCH Program provides specific health-care services to children, youth, and families (Bergeisen, 1991) to promote health services of such quality and availability to children, youth, and the family that participants will have full opportunity to attain and maintain optimal physical and mental health and to evaluate and improve services.

Indian Health Service Mental-Health Program

In fiscal year 1988 the per capita budget for mental-health services for persons of all ages in IHS areas ranged from $6.00 per person in California to $23.30 per person in the Billings, Montana, and Portland, Oregon, areas. As of April 1989, IHS reported that the 251 staff in the IHS areas were supported by mental-health categorical funds, with 198 providing direct care (U.S. Department of Health and Human Services, Public Health Service, Indian Health Service, 1989a). In actual practice, 80% of the service units have a mental-health presence and 20% do not (U.S. Department of Health and Human Services, Public Health Service, Indian Health Service, 1989a).

Additionally, only seventeen (9%) of the 198 direct-care professionals were trained to work with children or adolescents, while children ages 19 and younger account for approximately 43% of the Indian population (U.S. Department of Health and Human Services, Public Health Service, Indian Health Service, 1989a). The resources to provide mental-health services for adolescents are clearly inadequate.

Indian Health Service Alcoholism/Substance Abuse Program

The Alcoholism/Substance Abuse Program Branch (A/SAPB) of the IHS was established in March 1978. Currently, IHS funds 309 programs on Indian reservations and in urban communities (U.S. Department of Health and Human Services, Public Health Service, Indian Health Service, 1991). The most extensive summary of the status of IHS alcoholism programs can be found in Peake-Raymond and Raymond's (1984) report. Their identification and assessment of model programs led to the conclusion that virtually no alcoholism services were designed for Indian adolescents, and little coordination or continuity of care existed among alcoholism, social service, and mental-health programs.

The development of a youth-services component became a priority for the A/SAPB. In fiscal year 1987, IHS developed three elements to its youth-services component: prevention, outpatient treatment, and residential treatment. That same year, 445 Indian youths were treated as outpatients, and 147 were treated in residential facilities. By fiscal year 1988, IHS began the operation of two twenty-four-bed regional adolescent substance-abuse treatment centers. There are plans to establish residential centers for Indian adolescents in each of the twelve IHS areas (U.S. Department of Health and Human Services, Public Health Service, Indian Health Service, 1988) and purchase care in non-IHS facilities on a contract basis.

HEALTH-CARE UTILIZATION

Indian adolescents living on or near reservations have theoretical access to a complete range of care provided by IHS, yet, when asked, nearly 8% responded that they had no usual source of care (University of Minnesota, 1989a).

When health-care utilization was explored, approximately 54% of adolescents reported having had a physical and a hearing examination within the last two years. Just under half (49.2%) had a dental examination in the last year, and almost two thirds (68.1%) had received an eye examination in the last two years. Low utilization rates by Indian youth may be due to transportation problems to health facilities, inadequate coordination of health visits between the educational and health systems, or a perception on the part of youth that existing services are not responsive to adolescent needs.

Tribal Health Programs

In fiscal year 1985, 174 IHS-funded health programs were partially or wholly administered by Indian nations, an action facilitated by the Indian Self-Determination and Education Assistance Act of 1975. Each program is negotiated individually; thus, the scope of programs and resources varies considerably (U.S. Department of Health and Human Services, Public Health Service, Indian Health Service, 1988), and most are not large enough to have special programs for adolescents.

Urban Indian Health Programs

The majority of health programs for urban Indians were developed in the late 1970s, a consequence of the Indian Health Care Improvement Act of 1976. In 1988 there were thirty-five such programs that encompassed forty metropolitan areas in twenty states (American Indian Health Care Association, 1988). These programs differ from reservation-based health programs in that they emphasize increasing access to existing services funded by other public and private sources rather than provide or pay for services directly. Thus, it is difficult for urban programs to offer age-specific or culturally specific health services.

Bureau of Indian Affairs

The BIA is the federal agency with primary responsibility for working with Indian tribal governments and Alaska Native village communities and is charged with encouraging and supporting tribal efforts to govern their own communities. The BIA deals with Indian tribes as sovereign nations in a government-to-government relationship. The agency collaborates with tribal governments to provide a variety of social services, police protection, and economic development.

One of the agency's principal responsibilities is the provision of educational programs to supplement those provided by public and private schools. Bureau of Indian Affairs educational grants are also available for Indian college students, vocational training, adult education, gifted and talented students programs, and single-parent programs. More education programs have come under tribal control with the passage of two major laws: the Indian Self-Determination and Education Assistance Act and the Education Amendments Act. The implementation of these laws resulted in decision-making powers for Indian school boards, local hiring of teachers and staff, direct funding to the schools, and increased authority for the Indian education programs within the bureau.

In 1988, the BIA reported that 19.2% of all Indian children were enrolled in day and boarding schools funded by the BIA (U.S. Department of the Interior, Bureau of Indian Affairs, 1988). Schools are furnished with curriculum materials and technical assistance to develop and implement programs dealing with alcohol and substance abuse, with special emphasis on identification, assessment, prevention, and crisis intervention through the use of referrals and additional counselors at the schools. Boarding schools in particular depend on BIA personnel to screen for and intervene with students who experience social and emotional problems.

Child protection and family preservation services provided by tribes under the Indian Child Welfare Act have highlighted the unique needs of Indian adolescents who experience abuse and neglect. Unfortunately, mental-health and welfare resources are often missing and the families of adolescents are often given little more than crisis services (U.S. Department of the Interior, Bureau of Indian Affairs, and U.S. Department of Health and Human Services, Public Health Service, Indian Health Service, 1989). The law enforcement and criminal-justice systems, also under the purview of the BIA, also encounter health issues, especially in the detention and diversion of Indian adolescents involved with alcohol and substance abuse.

Socioeconomic and Cultural Influences on Indian Adolescent Health

As has been stated before, there is enormous and wonderful diversity within "Indian Country." Even tribal groups within the same geographical region have a unique set of social, religious, economic, and legal-political relations with other tribes, other races of color, and Euro-American cultures.

Despite the richness of Indian cultures, numerous social, political, and economic forces have eroded the integrity of these peoples. Many tribes share a culture of poverty and lower-class status.

The task of separating beliefs and behaviors arising out of poverty and cultural oppression from those originating in Indian culture is becoming increasingly difficult. For example, some believe that using alcohol to the point of intoxication is the "Indian way" or that any use of tobacco products is sanctioned by Indian culture because tobacco is a sacred and special gift to the Indian people. The acceptable frequency, mode, and circumstances of tobacco use in ritual and prayer are not communicated clearly, leading to the erroneous conclusion that daily use of cigarettes is culturally appropriate. Indian adolescents may be particularly at risk if they, as part of their search for identity, embrace such values and behaviors as part of the Indian culture.

Other beliefs and practices viewed as normative for Indians may need to be examined and modified. For example, piercing of the flesh in the Sun Dance is usually done with a common knife. Before the AIDS epidemic, there was little concern about this practice. However, today's spiritual leaders are facing a possible change of this aspect of the Sun Dance. Another example is associated with visiting and accepting the hospitality of the host(s). A person who is trying to adhere to a restricted diet (e.g., for hypertension or diabetes) can be caught in the dilemma of showing respect to the host(s) by accepting coffee and doughnuts.

STRENGTHS AND UNIQUE CULTURAL ISSUES

Contemporary Indian adolescents are more likely to hear positive and non-stereotyped messages about their Indian heritage than their parents' generation. Social scientists and humanities scholars are more likely to balance the focus on trauma and negative outcomes with a focus on the strengths and resiliency of Indian lifeways and beliefs. Writers also describe the complexity and rich diversity that exists from tribe to tribe or from clan to clan. Nonetheless, many Indian adolescents are likely to have ambivalent feelings about their Indian identity.

At the grass-roots level, Indians have begun to identify culturally congruent values and behavior that enhance life for the individual, the family, and the community. One of the most frequently heralded values is that of interconnectedness and collective interdependence: "The honor of one is the honor of all and the hurt of one is the hurt of all." In many Indian communities, the isolated Indian youth is given the message that each is a valuable part of the community and is encouraged by family, kin, and friends to become integrated into some aspect of the tribal community.

Honoring the central place of spirituality is another overarching value that is believed to promote strength at the individual and collective levels. Many tribal belief systems actively teach youth to respect the Creator and the created, including their own physical and spiritual selves. Various forms of ritual and prayer powerfully affirm the youth's self-esteem and abilities. Healing involves bringing balance and wholeness to all dimensions of the distressed person, that is, the physical, emotional, spiritual, mental, and social.

Indian families are generally larger, more inclusive, and more flexible in structure than non-Indian nuclear families. The extended family unit has a critical role in socializing children so that they learn and practice skills that are useful and meaningful in Indian and non-Indian societies. The insidious way the strengths of the Indian family system have been compromised in the past few generations has become clearer. Many formal and informal leaders of Indian communities are identifying ways to support the family unit. It is clear that many Indian youth desire to receive guidance about beliefs and practices that honor their Indian heritage.

Several tribes are successful in balancing development of economic progress by managing natural and human resources while also maintaining progress in cultural preservation, and this success has contributed to life-enhancing programs within their communities. Other tribes that are not so well off are at a disadvantage in pursuing these same goals, for all tribes face the daunting challenge of working within the federal bureaucracy, which can severely restrict their course of action. Coalitions that unite diverse tribes around common concerns are crucial for Indian and Native communities to benefit by both economic and cultural revitalization.

Implications and Recommendations
for Program Development

Indian and Native youth face major health issues, and a number of innovative programs have been and are being designed to address some of these issues.

SUBSTANCE USE

Without question the use of alcohol, tobacco, and illegal drugs by Indian adolescents is among the most worrisome of problems. For Indian males especially, substance abuse greatly heightens the risk for vehicular and other accidents, violence, and self-inflicted injuries. In the ninth grade, alcohol and illegal drug use rates take a sharp upward turn for Indian males, so prevention and early-intervention strategies, especially for Indian males in the sixth through eighth grades, are essential.

The National Association for Native American Children of Alcoholics (NANACOA), a grass-roots organization founded in 1988, focuses on breaking the unhealthy, multigenerational cycle of alcohol abuse and addiction. This group works with many Indian families and communities to heal emotional and spiritual pain through information dissemination, workshops, and conferences. Attention is given to the resiliencies and strengths of Native American peoples and their cultures. Late in 1992, NANACOA was awarded a contract to develop a national public-health campaign directed at American Indian youth. One of its latest initiatives will more systematically target the children and adolescents of alcoholic parents by providing special programs at the annual conference.

EMOTIONAL DISTRESS

It is also extremely important to develop strategies that acknowledge and strengthen resiliencies in Indian youth to mitigate the negative effects of stress. Family and community factors that strengthen the support of Indian youth also need to be explored, acknowledged, and supported.

Several groups are involved in such efforts. One strong program is the United National Indian Tribal Youth (UNITY), a national nonprofit organization designed to serve the individual and collective needs of American Indian and Alaska Native youth. The mission of UNITY is to foster the spiritual, mental, physical, and social development of Indian and Native youth and to allow Indian youth to have a voice in helping shape the future of all Indian and Native communities.

The activities of UNITY focus on leadership development and the development of effective tribal, village, and community youth councils. Affiliated youth councils interact and work cooperatively to address their concerns. They also have been involved in needs assessments and have provided testimony to Congress on their views of the needs of Indian adolescents. At a UNITY conference in 1987, participants identified their most pressing needs as alcohol, drug, and other substance abuse; suicide; teenage pregnancy; preservation of tribal culture and traditions; communication between themselves and tribal government officials; funding for higher education; motivation and self-esteem; school dropout rates; lack of recreational facilities; and unemployment.

The Earth Ambassadors and the Spirit of the Rainbow Development Program were established recently by the University of Lethbridge, Alberta, to identify key principles and strategies needed to implement effective youth programs in Indian communities. These programs recommended a long-term process whereby a core group of adults from the community commit to ongoing aid, suppport, and counseling of Indian youth by youth leaders.

ACCESS TO AND UTILIZATION OF HEALTH SERVICES

Health-care services specific to Indian adolescents are almost nonexistent nationally, and even where they do exist, utilization rates are far lower than those of mainstream teenage populations.

The network of teen centers developed by the University of New Mexico Department of Pediatrics is the flagship program focused on adolescent health within the IHS. It is modeled after school-based health centers with the following guidelines:

• the program must be accessible;
• services must be free of charge to adolescents, comprehensive, and provided by a multidisciplinary staff based on the perceived needs of both adult and teenage members of the community;
• adolescents should be involved in the planning and implementation of the program;
• the community should take part in appropriate aspects of the program both to support program efforts and to become part of the "change" in the community;
• the efforts need to be a partnership between the community, health professionals, and the funding source(s).

Activities of the New Mexico Indian teen centers include physical examinations, pregnancy testing, family planning, mental-health counseling, alcohol abuse evaluation, counseling and education, suicide prevention programs, health education and promotion, strategies aimed at reducing school absenteeism and truancy, and sponsorship of traditional and innovative activities related to health promotion and disease prevention.

The programs highlighted in this section all attempt to consider the unique situations and cultural values of American Indians and Alaska Natives in their design. It is heartening to see such attention being paid to these important aspects of Indian and Native lives. More of such programming, as well as more research on and sensitivity to the specific needs of these communities, is needed to improve their physical and mental health.

References

Ackerson, L. M., Dick, R. W., Manson, S. M., & Baron, A. E. (1990). Properties of the inventory to diagnose depression in American Indian adolescents. *Journal of the American Academy of Child and Adolescent Psychiatry, 29,* 601–607.

American Alliance for Health, Physical Education, Recreation and Dance, American School Health Association, Association for the Advancement of Health Education, and Society for Public Health Education. (1988). *National Adolescent Student Health Survey.* Unpublished preliminary results, 9 August.

American Indian Health Care Association. (1988). *Mental health services delivery: Urban Indian health programs.* Unpublished report. St. Paul MN.

American Psychiatric Association. (1987). *Diagnostic and statistical manual of mental disorders* (3rd ed.). Washington DC: Author.

Beauvais, F., Oetting, E. R., Wolf, W., & Edwards, R. (1989). American Indian youth and drugs, 1976–87: A continuing problem. *American Journal of Public Health, 79,* 634–636.

Bechtold, D. W. (1988). Cluster suicide in American Indian adolescents. *American Indian and Alaska Native Mental Health Research, 1* (3), 26–35.

Bechtold, D. W., Manson, S. M., & Shore, J. H. (1994.). *Psychological Consequences of Stress Among Native American Adolescents.* In R. Lieberman and J. Waeger (Eds.), *Stress and Psychiatry* (pp.101–116). New York: Plenum.

Beiser, M., & Attneave, C. L. (1982). Mental disorders among Native American children: Rate and risk periods for entering treatment. *American Journal of Psychiatry, 139,* 193–198.

Bennet, F. C., Ruuska, S. H., & Sherman, R. (1980). Middle ear function in learning–disabled children. *Pediatrics, 66,* 253–260.

Bergeisen, L. (1991). *Maternal and child health program of the Indian Health Service.* Unpublished manuscript.

Blum, R. W., Harmon, B., Harris, L., Bergeisen, L., & Resnick, M. (1992). American Indian–Alaska Native youth health. *Journal of the American Medical Association, 267,* 1637–1644.

Brown, E. F. (1973). A comparative study of Alaskan Native adolescent and young adult secondary school dropouts. In B. E. Oviatt (Ed.), *A perspective of the Alaskan Native School Dropout.* Salt Lake City: Social Service Resource Center of Utah. (ERIC Document Reproduction Service No. ED116876).

Bureau of the Census (1992). *1990 census of population: General population characteristics* (1990 CP-1-1). Washington DC: U.S. Government Printing Office.

Centers for Disease Control. (1988). *Advance report of final natality statistics for 1986. National Center for Health Statistics Monthly and Vital Statistics Report, 37* (Suppl.) (3).

Cockerham, W. C., Forslund, M. A., & Raboin, R. M. (1976). Drug use among white and American Indian high school youth. *International Journal of the Addictions, 11* (2), 209–220.

Corwin, S. (1978). *URRD needs assessment report, no.78-4.* Seattle: Seattle Public School Department of Management Information Services. (ERIC Document Reproduction Service No. ED209382).

Development Associates. (1983). *Final report: The evaluation of the impact of the Part A Entitlement Program funded under Title IV of the Indian Education Act.* Arlington VA: Author.

DiSarno, N. J., & Barringer, C. (1987). Otitis media and academic achievement in Eskimo high school students. *Folia Phoniatrics, 39,* 250–255.

Dise-Lewis, J. E. (1988). The life events and coping inventory: An assessment of stress in children. *Psychosomatic Medicine, 50,* 484–499.

Dougherty, D. (1989). Office of Technology Assessment, U.S. Congress. *Indian health,* testimony before the Special Committee on Investigations, Select Committee on Indian Affairs, Senate, U.S. Congress.

Fischler, R. (1985). Child abuse and neglect in American Indian communities. *Child Abuse and Neglect, 9,* 95–106.

Forslund, M. A., & Cranston, V. A. (1975). A self-report comparison of Indian and Anglo delinquency in Wyoming. *Criminology, 13,* 193–197.

Forslund, M. A., & Myers, R. E. (1974). Delinquency among Wind River Indian reservation youth. *Criminology, 12,* 97–106.

Hanks, G. A. (1973). Dependency among Alaska native school dropouts. In B. E. Oviatt (Ed.), *A perspective of the Alaskan Native school dropout.* Salt Lake City UT: Social Service Resource Center of Utah. (ERIC Document Reproduction Service No. ED116876).

Helfer, R., & Kempe, C. (1987). *The battered child* (4th ed.). Chicago: University of Chicago Press.

Horton, J. M., & Annalora, D. J. (1974). Student dropout study of Fort Wingate, New Mexico, high school. *BIA Education Research Bulletin 3* (2). (ERIC Reproduction Service No. ED096-084).

Howie, V. M., Ploussard, J. H., & Stoyer, J. (1975). The "otitis-prone" condition. *American Journal of Diseases of Children, 129,* 676–678.

Indian Center. University of Nebraska–Lincoln, Department of Sociology, Bureau of Sociological Research. (1986). *The native American adolescent health project: Report on interview surveys of runaways, parents, community leaders, and Human Service workers.* Unpublished report, Lincoln NE.

Jensen, G. F., Straus, J. H., & Harris, V. W. (1977). Crime, delinquency, and the American Indian. *Human Organization, 36,* 252–257.

Manson, S. M., Ackerson, L. M., Dick, R. W., Baron, A. E., & Fleming, C. M. (1990). Depressive symptoms among American Indian adolescents: Psychometric characteristics of the CES-D. *Journal of Consulting and Clinical Psychology, 2,* 231–237.

May, P. A. (1983). *A survey of the existing data on mental health in the Albuquerque area* (Contract No. 3-200423). Albuquerque NM: Office of Mental Health Programs, Indian Health Service.

May, P. A., Hymbaugh, K. J., Aase, J. M., & Sarnet, J. M. (1983). Epidemiology of fetal alcohol syndrome among American Indians of the Southwest. *Social Biology, 30*, 374–387.

National Center for American Indian and Alaska Native Mental Health Research. (1989a). *Indian boarding school project.* Unpublished preliminary data.

National Center for American Indian and Alaska Native Mental Health Research. (1989b). *College student life transitions.* Unpublished preliminary data.

Native American Rehabilitation and Training Center. (1979). Unpublished program report. Tucson: University of Arizona.

O'Connell, J. C. (Ed.) (1987). *A study of the special problems and needs of American Indians with handicaps both on and off the reservation.* Report prepared for the Office of Special Education and Rehabilitative Services, U.S. Department of Education, Washington DC.

Paradise, J. L. (1980). Otitis media in infants and children. *Pediatrics, 65*, 917–943.

Peake-Raymond, M. P., & Raymond, E. V. (1984). *Identification and assessment of model Indian Health Service alcoholism projects.* Unpublished report submitted to the U.S. Department of Health and Human Services, Public Health Service, Health Resources and Services Administration, Indian Health Service, Rockville MD.

Piasecki, J. M., Manson, S. M., Biernoff, M. P., Hiat, A. B., Taylor, S. S., & Bechtold, D. W. (1989). Abuse and neglect of American Indian children: Findings from a survey of federal providers. *American Indian and Alaska Native Mental Health Research, 3* (2), 43–62.

Squires, B. D. (1978). *Bridging the gap: A reassessment. Mimeo report.* St. Paul: Minnesota State Advisory Committee to the U.S. Commission on Civil Rights.

Stewart, J. L. (1975). The Indian Health Service hearing program: An overview. *Hearing Instruments, 26* (1), 22–23, 26.

Szasz, M. (1974). *Education and the American Indian.* Albuquerque: University of New Mexico Press.

U.S. Congress. Office of Technology Assessment. (1986a). *Indian adolescent mental health* (OTA-H-446). Washington DC: U.S. Government Printing Office.

U.S. Congress. Office of Technology Assessment. (1986b). *Indian health care* (OTA-H-290). Springfield VA: National Technical Information Service.

U.S. Congress. Office of Technology Assessment. (1986c). *Children's mental health:*

Problems and services (OTA-BP-H-33). Washington DC: U.S. Government Printing Office.

U.S. Congress. Office of Technology Assessment. (1987). *Special report: Clinical staffing in the Indian Health Services*. Washington DC: U.S. Government Printing Office.

U.S. Congress. Office of Technology Assessment. (1989). Unpublished mortality data from U.S. Department of Health and Human Services, Public Health Service, Indian Health Service.

U.S. Congress. Senate. Select Committee on Indian Affairs. Special Committee on Investigations. (1989). *Final report and legislative recommendations* (Report 101-216). Washington DC: U.S. Government Printing Office.

U.S. Department of Health and Human Services. Public Health Service. Indian Health Service. (1988). *Public Law 99-570 report*. Rockville MD: Author.

U.S. Department of Health and Human Services. Public Health Service. Indian Health Service. (1989a). *A national plan for Native American mental health services* (10th draft). Unpublished report.

U.S. Department of Health and Human Services. Public Health Service. Indian Health Service. (1989b). [IHS hospital discharge data]. Unpublished data.

U.S. Department of Health and Human Services. Public Health Service. Indian Health Service. (1991). *Trends in Indian health—1991*. Rockville MD: Author.

U.S. Department of the Interior. Bureau of Indian Affairs. (1988). *Report on BIA education: Excellence in Indian education through effective school process*. Washington DC: U.S. Government Printing Office.

U.S. Department of the Interior, Bureau of Indian Affairs, & U.S. Department of Health and Human Services, Public Health Service, Indian Health Service, National Oversight Committee on Child Protection. (1989, April). *Forum on child protection in Indian country: A report*. Unpublished report.

University of Minnesota. Adolescent Health Program. (1987). [Minnesota adolescent health survey]. Unpublished data.

University of Minnesota. Adolescent Health Program. (1989a). *The state of adolescent health in Minnesota*. Unpublished report.

Wax, M. L., & Wax, R. H. (1974). *Dropout of American Indians at the secondary level*. Paper presented at the University of Wisconsin-Milwaukee. (ERIC Document Reproduction Service No. ED018289).

Weibel, O. J. (1984). Substance abuse among American Indian youth: A continuing crisis. *Journal of Drug Issues, 14*, 313–335.

Wichlacz, C. R., & Wechsler, J. G. (1983). American Indian law on child abuse and neglect. *Child Abuse and Neglect, 7,* 347–350.

Young, W. R. (1981). *New Mexico dropout study.* Santa Fe: New Mexico State Department of Education. (ERIC Document Reproduction Service No. ED207776).

Zinkus, P. W., & Gottleib, M. I. (1980). Patterns of perceptional and academic deficits related to early chronic otitis media. *Pediatrics, 66,* 246–253.

5

Health Issues of
Asian Pacific American Adolescents

Nolan Zane and Stanley Sue

Asian Pacific American (APA) groups are the fastest-growing ethnic-minority populations in the United States, but little is known about the health status and service needs of the youth (i.e., those ages 10 to 18). This chapter examines the health status and needs of different APA groups; cultural influences on risk and protective factors for health; cultural factors that affect utilization and effectiveness of health and related services; and program and policy changes that may better meet the needs of APA youth and their families.

Population Characteristics of APAs

In 1980, APA population exceeded 3.7 million, easily doubling the 1.5 million figure in 1970 (U.S. Bureau of the Census, 1989). Similarly, from 1980 to 1990 the population almost doubled to 7.3 million, counting for 2.9% of the U.S. population (*Asian Week*, 1991). These increases can be attributed largely to immigration and, secondarily, to births. More than 50 APA groups have been identified by the U.S. Bureau of the Census, with the largest groups being Chinese, Filipino, and Japanese. Table 5.1 shows the 1990 distributions of the largest APA groups.

The diverse nature of APAs is also revealed by the proportion of the population born in other countries. The vast majority of Vietnamese, Koreans, Asian Indians, Filipinos, and Chinese in the United States were born overseas. However, Samoans, Japanese, Guamanians, and Hawaiians were largely born in the United States (U.S. Bureau of the Census, 1989). About 70% of APAs live in just five states—namely, California, Hawaii, New York, Illinois, and Texas.

Asian Pacific Americans tend to be young, although their age range

Table 5.1 Distribution of Asians in the United States, 1990

Group	Number	Percentage
Chinese	1,645,472	22.6
Filipino	1,406,770	19.3
Japanese	847,562	11.7
Asian Indian	815,447	11.2
Korean	798,849	11.0
Vietnamese	614,547	8.4
Hawaiian	211,014	2.9
Lao	149,014	2.0
Cambodian	147,411	2.0
Thai	91,275	1.3
Hmong	90,082	1.2
Samoan	62,964	0.9
Guamanian	49,345	0.7
Tongan	17,606	0.2
Total APA population	7,273,662	95.4

Source: U.S. Census, 1990.

varies among the different groups. A slightly higher proportion of APAs, 30.2%, are under the age of 18, compared with 28.2% for the entire nation. The percentage of APAs under age 18 living with their parents exceeds that of the national average, 85% to 77%, respectively.

The bimodal demographic characteristics revealed by the U.S. Bureau of the Census (1989) are important to note. Substantial differences exist on characteristics, such as percentage of high school graduates ages 25 years and older (75% to 66%) and college graduates (33% to 16%), but a greater percentage of APAs (5.3% to 2.4%) have fewer than six years of schooling. Median family income is $22,700 (compared with $19,900), although poverty levels were similar (13% to 12%). The dropout rates for Filipinos are substantially higher than those for other Asian groups and White Americans. Thus, the extent of specific health risk factors such as dropout rate may also be quite different depending on the Asian group studied.

Several implications can be drawn from these statistics. First, APAs differ from the general population in many demographic characteristics. Findings concerning health needs and services based on the general U.S. population may not be generally applicable to this population. Second, APAs constitute an extremely diverse population. For example, some groups, such as Japanese Americans, are likely to be highly acculturated relative to recent arrivals to the United States, such as the Vietnamese, over 90%

143

of whom were foreign born. Third, most groups exhibit a great deal of within-group variability. For example, the majority of Chinese are foreign born, but a substantial proportion of them (37%) are American born. Moreover, foreign-born Chinese come from different parts of the world (e.g., mainland China, Taiwan, Hong Kong) and speak different dialects of Chinese.

Any discussion of the cultural tendencies among APAs must consider important individual differences that exist within this population (e.g., acculturation level, education level). Cultural factors should be interpreted as a set of contextual variables for understanding the health behaviors and practices of APAs, rather than as stereotypic statements about how APAs live and function.

Scope of Analysis

Previous investigators have pointed to several problems in examining the health issues of the APA population (Kitano & Daniels, 1988; Leong, 1986; Sue & Morishima, 1982). First, relatively few empirical investigations in this area have been devoted to APAs. For example, in an analysis of grants and contracts funded by the National Institute of Drug Abuse, the Alcohol, Drug Abuse, and Mental Health Administration found that not a single award had been made to study substance abuse among APAs over a ten-year period (Alcohol, Drug, and Mental Health Administration, 1984). An examination of annual reports on health and vital statistics published by the U.S. Department of Health and Human Services and the National Center for Health Statistics reveals little information on APAs, except in a few special reports. If ethnic or racial statistics are presented, they typically include White, Black, and "other" Americans. Second, many of the studies that have been conducted lack adequate sample sizes or focus on unrepresentative samples. Third, most investigations have included different groups within the rubric of "Asian Pacific Americans" so that differences among the groups are masked, or researchers may study one particular group and be unable to draw conclusions concerning other APA groups. Fourth, the great growth rate of the APA population is largely the result of immigration. Few studies have been conducted to determine the needs of newly arrived groups such as the Southeast Asian refugees. Even fewer investigations have been conducted on APA adolescents. One must rely on inferences drawn from the available evidence, which may be quite indirect because the data constitute primarily adult samples.

Health Status and Health Needs

Little in the way of empirical research can be found on the incidence and prevalence of the health problems of various APA groups; data on adolescents are virtually nonexistent. The extent of morbidity and mortality for adolescents can only be inferred from data on adults. Available statistics on mortality rates for 1980 reveal some interesting findings (see Yu, 1987). The age-adjusted mortality rates per 1,000 population in the United States is 3.5 for Chinese, 2.9 for Japanese, 5.6 for Whites, 5.8 for American Indians and Alaska Natives, and 8.3 for Blacks. Thus, two APA groups show relatively low mortality rates. Death rates are high for ages 0–5 years and drop to a minimum for ages 5–14; after age 14, the rates increase with age for the entire population. In every age group, the largest APA groups have lower rates than those for Whites.

Yu (1987) also examined the leading causes of death. Heart disease, cancer, cerebrovascular disease, and accidents were the first four leading causes for Chinese, Japanese, Filipinos, and Whites. The fifth cause of death was pneumonia and influenza (Chinese, Japanese, and Filipinos) and chronic obstructive pulmonary disease (Whites). While previous studies of the general population reveal that social class and mortality are negatively related, no analysis of this relation has been performed for APAs. Yu did find that the mortality rate for foreign-born APAs was much higher than for native-born APAs in all age ranges. It is not clear why nativity is related to mortality, although factors such as the premigration health of immigrants or differences between foreign- and native-born APAs in socioeconomic levels, stressful life experiences, adjustment, available resources, cultural practices, and diets are likely to be involved.

For the past three decades, APAs have suffered from a pervasive stereotype concerning their extraordinary physical and mental health and social adjustment. Statistics on low divorce, crime, and juvenile delinquency rates coupled with high educational attainments and family incomes have obscured the within-group differences among Asians and their health problems. Some of the statistics are clearly misleading (Sue & Morishima, 1982). For example, many medical practitioners are often unaware of the health-risk status of Southeast Asian refugees. Compared with the general population, refugees are at higher risk for developing tuberculosis (14–70 times) and have a greater proportion of chronic carriers of hepatitis B, a major risk factor for primary hepatoma and cirrhosis (Lin-Fu, 1988; Ng,

1989). This population also has a higher prevalence of certain disorders seldom seen in the United States, including alpha and beta thalassemia, hemoglobin E disorders, nocturnal sudden death syndrome, cholera, malaria, and leprosy (Hoang & Erickson, 1985). Refugee infants and children are known to have a high incidence and prevalence of baby-bottle tooth decay and dental caries.

Mental-health problems of APAs have also been underestimated, as APAs tend to underutilize Western mental-health services. Once in treatment, they show high levels of disturbance and terminate therapy prematurely (Brown et al., 1973; Kitano, 1969; Los Angeles County Department of Mental Health, 1984; Shu, 1976; Sue & McKinney, 1975; Sue & Sue, 1971, 1974). The few available surveys reveal that APAs have high mental-health needs (Gong-Guy, 1987; Kim, 1978; Peralta & Horikawa, 1978; Prizzia & Villanueva-King, 1977). Moreover, studies of college students have also suggested that many experience major adjustment problems (Leong, 1986; Sata, 1983). Certain groups such as Southeast Asian refugees and immigrants have extremely high levels of depression and other disorders (Liu & Cheung, 1985; Owan, 1985).

Health Needs of Specific Asian Groups

One major study (Zane et al., 1987) on the health needs of various APA groups was conducted in Los Angeles. The investigation used key informant interviews and community forums with leaders and service agency personnel from the Cambodian, Chinese, Japanese, Korean, Lao, Filipino, Thai, Tongan, and Vietnamese communities. This research provided some insights into important Asian group similarities and differences with respect to their health-care needs and service-delivery issues. For instance, there was a great need for mental-health services among the Southeast Asian populations. A recent study on the Southeast Asians in California found that Cambodians, Lao, and Vietnamese were 3½, 3½, and 2 times, respectively, more likely than the general population to need inpatient or outpatient mental-health care (Gong-Guy, 1987). Many Southeast Asians had suffered great physical and psychological trauma experienced during their migration that placed them at greater risk for developing physical and mental-health problems. A significant number of Vietnamese (16.5%) and Lao (13.4%) had suffered the death of a close family member, whereas close to two thirds of the Cambodians had experienced this type of loss. However, there were important differences among the Southeast Asian groups with respect to other human-service needs. Cambodians were concerned about overcrowded and poor sanitary living conditions that fostered illness and disease, whereas the Vietnamese placed great priority on the need for low-cost health-care clinics and health education programs.

Most Asian groups considered low-cost health services staffed by bilingual, bicultural care providers to be a high priority health need, but these services were emphasized by the Chinese, Koreans, Thai, Tongans, and Vietnamese. Concerning specific services for youth, the Japanese, Filipino, Korean, and Thai communities tended to emphasize the need for substance-abuse interventions and family-focused mental-health programs addressing intergenerational and identity issues. Even within this domain, important intergroup differences were found. For example, the Korean community members indicated that family counseling services would be especially beneficial for one youth subgroup, adopted Korean children. It is no surprise that the Zane et al. (1987) findings indicate that, while there may be some overlap in the health needs among different Asian American groups, there also exists important inter-Asian differences that must be considered in delivering appropriate health care to these communities.

Risk Factors

DIETARY HABITS

Particularly for immigrants and refugees, dietary habits are significantly affected by social and economic factors. For example, Fishman, Evans, and Jenks (1988) noted that the average immigrant household typically lacks the presence of extended family members. Thus, dietary decisions are often made by young Asian parents with relatively little knowledge of nutritional value and no elder guidance to maintain traditional diets. Mainstream nutritional educational campaigns have minimal effect because most of these prevention efforts are conducted in English by nonbilingual health educators using nontraditional foods as models.

Studies of the dietary patterns among APA groups have found diets that are very high in sodium (Caplan, Whitmore, & Dui, 1984; Chew, 1983). Popular foods include bean sauces, dried shrimp and salted fish, pickled vegetables, and monosodium glutamate (Chew, 1983). Sodium restriction, of obvious importance in moderating hypertension risk, may be difficult to accomplish within the framework of traditional Asian food practices (Asian/Pacific Task Force on High Blood Pressure Education and Control, 1984; Chew, 1983).

Dairy products are also used to a much lesser extent among Asian and Pacific Islander groups than among the general U.S. population (Suitor & Crowley, 1984). Asian families often live in communities where the traditional sources of dietary calcium in Asian diets (tofu, green leafy vegetables, fish) are not available or are supplanted by conveniently or economically available foods that are low in calcium, which compounds the problem (Kim, Kohrs, & Twork, 1984). Given the need for dietary calcium in the formative years, this pattern points to high risk for immigrant and refugee youth. Nutrition information on the content of foods commonly used in the United States is important because immigrant adolescents are typically the most likely to adopt a Western diet.

Some data suggest a greater prevalence of linear growth stunting among APA children in comparison with either national standards or to the prevalence of growth stunting among White children (Centers for Disease Control, 1983). These comparisons were made from a population of low-income children who had received publicly funded services. For APA children less than 2 years old, the prevalence of low height for age was 17%–20% in 1979–1981, compared with the expected 5% prevalence of growth stunting for the national sample and the 9% prevalence among White children for the five-year period 1977–1981. For APA children 2–5 years old, even greater differences in growth stunting rates were found—33%–37% during 1978–1981 compared with the expected 5% normative prevalence and 9% prevalence for White children. No discernible patterns of risk were evident, however, based on the hemoglobin or hematocrit data. On the other hand, one study that controlled for the height and weight of the parents noted no stunting in the Asian children (Yip, Stanlon, & Trowbridge, 1992).

Griego (1989) found that Asian and Latino children have health problems similar to those previously found among White and Black children. Many were overweight and had low cardiovascular endurance and high cholesterol levels. In this Los Angeles sample, 38% of the Asian and Latino children had above-normal cholesterol levels for children, and 13% had cholesterol levels above normal for adults. By current health standards, 40% of the boys and 45% of the girls were moderately to severely obese. Investigators predicted that these poor health trends will continue until better health education and physical education programs are developed for children and parents.

SMOKING

Most studies have found that the smoking prevalence for APA males is similar to or greater than the rate of the general male population, but APA females tend to have lower rates than those found in the general female population. For example, a National Health Interview Survey of the Vietnamese population in California found that 35% of the males and 1% of the females were current smokers, compared with the general U.S. population rates of 22% and 19%, respectively (Centers for Disease Control, 1992). No prevalence studies have examined smoking among APA youth. However, for the most part, smoking patterns follow patterns observed in the Asian country of origin (Frerichs, Chapman, & Maes, 1984), and studies in East Asia have consistently found that Asian men begin smoking at an early age.

One study examined smoking among Chinese adolescents in Beijing and found that, by the early age of 10–11, 8.2% of the boys were smoking (Ye & Lin, 1982). This rate increased to 34% by the ages of 18–19. Given this trend, smoking may become an increasing health problem for recent immigrant youth. For example, Yee and Thu (1987) found that 45% of the Vietnamese in their sample reported trouble with drinking alcohol and/or smoking tobacco, although other drugs were not seen as problematic. Moreover, a significant number of those respondents viewed alcohol and smoking as acceptable ways to cope with stressful situations and to alleviate problems associated with stress.

STRESS

The unique needs of recently arrived Asians, who have been uprooted from their home culture and perhaps endured life in refugee camps with little or no preparation for the lifestyle facing them, have often been overlooked (Sue and Morishima, 1982). Numerous physical and mental-health problems have been linked to trauma from the migration and the resettlement camp experiences. Adolescent refugees often suffer from a delayed onset of chronic posttraumatic stress disorder syndrome and depressive disorders. Frequently, these problems are first manifested in the form of physical and medical complaints (Kinzie; 1985).

ALCOHOL AND SUBSTANCE USE AND ABUSE

In their review of the substance use research on Asian populations, Zane and Sasao (1992) concluded the following: alcohol use has apparently been underestimated, particularly for certain Asian groups such as Japanese and Filipino males; some evidence suggests that the use of barbiturates may be a major substance-abuse problem for older Asian groups; cultural factors appear to play an important role in either limiting or enhancing substance use among certain Asian groups; and past research has not indicated which Asian groups are being studied. More important, Zane and Sasao note that the Asian groups that appear at greatest risk for developing substance-abuse problems have seldom been studied. Present estimates are likely to grossly underrepresent actual substance use and abuse among APAs because many of the groups with the highest social risk factors (i.e., Southeast Asian refugees, Koreans, and Filipinos) are also the fastest-growing groups in the Asian population. Whereas Japanese and Chinese Americans constituted the largest groups in 1970, by the year 2000, the Filipinos will be largest group, followed by the Chinese, Vietnamese, Korean, Indian, and Japanese. These population shifts will undoubtedly be associated with significant changes in patterns of substance use and abuse.

Protective Factors

FAMILY SUPPORT

The most recently arrived Asian immigrants and their families must adapt to the effects of urbanization, role changes in the family, cultural conflicts, and acculturation pressures (Hoang & Erickson, 1985). Strong kinship and family ties are not only culturally consonant; they also provide the economic and social support needed for adjustment to a new culture. Males tend to serve as the heads of the household within family contexts in which age, experience, and seniority are respected and shape the hierarchy of role relationships (Shon & Ja, 1982). Therefore, those physical and mental-health programs that have promoted family decision making have tended to be more successful. Similarly, health education campaigns that have emphasized the network of supportive family relationships appear to have been especially effective for immigrant groups (Zane et al., 1987).

Community networks also have a powerful influence on health information and associated behavior change (Weaver, 1976). Subgroup communities or ethnic enclaves are frequently self-contained (e.g., Chinatowns and Koreatowns) with residents being predominantly immigrants and the elderly (Gould-Martin & Ngin, 1981). These ethnic communities tend to be quite cohesive and provide individuals with familiar, stable, and supportive environments. Residents generally do not travel beyond community boundaries for services and often encounter cultural and language barriers when they do. This support network can work against individuals seeking health services, especially when the person must seek help for a highly stigmatized disorder (e.g., AIDS, mental-health problems).

Cultural Factors Affecting Utilization and Effectiveness of Health Services

A number of factors affect the utilization and the effectiveness of health and related services. These factors involve accessibility (e.g., the ease of use, costs, location), availability, cultural and linguistic appropriateness, knowledge of available services, willingness to use services, the existence of alternative and competing services, and the nature of the health problems.

For APAs only one major study has examined the relationship between the use of services and social and health problems. Kim (1978) conducted a survey of problems and needs of Chinese, Japanese, Filipino, and Korean Americans (foreign and native born) in the Chicago area. Although the study was confined to respondents over the age of 18, the findings showed language and legal assistance services appeared to dominate as the highest-priority need for most Asian communities over such needs as mental-health service, employment service, vocational training, public aid, and bilingual referral service.

This study contributes to our understanding of APA adolescent health needs even though it was conducted with adults, for parents determine the kinds of services that their children use and socialize their children to the cultural attitudes and beliefs concerning health problems.

Most Asian cultures are "face" oriented, which means an individual's public actions and consequent sense of social integrity and status are tied to and directly reflect on one's family and other important kinship groups. Japanese *haji*, Filipino *hiya*, Chinese *mentz*, and Korean *chaemyun* are terms for the processes of loss of face or shame (Kim, 1978). The existence of certain problems in the family—such as juvenile delinquency and acting-out behaviors, mental-health disorders, AIDS, and poverty—is considered shameful and likely to bring loss of face or disgrace on the entire family (Sue & Morishima, 1982). Consequently, many APAs may avoid the juvenile-justice or legal system, mental-health agencies, health services, and welfare agencies.

Asian Pacific Americans are less likely to request outside help for emotional difficulties, turning first to their families for help and to outside agencies or mainstream services as a last resort (Tracey, Leong, & Glidden, 1986). Several consequences of the effects of shame and stigma can be hypothesized and appear to be supported clinically. Those behaviors (e.g., mental-health problems) that are likely to create shame and stigma are the ones that are most likely to be denied and services treating them underutilized. Thus, the need for services is not equivalent to the demand for services, and needs for certain services are likely not reflected in utilization patterns. If services are avoided and used as a last resort, problems may be exacerbated by the delay. Finally, a significant factor affecting service use by APA youth is the fact that a child's behavior is considered a reflection of the family upbringing. Therefore, parents may delay using services for their children if such services are needed for stigmatized problems.

In APA communities, there are great expectations for doing well in America for the sake of the family in the United States and in their native country. The personal networks in immigrant communities are often extensive and information about others flows quickly and widely. The development of physical or mental-health problems that may compromise a person's status can generate significant loss of face, and the need to seek outside help for such problems only exacerbates the shame for the entire family.

CONCEPTIONS OF HEALTH

The cultural orientations of APA populations can affect how health risks and problems are defined and identified, how symptoms are manifested once one becomes ill, the causes attributed to these problems, and the preferred modes of coping and seeking help (Leong, 1986). For example, Kitano (1969) found that Japanese schizophrenics were more likely to be withdrawn and to exhibit fewer acting-out behaviors than White schizophrenics. He attributed the differences in symptom patterns to cultural influences, such as the tendency for many Japanese to react to stress by becoming more stoic and to accept one's suffering (*ga-man*) without showing overt signs of agitation.

Many Asians perceive a unity between the mind and the body, and emotional disturbances may often be expressed in association with somatic symptoms. In a study of depression experienced by Whites, Blacks, and Chinese, Chang (1985) found ethnic differences in the patterns of symptomatology. Cognitive concerns characterized the White group; a mixture of affective and somatic complaints were found among Blacks; and Chinese were the most likely to exhibit somatic complaints. Similarly, Tung (1985) noted that somatic symptoms involving headaches, insomnia, fatigue, loss of memory, and poor appetite are quite common for many Southeast Asians with psychiatric problems. Some researchers (e.g., Kleinman, 1977; Marsella, Kinzie, & Gordon, 1973) have argued that this symptom pattern reflects a more culturally acceptable means of expressing emotional distress, since physical difficulties are less stigmatizing than having emotional or psychiatric problems.

Interpretations of the causes of disorders are also influenced by culture. In traditional Chinese culture, many physical afflictions are attributed to an imbalance of cosmic forces—yin and yang. The healing task restores balance through proper diet, exercise, and proper psychosocial relationships with others. Kinzie (1985) observed that many Southeast Asians believe illness to be caused by physiological factors or supernatural forces (e.g., the consequence of offending a deity or spirit). They may not differentiate between psychological, physiological, and supernatural causes of illness. The U.S. health-care system is predicated on the concept of discreet disease categories; consequently, many APAs may not consider mainstream services as the most credible or useful source of help.

Other Asian values affect health interventions. The desire for personal and familial self-sufficiency is especially strong, and a substantial fear or shame associated with dependency on outside help, particularly from non-family agents, exists (Shon & Ja, 1982). High value is also placed on personal, interpersonal, and environmental harmony. In traditional Asian households, children and youth are socialized to be in control of their feelings, needs, and impulses and not disrupt this harmony. Physical and emotional health are inseparable, as is the relation of the individual to the social and physical environment (Tung, 1980).

This holistic orientation suggests that health prevention concepts stressing balance and the avoidance of excess behaviors may be quite effective in many Asian communities. Highly credible interventions may also involve traditional approaches designed for actual restoration of balance. Since parents are responsible for the care of their adolescent children, they are likely to refer their children to those services that are consistent with their cultural beliefs. Those interventions that emphasize the service (and dependency oriented) nature of the program or incur public "face" loss during the process of providing care may be less effective and underutilized.

Utilization Patterns of Health Care
PHYSICAL-HEALTH SERVICES

In a review of data collected by the National Center for Health Statistics on visits to physicians by APAs, Yu and Cypress (1987) noted that, for both APAs and Whites, more females (60%) than males visited physicians. Interestingly, age differences were also found. Among those APAs who saw physicians, 30% were children under 15 years of age, compared with only 18% for Whites. One might expect to see this result, as the APA population is somewhat younger than that of White Americans. Another possible reason is that APA parents may be more concerned about their children's health than their own. The 45-years-and-over age group of APAs constituted only 29% of those who saw physicians, compared with 41% for Whites. One explanation for this pattern may be the relative younger age of APAs compared to Whites.

Yu and Cypress (1987) also examined the types of providers and services sought. Asian Pacific Americans were more likely than Whites to use pediatricians and less likely to see surgeons or psychiatrists, but more physician visits were made for preventive care than for Whites. Asian Pacific Americans were less likely than Whites to have problems with accidents, poisoning, and violence. Again, most of the findings do not specifically provide insight into the use of physician services by adolescents. They do suggest that APA users of mainstream health services tend to be relatively young and that important cultural differences exist in utilization patterns.

The extent to which alternatives to Western forms of medical treatment are used by different APA groups is unknown. In a study of the use of Western and Chinese medical-care systems among Chinese Americans, demographic variables, as well as identification with being Chinese, predicted the type of health care sought (Hessler et al., 1975). As expected, Chinese medicine was favored by those who were less acculturated to American society.

MENTAL-HEALTH SERVICES

Research on the utilization and treatment outcome of mental-health services reveals that few APAs use mental-health services, APA clients may avoid services until difficulties are severe and tend to be more disturbed than non-APA clients, and a high proportion of APA clients prematurely terminate treatment because they find the services to be ineffective or culturally incongruent (Sue & Morishima, 1982).

Zane and Sue (1991) reviewed the research and identified a number of factors that may contribute to these problems, including cultural differences in values (e.g., Lee, 1980), communication style (Chang, 1985), problem-solving preferences (Murase & Johnson, 1974), treatment expectations (Yuen & Tinsley, 1981), and mental-health beliefs (e.g., Sue et al., 1976). For example, differences between Asian and White cultures in the "language of emotion" (Chang, 1985) may adversely affect the working relationship between the client and the therapist. In Asian cultures, there is a tendency to convey affection through the use of gestures, often involving the exchange of material goods and services for the person's physical well-being. Also, metaphors are frequently used to communicate feelings; somatic terms often can be used to communicate affective states. Somatization tendencies among Asian clients may not reflect a denial of emotions or a lack of psychological sophistication but, instead, result from different display rules for problem expression (Cheung, 1982; Cheung & Lau, 1982; Cheung, Lau, & Waldmann, 1981; Kleinman, 1977; Marsella et al., 1973). In contrast, Western psychotherapy tends to rely on verbal expressiveness, open self-disclosure, and in-depth examination of emotional conflicts on the part of the client to resolve psychological problems. These aspects can conflict with the tendency by Asians to be less verbal and to refrain from the public expression of feelings (Kim, 1973).

BARRIERS TO SERVICE UTILIZATION

There is reason to believe that barriers exist in the delivery of services to APAS. Kim (1978) asked respondents to rate the most important characteristics of different service agencies. The most important were the availability of bilingual staff and the helpfulness of staff. Because of the large proportion of immigrants in this population, many APAs have limited English proficiency, which creates problems in knowing the sources of assistance, the services that are available, and the procedures and practices required to obtain effective and efficient care (Kim, 1978). Furthermore, immigrants are accustomed to services provided in a personal and informal manner. Health-care providers in Asia often function as friends, advisers, and advocates for their clients. The formality and regulations associated with health services in the United States may be contrary to what many Asians expect from a health-care provider.

As mentioned throughout this review, the research on APA adolescents is sparse. It is assumed that the research findings based on adult samples are to some extent pertinent to adolescents. They may have similar experiences with respect to racism and discrimination, cultural conflicts and adjustment, and the support and pressures involved with close social networks. Parents also help to determine adolescents' nutritional intake, health habits, place of residence, social patterns, and type of care sought.

But there are important differences to consider. Asian Pacific American adolescents, particularly if they are second generation, are more acculturated than their parents, are exposed to non-Asian peers in school, will experience different psychological issues such as ethnic self-identity, and are likely to follow higher health standards and practices than those found in Asian countries. Moreover, intergenerational conflicts are often exacerbated by these acculturation differences. Important differences may also be expected to occur between APA youth and their immigrant parents in diet (e.g., consumption of "fast foods") and the use of medical services (e.g., opposing use of folk healing services advocated by parents).

Implications and Recommendations for Adolescent Health Services

TYPES OF SERVICES NEEDED

The highly variant health needs and service issues among the different APA ethnic groups must be integrated into policies and programs. These differences appear to be especially marked between the predominantly recent immigrant (e.g., Korean) or refugee communities (e.g., Cambodian) and the predominantly early immigrant (e.g., Chinese) or American-born (e.g., Japanese) communities.

Affordable health services continue to be a high priority for many APA communities. Research has consistently found that recent immigrants, particularly Southeast Asian refugees, are at high risk for the development of health and mental-health problems (Sutherland et al., 1983; Van Deusen, 1982). Many APA families and individuals would benefit greatly from health education programs that promote disease prevention (e.g., tuberculosis, AIDS) and better nutrition practices. Accessible, community-based health-care clinics staffed by bilingual personnel can promote culturally responsive, appropriate health care to provide systematic health screening services (e.g., blood pressure exams) to reinforce a more preventive orientation toward health care.

With the increasing conflict between APA parents and youth over such issues as interracial marriage, drug use, discipline, truancy, and familial obligations, family counseling services are needed to help families negotiate these intergenerational tensions. Counseling would be especially beneficial for intercultural couples attempting to cope with problems arising from differences in communication style, cultural values, and role relationships. All APA communities would benefit from more mental-health outreach programs to reduce the shame and stigma of using mental-health and other related services (e.g., substance-abuse treatment). Kim (1985) has noted that family intervention can be an effective intervention tool with APAs, provided that the intervention is culturally matched to the clients.

Professionally staffed mental-health programs are needed to handle severe psychological problems and family crises with culturally congruent skills. A significant number of APA patients require careful monitoring of their psychotropic medications. Mounting evidence indicates that therapeutic levels of psychotropic drugs are achieved at significantly lower doses for Asians than for Whites (Lin & Finder, 1983). Toxic side effects may occur for Asians if they are given higher doses, resulting in patients discontinuing medication or being harmed if they do not discontinue using them (Lin, Poland, & Lesser, 1986).

ORGANIZATION OF SERVICES

A number of promising strategies for serving APA communities have been identified with respect to how services are organized, the population focus of such services, the type of prevention and outreach used, the links with other important service systems, the use of support services, and the development of culturally competent service providers. A multipurpose, multiservice center that provides both physical and mental health care has proved to be the most effective and culturally acceptable means of delivering these services to APA communities. Shame and loss are minimized if the center has multiple health and social services. These centers succeed because of convenience (several families can obtain services at one site), congruence with Asian values (the connection between physical and emotional health is treated holistically), and minimization of the stigma attached to seeking mental-health services (Sue & Morishima, 1982).

The recognition of the cohesive family unit as an important resource and support for Asians often generates recommendations to use family-based services and treatment approaches; however, for Asian adolescents at risk, a major problem may involve estranged family relations. The inclusion of family members must be considered carefully; Asian adolescents may be more willing to use health-care services without the involvement of family members.

ETHNIC-SPECIFIC PROGRAMS

Ethnic-specific programs frequently capitalize on culturally acceptable attitudes or practices to engage and treat clients. For example, the South Cove Community Health Center provides health services to low-income Asian immigrants and refugees in Boston, using bilingual and bicultural staff. The content works with natural support systems and establishes strong community interagency links.

The South Cove program also has incorporated several features that appear to be especially culturally responsive to APAs. Physical and mental-health services are provided together with a coordinated, holistic orientation that minimizes shame and stigma, and special efforts are made to gain and maintain family involvement to the point that the family serves as the primary system of support and intervention. These efforts support the Asian cultural values of filial piety and family obligations. Health-care staff often deliver services in community-based settings not primarily concerned with health care (e.g., restaurants, schools) or in the home to engage more effectively the youth's parents and other family members. Interventions are planned and implemented in ways that do not undermine the youth's identity with parents and cultural norms. Physical and mental-health problems are reframed and explained to make them compatible or at least less in conflict with folk medical beliefs and other cultural attitudes. The fact that many Asian families use Western medicine and indigenous healing systems concurrently is acknowledged and accommodated at South Cove. Services also take into consideration the parents' work schedules. Outreach and health care tend to be more proactive and aggressive than those found in mainstream health clinics. For example, health education sessions are often held in restaurants and scheduled around work hours because many fathers work in the restaurant industry.

In San Francisco, the Chinatown Child Development Center (CCDC) has designed mental-health services to be more acceptable to Chinese immigrant families (Chan-Sew, 1980). Traditionally, Chinese culture places a high value on the child's education and, particularly in the United States, education is considered to have great utility for survival and upward mobility. The CCDC programs capitalize on these attitudes by offering mental-health services in the context of educational experiences. The various types of mental-health services ranging from prevention to treatment are presented to Chinese immigrant families as a progression from general to more intensive education.

In addition to the usual outreach efforts, CCDC operates minimal-fee child-care services to initiate contacts with parents. Many parents are motivated to work with the program because of the chronic shortage of appropriate child-care facilities. The program then screens each child for the existence of mental-health problems and associated risks. An on-site mental-health education program enhances the continuity of service by offering parents classes and activities that address not only mental-health concerns, but also basic economic, language, and legal problems faced by immigrant families. Group counseling programs are offered to facilitate the development of support networks among the parents. Interaction between staff and parents is ongoing and more extensive than at most mental-health clinics, resulting in cooperative, trusting relationships between parents and health-care providers. Such relationships appear to have reduced the resistance to subsequent referrals of the children for diagnostic evaluations and outpatient mental-health treatment.

AGGRESSIVE PREVENTION AND OUTREACH PROGRAMS

Aggressive prevention efforts are required especially in the area of mental health because such services are devalued and those who seek help are stigmatized (Kim, 1978). Because physical-health services are more acceptable and familiar to APA clients, they can be used as an outreach tool for the dis-

semination of mental-health information. For example, mental-health education can be presented at health fairs as people are completing blood
pressure and other health screening exams. Videotapes of health education
programs could be made in different Asian languages and shown to various community groups. Public educational messages can focus on specific
health problems or psychological disorders such as depression and demonstrate the effect of these problems on daily functioning (e.g., they impair
performance at work or school). Part of this prevention effort would involve consultation by center staff with other human-service agency personnel for professional education on the mental-health issues and needs of
APAS. More accurate assessments can result in successful mental-health referrals and can address the issues of loss of face and stigma.

Care should be taken to tailor the outreach to specific APA communities
and to accommodate important cultural differences among APA cultures.
For example, outreach efforts by means of the television may be especially
effective in the Chinese community but not in other APA communities.
The use of community terminology is also important. For example, labeling services as psychological or mental health may be counterproductive
because many APAS associate psychological terms with extreme, bizarre,
and "crazy" behavior. Rather, mental-health problems should be defined
in terms of their effects on daily functioning (e.g., problems in working
with others, memory difficulties).

LINKS WITH SCHOOL SYSTEMS

Since school attendance is high for APA youth, integrating or linking services with the school system can greatly enhance the delivery of physical-
health and mental-health services to them. Linkage with schools not only
brings the services to the targeted population, but the efficiency of providing health services with educational ones may be especially appealing to
Asian parents given the great value placed on education in Asian cultures.

SUPPORT SERVICES

Bilingual APA professional staff are often called on to interpret, translate,
and perform case management functions for other service providers (Lee,
1980). As a result, their clinical services are not used efficiently, and they are
at higher risk for burnout as they attempt to satisfy the multiple demands

for their time. It is important that health centers provide an adequate system of support services that includes bilingual personnel for interpretation and full-time case managers so that the bilingual Asian clinical staff can focus on their clinical work.

HUMAN RESOURCE DEVELOPMENT PROGRAMS

There is a constant shortage of bilingual, bicultural APA service providers (Asian American Subpanel to the President's Commission on Mental Health, 1978). Scholarships for training health-care providers, as well as increased funding for careers in service delivery, are needed to recruit individuals for these careers. Human resource programs for the development of bilingual APA professionals should be established to address this personnel shortage. In these programs, community organizers could coordinate and monitor the professional and paraprofessional manpower resources available in the various APA communities. The resource program could also function as an information network that community-based agencies would use to assist them in the development of grants and contracts to initiate, enhance, or expand health services. Service providers working in APA communities are often underpaid, and salary levels should be made competitive enough to attract qualified and talented personnel.

Summary and Research Recommendations

Asian Pacific Americans represent the fastest-growing ethnic minority population in the United States. The population comprises more than fifty distinct groups. There are marked within- and between-group differences in histories, residence experience (involving immigrant, refugee, or American-born origins), cultural practices, acculturation levels, English proficiency, socioeconomic status, health needs, and service utilization patterns—differences that are obscured by popular stereotypes and by the lack of ethnic-specific research on these groups. Even less research has been conducted on APA adolescents.

The available evidence suggests that this population has a number of health needs that have been inadequately addressed by the American health-care system. There also seems to be little question that many APAs have experienced great life stress because of cultural conflicts, English-language limitations, prejudice and discrimination, and trauma experienced in their native countries and during immigration. These experiences may have especially adverse effects on adolescents, who must cope with such stressors during critical developmental periods. Intergenerational conflicts concerning independence versus obedience, achievement orientation, and ethnic identity between adolescents and parents or extended family members constitute additional sources of stress for APA youth.

Despite their needs for physical- and mental-health services, APA youth and their families have frequently avoided using mainstream health services because of both a lack of knowledge about how the U.S. health-care system functions and the unresponsiveness of the health-care system to their language, perceived needs from their worldview, and cultural traditions. Many Asian Pacific cultures are "face" oriented, and APAs may avoid using services for certain problems (e.g., substance abuse, mental health, and HIV/AIDS) associated with social stigma. Some APAs have different conceptions of health from the dominant Western paradigm and seek caregivers who provide services consistent with their conceptions, communication styles, coping styles, and role expectation.

In view of these problems, several recommendations should be considered. More ethnic-specific health research must be conducted, especially for adolescents, to discover the prevalence of health problems, the cultural values and behavioral patterns that affect health practices, and the intervention and prevention programs that could prove to be effective. The significant differences between and within APA groups must also be better understood. Additionally, gender and social-class differences in the incidence of disorders and response to treatment should be more thoroughly researched. In our review of the literature, very few studies considered the effect of either gender or social class on the health status of APAs; the impact of these important variables needs to be more fully explored.

Affordable and accessible health services must be provided, along with aggressive prevention and outreach programs. Such services should have bilingual and bicultural staff who can effectively communicate with different APA clients. The establishment of ethnic-specific multiservice centers involving a variety of physical- and mental-health and social services may improve utilization and the effectiveness of care. Finally, the recruitment and training of bilingual and bicultural personnel would greatly facilitate the delivery of effective health care to APA youth.

References

Administration for Alcohol, Drug, and Mental Health Administration. (1984). *List of publications on American Indians/Alaskan Natives, Asian/Pacific Americans, Blacks, and Hispanics resulting from ADAMHA-supported research on minorities 1972– 1981*. Washington DC: U.S. Government Printing Office.

Asian American Subpanel to the President's Commission on Mental Health. (1978). *Report to the President* (Vol. 3). Washington DC: U.S. Government Printing Office.

Asian/Pacific Task Force on High Blood Pressure Education and Control. (1984). *Social and cultural considerations in the treatment of hypertensives in selected Asian/ Pacific Islander populations*. Oakland CA: Asian Health Services.

Asian Week. (1991). *Asians in America—1990 Census*. San Francisco: Grant.

Brown, T. R., Huang, K., Harris, D. E., & Stein, K. M. (1973). Mental illness and the role of mental health facilities in Chinatown. In S. Sue & N. Wagner (Eds.), *Asian-American: Psychological perspectives* (pp. 212–231). Palo Alto CA: Science & Behavior.

Caplan, N., Whitmore, J. K., & Dui, Q. L. (1984). *Southeast Asian refugee self-sufficiency study*. Unpublished monograph. Washington DC: Office of Refugee Resettlement.

Centers for Disease Control. (1983). *Nutrition surveillance, 1981*. Washington DC: Department of Health and Human Services.

Centers for Disease Control. (1992). Behavior risk factor survey of Vietnamese: California, 1991. *Morbidity and Mortality Weekly Report, 41,* 69–72.

Chang, W. (1985). A cross-cultural study of depressive symptomatology. *Culture, Medicine, & Psychiatry, 9,* 295–317.

Chan-Sew, S. (1980, October). *Chinatown Child Development Center: A service delivery model*. Paper presented at the Conference on a Mental Health Service Delivery'Model for Chinese American Children and Families, San Francisco.

Cheung, F. M. (1982). Psychological symptoms among Chinese in urban Hong Kong. *Social Science & Medicine, 16,* 1339–1344.

Cheung, F. M., & Lau, B. W. K. (1982). Situational variations of help-seeking behavior among Chinese patients. *Comprehensive Psychiatry, 23,* 252–262.

Cheung, F. M., Lau, B. W. K., & Waldmann, E. (1981). Somatization among Chinese depressives in general practice. *International Journal of Psychiatry in Medicine, 19,* 361–374.

Chew, T. (1983). Sodium values of Chinese condiments and their use in sodium-restricted diets. *Journal of the American Dietetic Association, 82,* 397–401.

Fishman, C., Evans, R., & Jenks, E. (1988). Warm bodies, cool milk: Conflicts in the postpartum food choice for Indochinese women in California. *Social Science and Medicine, 26,* 1125–1132.

Frerichs, R. R., Chapman, J. M., & Maes, E. F. (1984). Mortality due to all causes and to cardiovascular diseases among seven race-ethnic populations in Los Angeles County, 1980. *International Journal of Epidemiology, 13,* 291–298.

Gong-Guy, E. (1987). *California Southeast Asian mental health needs assessment.* Oakland CA: Asian Community Mental Health Services.

Gould-Martin, K., & Ngin, K. (1981). Chinese Americans. In A. Harwood (Ed.), *Ethnicity and medical care* (pp.130–171). Cambridge: Harvard University Press.

Griego, T. (1989, October 19). Study finds poor fitness among many Asian and Latino children. *Los Angeles Times,* p.J5.

Hessler, R. M., Nolan, M. F., Ogbru, B., & New, P. K. (1975). Intraethnic diversity: Health care of the Chinese-Americans. *Human Organization, 34,* 253–262.

Hoang, G. N., & Erickson, R. V. (1985). Cultural barriers to effective medical care among Indochinese patients. *Annual Review of Medicine, 36,* 229–239.

Kim, B. L. C. (1973). Asian-Americans: No model minority. *Social Work, 18,* 44–54.

Kim, B. L. C. (1978). *The Asian-Americans: Changing patterns, changing needs.* Montclair NJ: Association of Korean Christian Scholars in North America.

Kim, K. K., Kohrs, M. B., & Twork, R. (1984). Dietary calcium intakes of elderly Korean Americans. *Journal of the American Dietetic Association, 84,* 164–169.

Kim, S. C. (1985). Family therapy for Asian Americans: A strategic-structural framework. *Psychotherapy, 22,* 342–348.

Kinzie, J. D. (1985). Overview of clinical issues in the treatment of Southeast Asian refugees. In T. C. Owan (Ed.), *Southeast Asian mental health: Treatment, prevention, services, training, and research* (pp.113–136). Washington DC: U.S. Government Printing Office.

Kitano, H. H. (1969). *Japanese-Americans: The evolution of a sub-culture.* Englewood Cliffs NJ: Prentice-Hall.

Kitano, H. H., & Daniels, R. (1988). *Asian Americans: Emerging minorities.* Englewood Cliffs NJ: Prentice-Hall.

Kleinman, A. M. (1977). Depression, somatization, and the new cross-cultural psychiatry. *Social Science and Medicine, 11,* 3–10.

Lee, E. (1980). Mental health services for the Asian-Americans: Problems and alternatives. In U.S. Commission of Civil Rights (Ed.), *Civil rights issues of Asian and*

Pacific-Americans: Myths and realities (pp.734–756). Washington DC: U.S. Government Printing Office.

Leong, F. T. L. (1986). Counseling and psychotherapy with Asian-Americans: Review of the literature. *Journal of Counseling Psychology, 33,* 196–206.

Lin, K. M., & Finder, E. J. (1983). Neuroleptic dosage in Asians. *American Journal of Psychiatry, 140,* 490–491.

Lin, K. M., Poland, R. E., & Lesser, I. M. (1986). Ethnicity and psychopharmacology. *Culture, Medicine, and Psychiatry, 10,* 151–165.

Lin-Fu, J. S. (1988). Population characteristics and health care needs of Asian Pacific Americans. *Public Health Reports, 103,* 18–27.

Liu, W. T., & Cheung, F. (1985). Research concerns associated with the study of Southeast Asian refugees. In T. C. Owan (Ed.), *Southeast Asian mental health: Treatment, prevention, services, training, and research* (pp.487–516). Washington DC: U.S. Department of Health and Human Services.

Los Angeles County Department of Mental Health. (1984). *Report on ethnic utilization of mental health services.* Unpublished manuscript.

Marsella, A. J., Kinzie, D., & Gordon, P. (1973). Ethnic variations in the expression of depression. *Journal of Cross-Cultural Psychology, 4,* 435–458.

Murase, T., & Johnson, F. (1974). Naikan, Morita, and Western psychotherapy. *Archives of General Psychiatry, 31,* 121–128.

Ng, J. (1989, September 15). Researcher: 17% of U.S. Asians afflicted by hepatitis B virus. *Asian Week,* p.4.

Owan, T. C. (1985). Southeast Asian mental health: Transition from treatment services to prevention—a new direction. In T. C. Owan (Ed.), *Southeast Asian mental health: Treatment, prevention, service, training, and research* (pp.141–167). Washington DC: U.S. Department of Health and Human Services.

Peralta, V., & Horikawa, H. (1978). *Needs and potentialities assessment of Asian American elderly in greater Philadelphia* (Report No. 3). Chicago: Asian American Mental Health Research Center.

Prizzia, R., & Villanueva-King, O. (1977). *Central Oahu community mental health needs assessment survey. (Part III): A survey of the general population.* Honolulu: Management Planning and Administration Consultants.

Sata, L. S. (1983). Mental health issues of Japanese-American children. In G. J. Powell (Ed.), *The psychosocial development of minority group children* (pp.362–372). New York: Brunner/Mazel.

Shon, S. P., & Ja, D. Y. (1982). Asian families. In M. McGoldrick, J. K. Pearce,

& J. Giordano (Eds.), *Ethnicity and family therapy* (pp. 208–228). New York: Guilford.

Shu, R. (1976). *Utilization of mental health facilities: The case for Asian Americans in California* (Occasional Paper No. 4). Chicago: Asian-American Mental Health Center.

Sue, S., & McKinney, H. (1975). Asian-Americans in the community mental health care system. *American Journal of Orthopsychiatry, 45,* 111–118.

Sue, S., & Morishima, J. K. (1982). *The mental health of Asian-Americans.* San Francisco: Jossey-Bass.

Sue, S., & Sue, D. W. (1971). Chinese-American personality and mental health. *Amerasia Journal, 1,* 36–49.

Sue, S., & Sue, D. W. (1974). MMPI comparisons between Asian- and non-Asian-American students utilizing a university psychiatric clinic. *Journal of Counseling Psychology, 21,* 423–427.

Sue, S., Wagner, N., Ja, D., Margullis, C., & Lew, L. (1976). Conceptions of mental illness among Asian and Caucasian American students. *Psychological Reports, 38,* 703–708.

Suitor, W., & Crowley, M. F. (1984). Promoting sound eating habits in different sociocultural situations. In *Nutrition principles and applications in health programs* (2nd ed., pp. 107–121). Philadelphia: Lippincott.

Sutherland, J. E., Avant, R. F., Franz, W. B., Monzon, C. M., & Stark, N. M. (1983). Indochinese refugee assessment and treatment. *Journal of Family Practice, 16,* 61–67.

Tracey, T. J., Leong, F. T. L., & Glidden, C. (1986). Help seeking and problem perception among Asian Americans. *Journal of Counseling Psychology, 33,* 331–336.

Tung, T. M. (1980). *Indochinese patients: Cultural aspects of medical and psychiatric care for Indochinese refugees.* Washington DC: Action for Southeast Asians.

Tung, T. M. (1985). Psychiatric care for Southeast Asians: How different is different? In T. C. Owan (Ed.), *Southeast Asian mental health: Treatment, prevention, services, training, and research* (pp. 5–40). Washington DC: U.S. Government Printing Office.

U.S. Bureau of the Census. (1989). *We, the Asian and Pacific Islander Americans.* Washington DC: U.S. Government Printing Office.

U.S. Bureau of the Census. (1993). *1990 Census of the Population, Asian and Pacific Islanders in the United States.* Washington DC: U.S. Government Printing Office.

Van Deusen, J. M. (1982). Health/mental health studies of Indochinese refugees: A critical overview. *Medical Anthropology, 6,* 231–252.

Weaver, J. L. (1976). *National health policy and the underserved: Ethnic minorities, women, and the elderly*. St. Louis: Mosby.

Ye, G.-S., & Lin, W.-S. (1982). Cigarette smoking among Beijing high schoolers. *Chinese Medical Journal, 95*, 95–100.

Yee, B. E. K., & Thu, N. D. (1987). Correlates of drug use and abuse among Indochinese refugees: Mental health implications. *Journal of Psychoactive Drugs, 19,* 77–83.

Yip, R., Stanlon, K., & Trowbridge, F. (1992). Improving growth status of Asian refugee children in the United States. *Journal of the American Medical Association, 267*, 937–940.

Yu, E. (1987). The health of Asian Americans. In W. Liu (Ed.), *The Pacific/Asian American Mental Health Research Center: A decade of review* (pp. 51–58). Chicago: Pacific/Asian American Mental Health Research Center.

Yu, E., & Cypress, B. (1987). Visits to physicians by Pacific/Asians. In W. Liu (Ed.), *The Pacific/Asian American Mental Health Research Center: A decade review* (pp. 59–64). Chicago: Pacific/Asian American Mental Health Research Center.

Yuen, R. K. W., & Tinsley, H. E. A. (1981). International and American students' expectations about counseling. *Journal of Counseling Psychology, 28*, 66–69.

Zane, N., Fujino, D., Nakasaki, G., & Yasuda, K. (1987). *Asian Pacific needs assessment study*. Los Angeles: United Way.

Zane, N., & Sasao, T. (1992). Research on drug abuse among Asian Pacific Americans. *Drugs and Society, 3/4*, 181–209.

Zane, N., & Sue, S. (1991). Culturally-responsive mental health services for Asian Americans: Treatment and training issues. In H. Myers, P. Wohlford, P. Guzman, & R. Echemendia (Eds.), *Ethnic minority perspectives on clinical training and services in psychology* (pp. 48–59). Washington DC: American Psychological Association.

6

Health and Related Services for Native Hawaiian Adolescents

Lawrence Miike

There is little specific information on the health services for Native Hawaiian adolescents residing in the state of Hawaii. Most of the available information is on adolescents in general or on Native Hawaiians in general, and much of that is descriptive. Nevertheless, the consistent undercurrent of this analysis is that the health and related problems of Native Hawaiian adolescents—and of Native Hawaiians of all ages—are those too often associated with low-income status, further aggravated by a clash between traditional Native Hawaiian culture and the predominantly Western-oriented society of the state of Hawaii.

Defining the Population

Various terminologies have been used to describe Native Hawaiians. Under federal statutes, "Native Hawaiian" refers to any person of Hawaiian ancestry. In the state of Hawaii, "native hawaiian" (*n* vs. *N*) refers to persons with at least 50% Hawaiian blood quantum for the purpose of determining eligibility for homestead rights on Hawaiian homelands. All other persons of Hawaiian ancestry are collectively known as "Hawaiian." Data from the state Department of Health, on the other hand, collectively refer to all persons of Hawaiian ancestry as "Native Hawaiians" and further break down the Native Hawaiians grouping into "Hawaiians" and "Part-Hawaiians," with "Hawaiians" in this instance referring to persons of 100% Hawaiian blood quantum.

For this analysis, the term "Native Hawaiian" will be used to describe collectively persons of Hawaiian ancestry, with additional categories of

"Hawaiians" and "Part-Hawaiians" in some of the data presentations. When the terms are used in different ways, such differences will be made explicit.

In the 1980 U.S. census, among 136,341 persons living in Hawaii who claimed some degree of Hawaiian ancestry (i.e., had one or more Native Hawaiian ancestors), 118,251 persons identified themselves as best fitting the ethnic category of "Hawaiians" (U.S. Bureau of the Census, 1983).

In contrast, the Health Surveillance Program (HSP) estimated that there were 175,909 Native Hawaiians living in Hawaii in 1980 (Oyama & Johnson, 1986). The HSP estimates are based on a questionnaire in which respondents are asked to identify the race or combination of races of their father or mother. "Hawaiians" are represented by respondents with both parents identified as "Hawaiian" only, and "Part-Hawaiians" are represented by respondents who have at least one parent with Hawaiian blood. The estimated Native Hawaiian population is the sum of respondents in these two groups. If we take the 1980 census and HSP results as rough proxies, then 118,251 of 175,909 Native Hawaiians residing in Hawaii (67%) think of themselves as principally of Native Hawaiian ancestry.

In 1984 a special survey sponsored by the Office of Hawaiian Affairs of the State of Hawaii (1986) was performed on persons identified as Native Hawaiian in the annual HSP. This survey was done to estimate the distribution of persons with different degrees of Hawaiian blood quantum in the overall resident Native Hawaiian population. Some 61.4% of Native Hawaiians were estimated to have less than half Hawaiian blood quantum, and "pure" Hawaiians made up 3.7% of the total.

The 1980 U.S. census also estimated that there were approximately 177,900 Native Hawaiians living in the United States, about 69% of them in Hawaii. Approximately 16% of Native Hawaiians born in Hawaii move elsewhere (U.S. Congress, Office of Technology Assessment, 1987).

Native Hawaiians represent nearly 20% of the population of the state of Hawaii. Clusters of predominantly Native Hawaiian communities are distributed throughout the islands of Hawaii. The establishment of health and related services specifically for Native Hawaiians is a recent policy issue in Hawaii; few quantitative analyses of services to Native Hawaiians are available. Therefore, the data and literature base as might exist for the Black, Hispanic, and Native American populations will not exist when we attempt to focus on a subpopulation of Native Hawaiians, such as adolescents.

Figure 6.1. Comparison of U.S., Hawaiian, and Part-Hawaiian age distribution

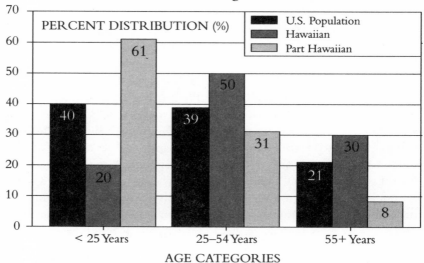

Source: U.S. Congress, Office of Technology Assessment, Health Program, "Current Health Status and Population Projections of Native Hawaiians Living in Hawaii," April 1987.

The Native Hawaiian Population in Hawaii

DEMOGRAPHY

Because of intermarriage with other ethnic groups, the "pure" Hawaiian population now makes up less than 5% of all Native Hawaiians and is significantly older and rapidly diminishing in numbers. The Part-Hawaiian population, on the other hand, is young and rapidly increasing in numbers. In the early 1980s, 40% of the U.S. population was less than age 25, compared to only 20% of Hawaiians but 61% of Part-Hawaiians. At the other end of the age spectrum, 21% of the U.S. population, 30% of Hawaiians, and only 8% of Part-Hawaiians were more than age 55 (see Fig. 6.1). By 1986, there were only an estimated 652 Hawaiians below age 18, compared with 92,930 Part-Hawaiians in this age group. Because of the great number of Part-Hawaiians compared to Hawaiians, the overall characteristics of the Native Hawaiian population will be nearly identical with that of the Part-Hawaiian population.

In 1987, 47% of Native Hawaiian marriages were with other Native Hawaiians. Native Hawaiians comprise the largest ethnic group of newborns. More than 29% of infants born in the state in 1987 were Part-Hawaiian, followed by 23.5% for Whites, 15.6% for Filipinos, and 12.5% for Japanese (State of Hawaii, 1987).

In 1986 Native Hawaiians made up 19.8% of the total state population of 1,032,454, second in numbers only to Whites (24.7%) and Japanese (22.1%) (see Fig. 6.2). Native Hawaiians resided among the various islands of the state in generally similar distributions as all other ethnic groups, although proportionately more Native Hawaiians live in "neighbor islands" (islands other than Oahu, the major population center of the state).

SOCIOECONOMIC INDICATORS

Native Hawaiians are overrepresented in the low-income categories, especially in the lowest-income category, and underrepresented in the higher-income categories compared with all other ethnic groups (State of Hawaii Department of Health, 1987). A higher proportion of Native Hawaiian families receive public assistance than non-Native Hawaiian families (18.4% vs. 8.2%), and a higher proportion of Native Hawaiians than non-Native Hawaiians are below the poverty level (15.4% vs. 9.1%) (Plett & Heath, 1987).

Native Hawaiian households show significant problems associated with the stress of poverty such as more child-abuse and child-neglect cases. Abuse is most often associated with family discord, lack of tolerance, loss of control, and neglect (Plett & Heath, 1987). Native Hawaiians also are disproportionately represented in crime statistices, constituting 35% of all juveniles arrested (State of Hawaii, Criminal Justice Data Center, 1985).

EDUCATION

The Native Hawaiian adolescent population is among the largest ethnic adolescent populations (State of Hawaii, Department of Education, 1989). The proportion of children who are Native Hawaiian increases in the lower grades and in less urbanized areas, indicating that the Native Hawaiian population in Hawaii is young and growing.

Native Hawaiians complete high school at a rate lower than that of all other groups except Samoans. School attendance by Native Hawaiians drops sharply after ages 16–17 (Barringer & O'Hagan, 1989).

A much lower percentage of Native Hawaiian students (20%) receive some college education, compared with nearly 40% of non-Native Hawaiian students in Hawaii (Plett & Heath, 1987). About 10.7% of Native Hawaiians have completed college or some other form of higher education, compared with 19% for Whites, 28.7% for Japanese, and 40.1% for Chinese (Barringer & O'Hagan, 1989). In 1980, only 9.9% of all Native Hawaiian students were in college, compared with 22.5% of all non-Native Hawaiian students (Plett & Heath, 1987).

On the basis of standardized tests, Native Hawaiian students persistently perform below the statewide averages. Additionally, the percent of Native Hawaiian students in the high range is lower than for students statewide, and the percentage of Native Hawaiian students performing in the high range decreases with advancing grade level.

HEALTH
Health Status

Mortality rates for Native Hawaiians are greater for the major causes of mortality, such as heart disease, cancer, cardiovascular disease, and diabetes (U.S. Congress, Office of Technology Assessment, 1987; see Fig. 6.2). Diabetes in particular is a special problem among Native Hawaiians, with age-adjusted prevalence rates twice those of all other ethnic groups combined in the state, and diabetes among Native Hawaiians is almost exclusively adult-onset, Type II (noninsulin dependent) diabetes mellitus (State of Hawaii Department of Health, 1989a).

About two thirds of patients with Type II diabetes are obese when the disease is first diagnosed, and Native Hawaiians have the highest obesity rates among the ethnic groups in Hawaii. Furthermore, the percentage of Hawaiian blood quantum is significantly correlated with an overweight state (U.S. Department of Health and Human Services, 1989).

Hawaii's residents generally engage in fewer high-risk behaviors than the U.S. population as a whole, yet they take the lead compared with other ethnic-minority groups in six high-risk categories: seat-belt nonuse, obesity, smoking, acute drinking, heavier drinking, and drinking and driving (State of Hawaii, 1987).

Native Hawaiians in the 15–24 age group have higher marriage rates than non-Native Hawaiians. Native Hawaiian mothers are three years younger on average, have higher birth rates in the lower-age groups, and have higher percentages of births in the higher birth orders (3+ births) than non-Native Hawaiian mothers (Plett & Heath, 1987). Native Hawaiian

Figure 6.2. Selected behavioral risk factors, morbidity and mortality

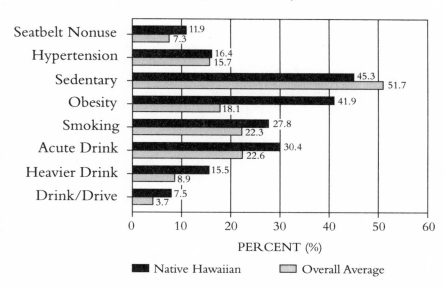

PERCENT (%)

■ Native Hawaiian   □ Overall Average

Source: State of Hawaii Department of Health, Health Promotion and Education Office Telephone Survey, 1987.

women also have the highest rate of illegitimate births in the state. Among Native Hawaiians, 5.9% of total births were to mothers 17 or younger, compared with 2.1% for all other ethnic groups; and 17.5% of total births were to mothers 19 or younger, compared with 7.5% for all other ethnic groups (Plett & Heath, 1987). In 1987, 45% (by the race of the mother) and 55% (by the race of the child) of all illegitimate live births were Native Hawaiian—the highest rate in the state (State of Hawaii, 1987).

In 1987 Native Hawaiians also had the highest infant death rate in the state. Infant deaths among Native Hawaiian mothers ages 15–17 were higher than for other ethnic groups (State of Hawaii, 1987).

Finally, Native Hawaiians have a physical impairment rate slightly higher than the average (155.6/1,000 vs. 152.5/1,000; range of 198.4/1,000 for Whites to 82.0/1,000 for Filipinos). Among impairment categories (vision, hearing, back and spine, upper extremity–shoulder, lower extremity–hip, and other), Native Hawaiians in the 5–17 age group had impairment rates above the rate for all ethnic groups for all impairment categories, with only Whites having higher rates (Oyama & Johnson, 1986).

In the 5–17 age group, hearing impairments are the most prevalent of any single impairment. Native Hawaiians and Whites have hearing impairment rates twice those of other ethnic groups (Woods, Oyama, & Johnson, 1987). Data were available for the ages 5–17 group and not for ages 10–18. Hearing impairments among Native Hawaiian children, most likely from untreated middle ear infections, have been recognized as a major problem and a probable contributor to poor school performance. In a study conducted at a private school limited to children of Native Hawaiian ancestry, preschoolers were screened for hearing dysfunctions. Only 22% of the children passed the hearing screening. Statistically significant differences in fall and spring test performance were found between those who passed the hearing tests and those who failed tests in vocabulary, language usage, general information, and quantitative concepts (Kamehameha Schools/ Bernice Pauahi Bishop Estate, 1983).

These findings have led to a project to produce a significant improvement in the educational achievement of Native Hawaiian preschool children within two years. The program consists of an enhanced hearing and speech screening procedure; a follow-up effort that ensures that every child who fails the screening receives appropriate medical care; the reduction of classroom ambient noise levels; the amplification of instructional communication; the implementation of special classroom teaching techniques and equipment (electronic speech trainers) designed to improve the communication competence of children experiencing moderate speech and hearing difficulties; and an individualized home and school communication therapy program for those children identified as most in need (Kamehameha Schools/Bernice Pauahi Bishop Estate, 1983).

HEALTH INSURANCE

A recent background paper prepared for the congressional Office of Technology Assessment concluded that 4.6 million adolescents, ages 10–18, or 15% overall, lacked public or private health coverage in 1987 (Kronick, 1989). Hawaii's residents, however, are better situated. The state's Prepaid Health Care Act of 1974 mandates employment-based health insurance, under which the employee may enroll in any of the usual range of health-insurance programs. As a result of this legislation, only an estimated 5% (with a range of 3%–7%) of the state's residents remain uninsured (State of Hawaii, 1989a).

The Prepaid Health Care Act extends only to employees who work more than twenty hours per week for any employer. The Hawaii Department of Health has noted that its preliminary school survey indicates that schools in predominantly "blue collar" or "working poor" areas seem to have more uninsured children (State of Hawaii, 1989a).

The proportion of Native Hawaians with annual incomes of less than $10,000 was twice their proportion of the state's population. Thus, Native Hawaiians who are eligible for public-assistance programs would be expected to be enrolled in public-assistance programs in greater proportion than the proportion of the total population that Native Hawaiians represent. While Native Hawaiians are indeed overrepresented in the Aid to Families with Dependent Children, General Assistance, and food-stamps programs, they are underrepresented as recipients of medical assistance (Medicaid) and aged, blind, or disabled assistance, for unknown reasons (Plett & Heath, 1987).

In June 1989 the State Health Insurance Program Act was enacted with the purpose of providing health-insurance coverage to the remaining uninsured state residents. Persons or families with incomes up to 300% of the federal poverty level are eligible to enroll in the State Health Insurance Program (SHIP), with a subscriber's premium dependent on income, family size, and number of members enrolled. Approximately 80% of SHIP costs is subsidized by the state. Preventive, maternity, inpatient and outpatient medical care, and emergency services are covered under this program, with a small copayment required for some services.

As of May 1991, there were nearly 12,000 SHIP enrollees. Whites (28% enrolled) and Native Hawaiians (23% enrolled) were overrepresented, compared with their state population (24% and 20%, respectively). Enrollees were predominantly rural dwellers, with 54% living in rural areas, compared with 14% of the state's residents. Nearly 63% reported family income below the federal poverty level, as compared with less than 10% for the state's population. Also, nearly one half had been without health insurance for at least one year. More than 15% reported never having health insurance, while another 25% had been without coverage for four to twelve months (Kaiser Permanente Center for Health Research, 1991).

Finally, the Native Hawaiian Health Care Act of 1988 was enacted to establish Native Hawaiian health-care systems concentrating on health promotion, disease prevention, and primary-care services. The services and service systems were intended to address health problems of particular severity among Native Hawaiians, to be under the control of Native Hawaiians, and to be provided in a culturally appropriate manner. The services of traditional Native Hawaiian healers may be provided; education in health promotion and disease prevention must be provided by health-care practitioners, community outreach workers, counselors, and cultural educators of Native Hawaiian ancestry whenever possible; interpreters must be provided for clients with limited ability to speak English; and health practitioners of Native Hawaiian ancestry must significantly participate in the planning, management, monitoring, and evaluation of health services at the community level. A statewide Native Hawaiian organization, Papa Ola Lokahi, was created to plan, develop, and establish the Native Hawaiian service systems.

Five islandwide, community-based Native Hawaiian health-service organizations have been recognized or established by Papa Ola Lokahi. Federal appropriations for service delivery became available beginning in the fall of 1991.

CULTURAL FACTORS

Cultural factors affecting Native Hawaiians have been examined in several studies in recent years. Hawaiian tradition involves family practices that include multiple parenting within an 'ohana [an extended family] group, early indulgence followed by a shift at age 2–3 to a primarily peer-directed socialization experience, socialization toward a group- and family-oriented values system, and learning experiences that emphasize modeling and mutual participation rather than verbal interaction (Kamehameha Schools/ Bernice Pauahi Bishop Estate, 1983). These practices are reflected in family size: the average Native Hawaiian household is 40% larger than the average non-Native Hawaiian household, and the average number of persons in Native Hawaiian families is 27% higher. Additionally, about 75% of Native Hawaiian children live in married-couple families, compared with 86% of non-Native Hawaiian children, and 93% of Native Hawaiians live in family households, compared with 86% of non-Native Hawaiian children.

The value placed on the family, while important for social cohesion, may put at risk Hawaiian youth within Western-oriented education systems. A study of Native Hawaiian adolescents (McNassor & Hongo, 1972, p. 281) concluded:

Self-disparagement in a significant number of ethnic Hawaiian youth on the Island of Hawaii is deeply imbedded in personality by age 18. These unpretentious, forthright children of an island people who value independence and freedom, warm, everlasting family ties, and autonomy of emotions are becoming strangers in their own land. In terms of intellectual ability in the performance of the school's academic tasks, they think they are inferior, incapable of success in liberal studies beyond high school. . . . The ethnic Hawaiian child, above all else, develops a particularly vital identification with many members of an extended family, and with everything that grows and lives on the land of his verdant island and on the ocean shelf surrounding it. In the communal life of the family, particularly in rural areas, the joys of today take precedence over planning for a vague, dubious future. . . . Hawaiian youth seem almost instinctively afraid of getting into school books. They hesitate to devour what is inside. This may be partly because books never have been vital to life goals of the family, to be sure, as well as because of reading difficulties in the early grades. But in a more profound way, the resistance to print stems from child-rearing practices emphasizing very early independence (by age 7 and 8 years), self-reliance, and learning from direct experience rather than from symbols.

Similar observations have been made by others:

Interaction between Hawaiian children and their teachers is impaired by cultural socialization practices that deemphasize certain patterns of verbal exchange. For example, direct questions to a child by an adult may be interpreted as displeasure or ridicule, and interactions with adults on a one-on-one basis may be unfamiliar since direct communication is ordinarily with peers rather than adults. Furthermore, while adults at home often do not expect immediate compliance with verbal requests, teachers do; and when adults are punitive or critical, a child's learned preference seems to be withdrawal or avoidance, a response that teachers find disconcerting. Finally Hawaiian youth may be further inhibited in school by the emotional neutrality of teachers, a characteristic that makes them less salient and results in reduced student attentiveness (Kamehameha Schools/Bernice Pauahi Bishop Estate, 1983). Western cultural characteristics of success in many areas (e.g., education, business) are diametrically opposed to Hawaiian cul-

tural or moral values. For example, Hawaiian values stress cooperative effort for mutual gain within a group and scorn individual ambi-
tion, personal accumulation, and competition. Scholastic achievement in most educational settings is impeded when aggressiveness
and individual striving are culturally unacceptable to students. (Kamehameha Schools/Bernice Pauahi Bishop Estate, 1983)

Finally, the authors of a needs assessment review for Hawaii's Child and
Adolescent Service System Program (State of Hawaii, 1989c) observed that
the cultural concept of health in Hawaiian and other Polynesian cultures is
defined and conceptualized differently in each cultural setting. For instance, the Hawaiian language has no word for mental health or illness. Instead, the Hawaiian cultural concepts of mental health are more holistic
than Western concepts and include physical and spiritual states. One of the
Native Hawaiian health organizations made these comments in its statement of philosophy:

The traditional Native Hawaiian society and system of wellness and
healing are based on a holistic view of man, physically and spiritually
connected to family, the spiritual world, and nature. The current
"Western" medical care system is high tech, low touch, scientific, usually delivered in impersonal and bureaucratic settings and premised on
one's ability to pay for services. The Native Hawaiian concept of caring was high touch, highly interpersonal, and often took place where
the individual lived. The services and help of traditional healers were
not dependent on one's having medical care insurance or an ability to
pay. (Kamehemaha Schools/Bernice Pauauhi Bishop Estate, 1989)

Hawaiians tend to use nonprofessional, lay, and informal sources of
mental-health care. In one survey of a predominantly Native Hawaiian
community, two thirds of all respondents had some knowledge of informal nonprofessional sources of care. These sources included *kahunas* (traditional healers, ministers, and friends). In another statewide survey of
Hawaiians reported in this chapter, 78% of all respondents reported participating either frequently or occasionally in *ho'oponopono* (a traditional Hawaiian problem-solving process). Help for personal and psychological
problems was most often sought from ministers and religious organizations (State of Hawaii, 1989c).

The very meaning of what it means to be "Hawaiian" is being trans-
formed by extensive intermarriage with other racial groups (Kamehameha

Schools/Bernice Pauahi Bishop Estate, 1983). There is a lack of consensus over the notion of biculturalism—whether a blend of two or more cultures should be embraced in several ethnic identities, ethnic identity should be exclusively retained, or cultural background should be eradicated completely in the interest of assimilation into a larger society. Additionally, many Hawaiian service agencies, social organizations, and political factions set "Native" Hawaiians (of 50% or more aboriginal blood) apart from "Part-Hawaiians" (of less than half blood quantum). Thus, traditional Native Hawaiian culture and values are harder to maintain because of institutional and social factors. Hawaiians struggle to maintain the strength in the "Hawaiian" way, such as cooperative effort, group well-being as the source of individual well-being, and strong family affiliation.

INTEGRATING CULTURAL FACTORS INTO HEALTH CARE

The Native Hawaiian Health Care Act provided Native Hawaiians in Hawaii the opportunity to infuse Hawaiian definitions of health and Hawaiian health practices into Western-oriented health care. The issues the Native Hawaiian community and Native Hawaiian traditional practitioners must resolve to accomplish these objectives are beyond the scope of this analysis, but a flavor of the tasks can be provided.

Three Native Hawaiian health organizations state that Native Hawaiians do not use the available health-care system because of its method of delivery. One noted that they instead rely on traditional Hawaiian healing methods such as *ho'oponopono*, *la'au lapa'au* [herbal medicine], *lomilomi* [massage], and *haha* [palpation], and seeking the advice of the Native Hawaiian health practitioner or *kahuna* rather than the medical doctor. Native Hawaiians believe the healing process begins in the mind, and the traditional practitioner looks to the source of the problem, seeking to return the troubled individual to a state of *lokahi* [harmony, or unity in all aspects of life].

These principles are often in direct conflict with the Western values of specialization, competition, materialism, economic gain, and emphasis on the individual. Conflicting values directly affect the health-seeking behaviors of Native Hawaiians, who must negotiate Western systems of health care. Therefore, several of these agencies intend to provide services that acknowledge cultural underpinnings by doing the following (Na Pu'uwai, 1991):

• Acknowledge and accommodate preferences for traditional healing practices and incorporate traditional health practices and practitioners in the spectrum of health care when appropriate.

• Collaborate with the client's *'ohana* in the assessment and management of any client to facilitate the healing process and respect the existing support network. This would also include recognition of the designated roles that specific *'ohana* members play.

• Recognize that *pule* [prayer] is integral to the healing process for many Native Hawaiians and accommodate its use in client management and all aspects of daily life, as well as in the community at large.

Whether such health-care services—created through an act of the United States Congress, administered by the federal Department of Health and Human Services, and patterned on the federal community health center program—can in fact be "culturally relevant" will soon be tested. The proof will be in the small details of program implementation. For example, Hui Malama Ola Na 'Oiwi's service delivery grant application contained the following statement (1991):

> The Hawaiian tradition on payment is through barter. At one community meeting, participants asked if they could trade their in-kind services for Hui Malama services, i.e., to clean the office to pay for a Doctor's visit. At that time, we could not respond. The point is cultural bartering is appropriate. The second method of "paying" is to leave a calabash at the door so those who wish to contribute will do so, but no embarassment is caused to others who are unable to do so. . . .
> Hui Malama will accept all contributions of goods, services or through the calabash.

We should follow with interest how the Department of Health and Human Services will reconcile these methods of payment with the statute's requirement of a sliding-fee scale for services.

Health-related Services for Adolescents and for Native Hawaiians

In general, the state of Hawaii has a wide range of health and social-services programs, and the Prepaid Health Care Act and State Health Insurance Program are representative of the State's commitment toward improving the social welfare of its residents.

There is a large variety of services for adolescents, and services specifically for Native Hawaiians as a group are increasing. There is still a paucity of services for Hawaiian adolescents, but the necessary infrastructures to serve their particular needs are gradually being put into place.

The federal mental health and alcohol and drug abuse block grant to the state of Hawaii has a mandatory 17% of funding set aside for Native Hawaiians for drug abuse programs. The 1989 drug abuse disbursements for programs directed at Native Hawaiians actually equaled 28% of funds. The Native Hawaiian Health Care Act of 1988, as described previously, has also created Native Hawaiian health-services delivery systems to provide health promotion, disease prevention, and primary-care services. Pregnancy and infant-care services, family-planning services, immunizations, prevention and control of otitis media and other infectious diseases, control of sexually transmittable diseases, reduction in the misuse of alcohol and drugs, and mental-health care should all be beneficial to Native Hawaiian adolescents.

Many programs are being implemented at the state level. A state Office of Hawaiian Health has been established; its mission is to ensure culturally sensitive and relevant health services and an advocacy program for Native Hawaiians within the Department of Health (State of Hawaii, 1989b).

The Hawaii state legislature has created a task force to examine the provision, coordination, quality, and effectiveness of services for the health and welfare of Native Hawaiians. Specific analyses are to be made of educational services for Native Hawaiian youth (ages 3–19) with special attention to school dropouts, juvenile offenders, and pregnant teenagers. An Office of Youth Services was also created within the Department of Human Services to examine currently available services for youth (W. Rubin, personal communication).

Additionally, the Maternal and Child Health Network of the Hawaii Department of Health was initiated to develop a health network to improve the health status of youth from 10–19 years old. The network particularly planned to establish a permanent unit for adolescent health within the Department of Health (for policy and systems development) that would coordinate adolescent health services at the state level and case management systems for local delivery of health services (State of Hawaii, 1989b).

The Center for Youth Research of the Social Science Research Institute of the University of Hawaii at Manoa is also in the process of developing a computerized, comprehensive information system covering all available youth and family-related services in the state, with the primary purpose of making its database available to all youth and family-related agencies in Hawaii, the Pacific Basin, and the continental United States (University of Hawaii, 1988).

One activity specifically targeted to Native Hawaiian adolescents is a three-year pilot program funded by the U.S. Department of Education that has been established for the Native Hawaiian Drug Free Schools/Communities Program. The project is intended to develop a kindergarten through grade twelve curriculum, educational programs and materials, and resource and referral services appropriate for Native Hawaiian communities.

Other adolescent services or activities with a large proportion of Native Hawaiians in their client population are those in the Waianae and Waimanalo communities on Oahu, two predominantly Native Hawaiian communities.

In sum, there are parallel efforts proceeding statewide to coordinate programs either solely or substantially providing health and related services to adolescents and to establish federally mandated and supported health promotion, disease prevention, and primary medical care services to Native Hawaiians.

Within the adolescent programs, because of state legislature interest and the establishment of the Office of Hawaiian Health within the state Department of Health, activities directed at Native Hawaiians should expand. Several of the service components in the Native Hawaiian health care system will have adolescents as the primary target group. It will be important to see whether the intent of federal and state legislation—to raise the comfort level of Native Hawaiians in using a Western-based health system by placing it in their control and infusing it with traditional Native Hawaiian healing practices—can substantially reverse the poor health and health practices of Native Hawaiians residing in Hawaii.

Conclusions

Native Hawaiian adolescents must surely be affected by fundamental changes in their culture, by the ambivalence that their adult role models are manifesting, and by the accelerated pace of urbanization of their islands. Many Native Hawaiian adolescents must feel that they are "strangers in their own land" (McNassor & Hongo, 1972) and may need special programs to serve their physical- and mental-health needs.

The 1986 Hawaii Child and Adolescent Service System Program Needs Assessment (State of Hawaii, 1986) recommended interventions that encompass an ecological approach for training providers in ethnocultural issues, funding ethnocultural research, and particularly developing creative intervention programs for child abuse and neglect. The Task Force for Services to Hawaiians should provide a blueprint specifically for Native Hawaiian adolescents, while the Native Hawaiian Health Care Act of 1988 provides a specific vehicle for health promotion and disease prevention services to Native Hawaiians of all ages.

Thus, in Hawaii, even though proven culturally appropriate health and related services for Native Hawaiian adolescents may not yet exist, there is at least promising infrastructure developments on which such future services can be based. The Native Hawaiian traditions of "learning by doing," peer-directed socialization, and cooperative effort for mutual gain within a group are positive attributes for dealing with the problems of drug and alcohol abuse and for reducing the high-risk health behaviors that plague the Native Hawaiian community. The inclusion and integration of traditional Native Hawaiian healers and healing practices in the forthcoming Native Hawaiian health-care systems—practices that many Native Hawaiians still use, in addition to their use of Western-based medicine—are further positive attributes in dealing with personal and psychological problems and in child abuse and neglect.

Finally, the charge to the authors of the Office of Technology Assessment–commissioned papers on ethnic minority adolescents included evaluation of service needs of adolescents, with a careful analysis and fine differentiation of needs at various ages and stages of development, so that a developmental perspective within the age boundaries (10–18) could be formulated; and implications for federal policy with respect to appropriate utilization, effectiveness, coordination, and continuity of care between targeted services and traditional services.

Unfortunately, the information needed about Native Hawaiian adolescents is simply not available. Moreover, from the information on hearing loss presented in this analysis, it is evident that interventions must begin before the adolescent years. There are also indications that other educational interventions must begin in the elementary school years, or many

Native Hawaiian students will be irretrievably lost by junior high school (Kaiser Permanente Center for Health Research, 1991; Kronick, 1989). These interventions quite clearly must include parental involvement. In fact, one of the major activities of Ho'ola Lahui Hawai'i, one of the five Native Hawaiian health organizations, is to focus on Native Hawaiian children in kindergarten through sixth grade as a means of reaching parents not only for their children's health needs but for their own health needs as well (Ho'ola Lahui Hawai'i, 1991).

Despite the special circumstances needed to deal with Native Hawaiians, federal policy can be used to increase general support for ethnic-minority adolescents through the traditional federal method of financing resources development. For example, resources could be increased in the areas of professional training (e.g., scholarship and loan programs for ethnic minorities in adolescent services and studies); interdisciplinary research (cultural, health, social); and biomedical and health services research (e.g., among Native Hawaiians, the high incidence of diabetes and cancer; use of traditional medicine compared with Western health care). Special emphasis could be given to the training of health-services researchers in minority adolescent issues.

Such programs and activities already exist, although none are specifically directed at adolescents. There are health scholarships for specific ethnic minorities (such as American Indians/Alaska Natives and Native Hawaiians), which are tied to service payback among their own people. The National Center for Health Services Research and Health Care Technology Assessment convened a conference to encourage research in primary care, aimed at young investigators in the field of general pediatrics, general medicine, family medicine, and nursing. A major focus of research is the development of services for disadvantaged and underserved populations, primarily those of ethnic minorities and the poor (J. Mayfield, personal communication). At the National Cancer Institute, the Special Populations Branch is exclusively devoted to research issues concerning populations with special cancer problems, including Alaska Natives, American Indians, Asian Americans, Blacks, blue-collar groups, the elderly, Hispanics, low-income groups, and Native Hawaiians (U.S. Department of Health and Human Services, undated). And of course, within the Department of Health and Human Services is the Office of Minority Health.

If activities directed at ethnic adolescents are scattered among various agencies, the balkanization of programs for ethnic-minority adolescents may be an important concern. On the other hand, unless there are specific activities and substantial funds devoted to ethnic-minority adolescent issues in the relevant agencies, there will be much "coordination" but little commitment. There are precedents for more substantial organizational efforts that are age specific, such as the Maternal and Child Health Block Grants and the National Institute of Aging. It thus seems appropriate to have an "Administration on Adolescents," an "Office on Adolescents," or even a "National Institute for Adolescent Health," each with a branch or division on ethnic minorities. Such major new efforts are tried and true methods of focusing attention and providing substantial resources to a particular problem area. Perhaps the time has come for such major efforts to deal with the health and related problems of ethnic adolescents—and, indeed, all adolescents.

References

Barringer, H., & O'Hagan, P. (1989). *Socioeconomic characteristics of Native Hawaiians*. Honolulu: Alu Like.

Ho'ola Lahui Hawai'i (1991). *Grant proposal for: Native Hawaiian Health Care Act of 1988, Public Law 100-579*. (Available from P.O. Box 742, Waimea, Kaua'i HI 96796)

Hui Malama Ola Na 'Oiwi (1991). *Proposal to deliver community-based primary care services to Native Hawaiians of Hawai'i County*. (Available from 305 Wailuku Drive, Suite 3, Hilo HI 96720)

Kaiser Permanente Center for Health Research. School of Public Health. University of Hawaii at Manoa, & Hawaii Medical Service Association Foundation (1991, September). *The State Health Insurance Program of Hawai'i: From legislative priority to reality*. (Submitted to Department of Health, State of Hawaii)

Kamehameha Schools/Bernice Pauahi Bishop Estate (1983, July). *Native Hawaiian Educational Assessment Project*. Honolulu: Author.

Kamehameha Schools/Bernice Pauahi Bishop Estate. Center for Development of Early Education (1989, March). *A proposal for a research and demonstration hearing screening and follow-up program for Hawaiian children*. Honolulu: Author.

Kronick, R. (1989, July). *Adolescent health insurance status* (Publication No. OTA-BP-H-56). Background paper prepared for Office of Technology Assessment's Project on Adolescent Health; U.S. Congress, Office of Technology Assessment. Washington DC: U.S. Government Printing Office.

McNassor, D., & Hongo, R. (1972). *Strangers in their own land*. Paper presented at the Claremont Reading Conference, Claremont Graduate School, Claremont CA.

Na Pu'uwai (1991, July). *Native Hawaiian health care system for Moloka'i, Kalaupapa, and Lana'i.* Kaunakakai, Moloka'i HI: Author.

Oyama, N., & Johnson, D. B. (1986). *Hawaii Health Surveillance Program survey methods and procedures.* Honolulu: Hawaii State Department of Health, Research and Statistics Office.

Plett, J. D., & Heath, R. W. (1987, October). *Hawaiian early childhood data book.* Honolulu: Kamehameha Schools/Bernice Pauahi Bishop Estate.

State of Hawaii. Criminal Justice Data Center. (1985). *Crime in Hawaii: 1984.* Honolulu: Author.

State of Hawaii. Department of Education. Office of Program Evaluation and Planning. (1989, November). [Analysis of data tapes, Kamehameha Schools/ Bishop Estate]. Unpublished data.

State of Hawaii. Department of Health. Maternal and Child Health Branch. (1986, August). *Hawaii Child and Adolescent Service System Program: Needs assessment.* Honolulu: Hawaii Child and Adolescent Service System Program.

State of Hawaii. Department of Health. Research and Statistics Office. (1987). *Statistical report.* Honolulu: Author.

State of Hawaii. Department of Health. Director's Office. (1989a, June). *Universal primary and preventive health care for Hawaii.* Honolulu: Deputy Director for Health Resources.

State of Hawaii. Department of Health. Health Resources Administration. (1989b, June). *Statement of function.* Unpublished report.

State of Hawaii. Department of Health. Maternal and Child Health Adolescent Network. (1989c, June). *Summary of progress: Report for maternal and child health improvement projects.* Honolulu: Department of Health.

State of Hawaii. Office of Hawaiian Affairs. (1986, June). *Population survey/needs assessment, Final report.* Honolulu: Office of Hawaiian Affairs.

University of Hawaii–Manoa. Social Science Research Institute. Center for Youth Research. (1988). *Annual report: 1987–88.* Honolulu: University of Hawaii.

U.S. Congress. Office of Technology Assessment. (1987, April). *Current health status and population projections of Native Hawaiians living In Hawaii.* Washington DC: U.S. Government Printing Office.

U.S. Bureau of the Census. (1983). *1980 Census of Population: General Social and Eco-*

nomic Characteristics, PC80-1-C1. Washington DC: U.S. Government Printing Office.

U.S. Department of Health and Human Services, National Institutes of Health, National Institute of Diabetes and Digestive and Kidney Diseases. (1989). *Efforts to combat diabetes in Native Hawaiians*. (Draft). Bethesda MD: Author.

Woods, D. W., Oyama, N., & Johnson, D. (1987). *Technical report: A report on the prevalence of impairments in Hawaii 1981–1983*. Honolulu: John A. Burns School of Medicine, University of Hawaii, Rehabilitation Hospital of the Pacific.

7

The Federal Government's Role in Improving the Health of Poor and Ethnic-Minority Adolescents

Denise Dougherty and Kerry B. Kemp

Available evidence suggests that roughly 5 million adolescents ages 10–18 live in poverty and that 9 million Black, Latino, Asian Pacific, Native American, and other potentially marginalized ethnic-minority adolescents are disproportionately at high risk for selected health problems (U.S. Congress, Office of Technology Assessment, 1991a, 1991b, 1991c; see other chapters in this volume).

As also noted in other chapters in this volume, poor and ethnic-minority adolescents may encounter a variety of barriers to access to appropriate health care. Some of these barriers are experienced to a greater or lesser degree by many nonpoor nonminority U.S. adolescents—for example, a lack of health insurance, limited availability of health-care providers who are competent and willing to treat adolescents, and legal requirements for parental consent or notification. But some of the poor and ethnic-minority adolescents confront additional barriers to access, including financial inability to purchase health services out of pocket and cultural and linguistic differences with health-care providers and researchers (Bergeisen, 1989; Miike, 1989; Ooms and Herendeen, 1990; Spencer and Dornbusch, 1990; other chapters, this volume).

The federal government has developed a multitude of programs and policies that directly or indirectly affect the health of poor and ethnic-minority adolescents. Direct programs include those that provide subsidies or services to adolescents or their families; indirect programs include support for research on health issues affecting poor and/or ethnic-minority adolescents. This chapter reviews the major federal programs related to the health of poor and/or ethnic minority adolescents and is based largely on a review of federal programs conducted as part of a congressional study of adolescent health, for which we were project director and editor, respectively. The survey and overall study were conducted by the Office of Technology Assessment (OTA), a congressional support agency that provides congressional committees with objective analyses of the emerging, difficult, and often highly technical issues of our time. The OTA surveyed numerous executive-branch agencies with potential activities in adolescent health policies, including cabinet departments and the so-called independent agencies (e.g., the Consumer Product Safety Commission, the Corporation for National Service, the National Transportation Safety Board). The agencies with the greatest federal investments in adolescent health were the Department of Health and Human Services (DHHS) and the Department of Education.

The OTA survey remains the most comprehensive analysis of federal efforts on adolescents ever conducted. Other efforts to discern federal spending on adolescents have focused on youth, including young adults, or on children and families, with some mention of programs whose target group is adolescents (U.S. Congress, Library of Congress, Congressional Research Service, 1992), making it difficult to grasp the level of federal effort on adolescents in general or on poor and ethnic-minority adolescents in particular. Nevertheless, the OTA survey results are limited in several respects. Agencies often combined activities affecting all children, or both adolescents and young adults, and could not separate their other activities and responsibilities from budgets and activities with an impact on adolescent health. Further, with the exception of efforts focused on Native Hawaiians and Native Americans, few federal efforts were limited to ethnic-minority adolescents. Poor and low-income people (variously defined, but usually specified as those with family incomes below the federal poverty level [approximately $14,764 for a family of four in 1993]) were more typically a focus of federal programs than were poor adolescents per se; agencies differed in whether they could calculate particular program funds associated with adolescents. Finally, OTA's survey was conducted in 1989–1990, making its results somewhat dated.

This chapter also summarizes major legislative and executive-branch changes that occurred since the release of the OTA report in April 1991. Figure 7.1 illustrates the relationship between the agencies described in this chapter. Whereever possible, we update agencies' budget figures and adolescent program participation statistics.

Major Federal Programs Related to the Health of Poor or Ethnic-Minority Adolescents

Because the OTA study broadly defines adolescent health and health problems to include physical, social, and mental aspects of health and aspects of well-being rather than merely the presence or absence of problems (U.S. Congress, Office of Technology Assessment, 1991a, 1991b, 1991c), it surveys a wide range of federal agencies. This summary focuses first on activities of the DHHS, which has the greatest share of the federal budget for adolescent health, and then on the U.S. Departments of Education, Agriculture, Justice, Labor, and Housing and Urban Development, and the independent agency the Corporation for National Service (formerly ACTION).

DEPARTMENT OF HEALTH AND HUMAN SERVICES

The DHHS administers a wide range of service, subsidy, and research programs related to health, welfare, and income security. The Health Care Financing Administration (HCFA) and the Public Health Service (PHS) have the major DHHS programs relevant to low-income and ethnic-minority adolescents' health. The Administration for Children and Families may also help improve the health of ethnic minority and/or poor adolescents through cash assistance and support for the provision of social services. The office of the Assistant Secretary for Planning and Evaluation and the inspector general's office in DHHS have recently become involved in issues surrounding school-based health centers, a promising approach to providing services to adolescents in need.

Health-Care Financing Administration and Medicaid

The largest single source of federal spending on adolescent health is the Medicaid program, a federally aided, state-administered program of medical assistance to very low-income people. The Medicaid program accounted for about three quarters ($3.3 billion) of DHHS spending on adolescents in 1989 (U.S. Congress, Office of Technology Assessment, 1991a, 1991c).

In fiscal year 1988, according to estimates by HCFA, an estimated 4.58

Figure 7.1. Agencies of the federal government with major roles
in the health of poor and ethnic minority adolescents

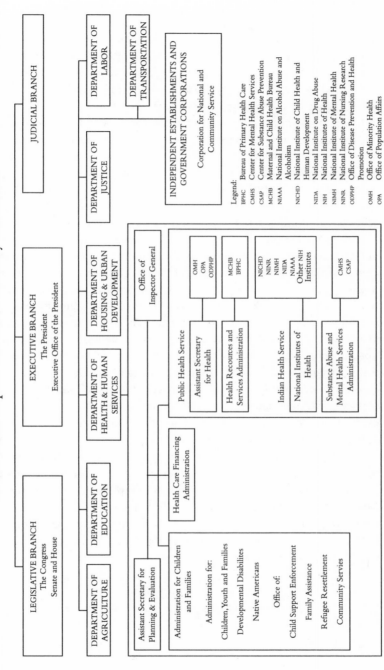

Source: Adapted from the Office of the Federal Register, 1993.

million U.S. adolescents ages 10–18 had Medicaid coverage at some point in time during the year, representing 17.1% of Medicaid enrollees. However, federal and state Medicaid expenditures on adolescents in that year accounted for approximately 6.9% of Medicaid expenditures (U.S. Congress, Office of Technology Assessment, 1991c).

Medicaid coverage as a source of access for poor and ethnic-minority adolescents is limited. As several authors in this volume have pointed out (e.g., Allen & Mitchell; Taylor & Katz), not all poor adolescents have been eligible for Medicaid. That situation is changing slowly as a result of a provision in the Omnibus Budget Reconciliation Act of 1990 gradually extending Medicaid coverage to individuals born after 30 September 1983 who live in families below 100% of the federal poverty level.

Even adolescents covered by Medicaid may experience financial and nonfinancial barriers to appropriate health care. Not all services are covered, not all physicians participate in the program (Yudkowski, Cartland, & Flint, 1990), and procedures for confidentiality can vary across states (Gittler, Quigley-Rick, & Saks, 1990). Services that states may opt not to provide to Medicaid beneficiaries include some that may be of particular importance to adolescents: case management; dental services; some diagnostic, screening, preventive, and rehabilitative services; prescription drugs; eyeglasses; physical, occupational, and speech, hearing, and language disorder therapies; services of psychologists and optometrists; clinic services; intermediate care facility services; inpatient psychiatric facility care for individuals under age 21; and other medical or remedial care (see Allen and Mitchell, in this volume).

There has been at least one minor expansion in benefits, however. In 1994, President Bill Clinton signed an executive order requiring states to use Medicaid to pay for abortions in cases of rape and incest. On the whole, Medicaid, in particular its Early Periodic Screening, Diagnostic and Treatment program for minors, is often viewed as a model for the types of benefits that should be included in a uniform benefit package as it applies to children and adolescents.

Public Health Service

Several PHS agencies administer programs that are specifically intended to help poor and ethnic-minority people, sometimes focusing on adolescents (see table 7.1):

Table 7.1 Partial List of Offices of the Department of Health and Human Services

	Functions
PHS Agencies:	
MCHB	Awards maternal and child health block grants
BPHC	Supports services in school-based centers; and administers urban, rural, and migrant health center
NICHD	Initiates several longitudinal studies on adolescents
NINR	Convened seven Priority Expert Panels to establish research and service needs for the next five years
NIMH	Funds research centers that do research and provide treatment for needs of particular ethnic groups
CMHS	Houses CSAP. Provides initiatives to improve the delivery of mental-health services to severely emotionally disturbed children and adolescents
CSAP	Provides national leadership for alcohol and drug abuse prevention
CDC	Coordinates surveillance, data collection and analysis, epidemiologic investigations, and laboratory research; provides technical assistance, grants, and cooperative agreements to state and local health departments; and collaborates with partners in many diverse organizations
OASH Agencies:	
OPA	Administers two Public Health Service Act programs important to poor and/or ethnic minority adolescents
ODPHP	Provides leadership for disease prevention and health promotion among all Americans by stimulating and coordinating federal activities
OMH	Focuses on addressing minority health needs with and through communities, and does not focus on specific age group
ACF Offices:	
ACYF	Administers programs that contribute to improving the health of poor and/or ethnic minority adolescents
ANA	Provides training and assistance to public and private Native American organizations in developing and administering projects to carry out locally determined social and economic development strategies
ORR	Provides funds to states for refugee and entrant assistance program

Note. Abbreviations as follows: ACF, Administration for Children and Families; ACYF, Administration for Children, Youth, and Families; ANA, Administration for Native Americans; BPHC, Bureau of Primary Health Care; CDC, Centers for Disease Control and Prevention; CMHS, Center for Mental Health Services; CSAP, Center for Substance Abuse Prevention; MCHB, Maternal and Child Health Bureau; NICHD, National Institute of Child Health and Human Development; NIMH, National Institute of Mental Health; NINR, National Institute of Nursing Research; OASH, Office of Assistant Secretary for Health; ODPHP, Office of Disease Prevention and Health Promotion; OMH, Office of Minority Health; OPA, Office of Population Affairs; ORR, Office of Refugee Resettlement; PHS, Public Health Service.

• the Health Resources and Services Administration (HRSA);
• the National Institutes of Health, which includes the Institute of Child
Health and Human Development (NICHD), the National Institute of Nursing Research (NINR), the National Institute of Mental Health (NIMH), the
National Institute on Drug Abuse (NIDA), and the National Institute on Alcohol Abuse and Alcoholism (NIAAA);
• the Centers for Disease Control and Prevention (CDC);
• the Substance Abuse and Mental Health Services Administration
(SAMHSA);
• the Office of Minority Health (OMH) and the Office of Population Affairs
(OPA) in the Office of the Assistant Secretary for Health (OASH);
• the Indian Health Service (IHS), which is discussed in detail by Fleming,
Manson, and Bergeisen (in this volume).

Health Resources and Services Administration. The HRSA has historically, if
somewhat informally, been heavily involved in the provision and improvement of health services to adolescents, although it has been difficult to say
how much of HRSA efforts benefit ethnic-minority adolescents. A more formal involvement came as a result of 1991 legislation in which the Division
of Maternal and Child Health was renamed the Division of Maternal, Infant, Child, and Adolescent Health and the Adolescent Health Branch was
added (J. Evans, personal communication).

The HRSA Maternal and Child Health Bureau (MCHB) sets aside 15% of
the MCHB appropriation for competitive awards to support Special Projects
of Regional and National Significance (SPRANS), including some SPRANS
grants focused on improving the provision of health services to ethnic-
minority and poor adolescents (Hutchins & Walsh, 1989; National Center
for Education in Maternal and Child Health, 1993a, 1993b).

In fiscal year 1994, the appropriation for the MCHB block-grant programs
was $679 million (U.S. Executive Office of the President, Budget, 1994);
but because the funds are in block grants without specific reporting requirements, it is impossible for MCHB to distinguish block-grant funds
spent by age group or ethnic group. The MCHB has used the SPRANS grants
to focus on adolescent health needs by funding direct service provision and
interdisciplinary training for specialists in adolescent health (Hutchins &
Walsh, 1989; National Center for Education in Maternal and Child Health,
1993a, 1993b). The interdisciplinary training programs for providers wish-
ing to work on adolescent health comprise a longstanding, prominent, and

worthwhile use of SPRANS funds (U.S. Congress, Office of Technology Assessment, 1991c), but none of these programs has been rigorously evaluated.

Most recently, under congressional directive, HRSA has taken a very active role in the expansion of school-based health services. For example, combining a $3.25 million appropriation for school-based primary care services designated for homeless and at-risk children and youth with $1 million in SPRANS funds, HRSA created a school health initiative called Healthy Schools, Healthy Communities (HSHC), to be managed jointly by HRSA's Bureau of Primary Health Care (BPHC) and MCHB (U.S. Department of Health and Human Services, Public Health Service, Health Resources and Services Administration, 1994). In addition, seven awards were to be made in August 1995 for partnerships between health, state mental health, and education departments in five states and staff training, both aimed at enhancing mental-health services for adolescents in schools (J. Evans, personal communication). The HRSA also contributed toward a National Assembly of School-Based Health Centers, which met in early 1995, and has contracted with the "Making the Grade" school-based health-center grant project funded largely by the Robert Wood Johnson Foundation (J. Evans, personal communication). The school-based health centers funded under HSHC were to be located in areas with large numbers of homeless children, or children broadly defined to be at risk of homelessness, and required to serve any student seeking services. The HRSA is funding an evaluation of HSHC (U.S. Department of Health and Human Services, Public Health Service, Health Resources and Services Administration, 1994); evaluators are to collect information on ethnic group and family income and conduct an evaluation of staff development.

In addition, the BPHC provided about $426 million in federal funds in fiscal year 1988 to urban, rural, and migrant health centers (formerly community and migrant health centers; U.S. Department of Health and Human Services, Public Health Service, Health Resources and Services Administration, Bureau of Health Care Delivery and Assistance, 1989). In 1989, 814,000 adolescents received medical care in community and migrant health centers; of these adolescents, 117,000 females ages 10–14 received family-planning services and at least 121,000 adolescents received dental care at an estimated cost of $33 million. About 13,000 students a year take part in HRSA's Health Careers Opportunity Program (U.S. Department of Health and Human Services, Public Health Service, Health Resources and

Services Administration, 1989), which provides direct financial assistance to disadvantaged students.

In 1993, HRSA and MCHB set goals for their adolescent health activities (National Center for Education in Maternal and Child Health, 1993a, 1993b). By mid-1995, several of the goals had been reached or exceeded, despite the fact that the MCHB was staffed by four professionals and a secretary. The MCHB has established a National Adolescent Health Work Group, a group of outside advisers that has met several times. It has funded a National Adolescent Health Information Center (NAHIC) at the University of California, San Francisco. The NAHIC is a five-year demonstration project designed to keep abreast of legislation and trends in adolescent health, to disseminate knowledge on adolescent health in a timely way, and to ensure that state adolescent health coordinators continue to be brought together to share information regularly. In addition, in late 1995, MCHB will expand its staff to include a medical officer and a nurse. In legislation passed in 1994, HRSA was given $300,000 to establish itself as the site of the Office of Adolescent Health. Unfortunately, MCHB is affected by a personnel ceiling and cannot use the funds to hire additional people. Instead, the director of MCHB will use part (approximately $75,000) of these funds to stimulate adolescent health activities at three off-site nonprofit organizations, the American Psychological Association, the American Bar Association, and the National Association of Social Workers (J. Evans, personal communication). (None of these professions is represented on the MCHB adolescent health staff.)

National Institutes of Health

The NIH comprises many of the nation's premier research institutes, providing grants for much of the health-related research work in academic institutions in the United States. Of the many research institutes and centers that make up NIH, the NICHD, the NINR, and the newly placed NIMH, NIDA, and NIAAA are the agencies with the most activities related specifically to poor and ethnic-minority adolescents.

National Institute of Child Health and Human Development. Although it would appear to be the agency with the most relevance to adolescent health, NIH's NICHD has traditionally spent little of its budget (6.9% in 1989) on adolescent health issues (U.S. Congress, Office of Technology Assessment, 1991a, 1991c). This money was mainly focused on biological facets of sexual development and adolescent pregnancy. Since 1992, however, NICHD implemented the Minority Youth Behavior Research initiative (being funded through the Office of Minority Health) and a congressionally mandated $22.5 million longitudinal study of adolescent general health and well-being (American Psychological Association, 1994).

The Minority Youth Behavior Research initiative provides grants to seven programs and one data center to develop, implement, and evaluate strategies for decreasing violence-related injuries and deaths, sexually transmitted diseases and unwanted or unintended pregnancies, and other problems in minority youth ages 10 through 24. Funded projects are located in widely dispersed settings, including schools and housing projects and urban and rural sites, and are well distributed geographically (e.g., the Fort Greene area of Brooklyn, New York; Durham, North Carolina; the inner suburbs of Chicago; the Great Lakes area of Wisconsin; Seattle, Washington). African American, Asian, American Indian, and Pacific Islander communities are represented. Grantees are required both to work closely with community organizations and to have a strong evaluation component, with at least some common data points for comparison across programs. Finally, the program can include the provision and evaluation of actual health services. Overall funding for the projects is relatively generous: $27 million over a five-and-a-half-year period.

The NICHD-funded survey called ADD HEALTH is the first nationwide comprehensive study focused on potential determinants of adolescent health (e.g., school, family, neighborhood, and community characteristics) and on ethnic minority adolescents' experiences and health. Richard Udry of the University of North Carolina–Chapel Hill is the lead investigator.

National Institute of Nursing Research. The NINR's Health Promotion for Older Children and Adolescents (defined as individuals ages 8–18) panel identified a range of specific research and service needs and opportunities for the five-year period beginning in 1994 (U.S. Department of Health and Human Services, Public Health Service, National Institutes of Health, National Institute of Nursing Research, 1993). Many of the areas identified focused on economically disadvantaged or ethnic-minority adolescents.

National Institute of Mental Health. The NIMH awarded $1.4 million in 1991 for a new Research Center on the Psychobiology of Ethnicity that will investigate, among other things, ethnic differences in how people respond to drugs for mental disorders, "culture-bound syndromes," and how different groups conceptualize psychiatric disorders (Holden, 1991).

Other NIH Institutes. In a 1993 report the NIH reported that various institutes had supported more than 485 research projects that dealt with the issues of adolescence in fiscal year 1992 (U.S. Department of Health and Human Services, Public Health Service, National Institutes of Health, National Institute on Child Health and Human Development, 1993). Apart from activities described above, NIH cited several activities of specific relevance to ethnic minority adolescents:

• a research program to develop and evaluate interventions for control of asthma among minority children (in the National Heart, Lung, and Blood Institute [NHLBI]);
• demonstration and education research projects designed to reduce the severity and/or incidence of asthma in urban minority children and adolescents (National Institute of Allergy and Infectious Diseases [NIAID]);
• a collaborative study on obesity prevention in Native Americans and Alaska Natives (NHLBI);
• support for research on new diagnostic procedures on childhood language impairment in multicultural populations (National Institute on Deafness and Other Communication Disorders);
• support for research on sickle cell disease and treatments for that disorder (National Institute of Diabetes and Digestive and Kidney Diseases [NIDDKD]);
• research on all aspects of obesity, which is noted as being particularly prevalent in the young female minority population (NIDDKD).

The NIH was not asked to specify research programs on minority adolescents, so it is likely that more adolescent projects than those specifically referring to minority adolescents (e.g., projects on HIV and AIDS in NIAID) could benefit ethnic-minority adolescents.

Centers for Disease Control and Prevention
The mission of the Centers for Disease Control and Prevention (CDC) is to promote health and quality of life by preventing and controlling disease,

injury, and disability among Americans of all ages. Thus, the CDC directs a wide range of activities, from surveillance of health problems and risk factors to implementation of prevention strategies, primarily through partnerships with state and local governments and other organizations. The CDC focuses on adolescents primarily through its Adolescent and School Health Programs (ASHP), but activities around such issues as unintended pregnancy and youth violence can all potentially benefit ethnic–minority adolescents (U.S. Department of Health and Human Services, n.d.).

The ASHP began as part of CDC's focus on HIV prevention and still supports fifty-four state/territorial and seventeen local education departments and twenty-three national organizations to provide education in HIV risk reduction to youth, including ethnic–minority adolescents. But ASHP has grown to support comprehensive school health program activities in jurisdictions that include states with large numbers of ethnic–minority youth, in particular African American and Latino adolescents (e.g., Arkansas, the District of Columbia, and Florida).

The CDC's work to prevent unintended pregnancy includes several studies of potentially influential factors and an effort to specify a theoretical model. Programs in California, New York City, Rhode Island, Florida, Maryland, North Carolina, and Kansas City target youth violence through a number of interventions, including conflict resolution education, mass media campaigns, community organizations, mediation programs, and crisis intervention. However, CDC's budget for youth violence prevention has been relatively small (estimated at a little over a million dollars in 1993) and particularly small for programs directed specifically at youth violence in minority communities (an estimated $10,000 in 1993) (U.S. Department of Health and Human Services, n.d.).

Substance Abuse and Mental Health Services Administration

The SAMHSA is a relatively new entity created by federal legislation in 1992. It is intended to replace the "services" programs of the former Alcohol, Drug Abuse, and Mental Health Administration (ADAMHA) and was budgeted $100 million for grants for comprehensive community mental-health services for individuals ages 21 and younger with severe emotional disturbances.

Projects funded by ADAMHA included several studies examining the effects of drug use on school dropout rates in minority communities, the etiology of substance abuse among high–risk Black adolescents, and cultural factors affecting vulnerabilities to substance abuse among Latino adolescents (U.S. Congress, Office of Technology Assessment, 1991a, 1991c).

The Center for Mental Health Services in SAMHSA houses the important Child and Adolescent Service System Program. This small-grant program was established in 1984 to ensure that mental health and related (child welfare, juvenile justice, mental health, and special education) services to severely emotionally disturbed children and adolescents from ethnic minorities are culturally competent. Cultural competence is defined as "a set of congruent behaviors, attitudes, and policies that come together in a system, agency, or amongst professionals and enables that system, agency, or those professionals to work effectively in cross-cultural situations" (Cross et al., 1989; Isaacs & Benjamin, 1991).

The Center for Substance Abuse Prevention (CSAP) awarded 130 demonstration grants in 1987 (most of which target adolescents), and 56% of those grants were targeted at minority groups (U.S. Department of Health and Human Services, Public Health Service, Alcohol, Drug Abuse, and Mental Health Administration, Office of Substance Abuse Prevention, 1990). Many of the projects incorporated strategies to enhance cultural competence, such as involving respected community members in the program, recruiting minority staff at all levels, encouraging the use of traditional cultural activities, and using culturally appropriate media and messages in drug and alcohol education efforts.

The activities of the OSAP had been criticized for paying inadequate attention to evaluating the programs it funded (U.S. Congress, Office of Technology Assessment, 1991b). A 1994 OTA study found that CSAP has been attempting to incorporate more stringent methodological criteria for evaluating the outcomes of demonstration projects (U.S. Congress, Office of Technology Assessment, 1994).

Office of the Assistant Secretary for Health (OASH)

Three OASH offices are particularly relevant to adolescents: the Office of Population Affairs (OPA), the Office of Disease Prevention and Health Promotion, and the Office of Minority Health.

Office of Population Affairs. The OPA administers the Title X family planning program and the Title XX adolescent pregnancy and parenting program. Title X is the major source of federal funding ($130 million appropriation in fiscal year 1990) for public and private nonprofit family-planning clinics that offer contraceptive and other reproductive-health services. Title X also supports family-planning research, training, information, and educational activities.

Title X programs may be particularly important to ethnic-minority adolescents. The OTA found that Black female adolescents tend to use family-planning clinics to obtain contraceptives more than they use private physicians (U.S. Congress, Office of Technology Assessment, 1991b). The provision of contraceptives to adolescents by Title X clinics has been controversial, but the courts have held that adolescents may obtain Title X family-planning services without parental consent or notification (U.S. Congress, Library of Congress, Congressional Research Service, 1989b). The extent to which ethnic-minority adolescents use Title X clinics is unknown, but most publicly supported family-planning clinics get some funds from the federal government. In fiscal year 1992, clinics that received Title X funds served more than 4.3 million clients, about one third (1.3 million) of whom were adolescents ages 15–19 (U.S. Congress, Library of Congress, Congressional Research Service, 1992).

The use of Title X funds for abortions for individuals of all ages has been prohibited by statute (§1008) and by regulations since the enactment of the Title X program (Family Planning Perspectives, 1991). From the early 1980s to 1992, health-care providers other than physicians accepting Title X funds were not allowed to mention the use of abortion as a possible alternative to childbearing (U.S. Congress, Office of Technology Assessment, 1991b); a signed executive order overturned this so-called gag rule. Title X continues to be controversial, however, and narrowly escaped a loss of directed federal funding in the summer of 1995, when one proposed amendment to the House Department of Health and Human Services appropriations bill was superseded by another amendment that preserved funding for the program (Morgan, 1995).

Title XX funds two types of Adolescent Family Life demonstration projects: those seeking to prevent adolescent pregnancy (primarily by encouraging abstinence from sexual activity) and those providing health and social services (including adoption) for pregnant or parenting adolescents. Title XX programs are not limited to low-income or ethnic-minority individuals, but Congress has suggested that service areas with a high proportion of low-income families should receive priority when grant applications are considered (Title XX, §2005).

In its fiscal year 1995 budget proposal, the Clinton administration proposed that adolescent family life programs be relabeled adolescent health programs, with funding of $6.8 million for fiscal year 1995 (decreases of $175,000 from estimated fiscal year 1994 spending, and $728,000 from fiscal year 1993 Office of Population Affairs spending; U.S. Executive Office of the President, 1994). Congress stipulated that an Office of Adolescent Health be created but did not appropriate the funding for it. The administration was expected to reallocate existing funds. As noted above, $300,000 was allocated to HRSA, to be used for creating an Office of Adolescent Health in the MCHB.

Office of Disease Prevention and Health Promotion. Healthy People 2000 was billed as an initiative to be implemented at many levels of government, by the private sector, and through individual citizens' activities (U.S. Congress, Office of Technology Assessment, 1991a), but the executive branch plays a key role in incorporating goals into federal requests for proposals, justifying federal agency activities, and tracking the nation's progress in meeting the goals (e.g., U.S. Department of Health and Human Services, Public Health Service, 1993, 1994).

In a December 1993 review of progress on Healthy People 2000 objectives related to adolescents and young adults, Office of Disease Prevention and Health Promotion representatives, several other DHHS agencies, the Department of Education, and several outside observers (including one of the authors of this chapter) discussed both recent data on the health status of adolescents and young adults and actions required to meet the objectives (U.S. Department of Health and Human Services, Public Health Service, 1993). Healthy People 2000 objectives for adolescents and young adults typically did not distinguish goals for different ethnic-minority groups, but participants were provided with some health status data that made such distinctions (i.e., differences in mortality and drug-use rates).

Only one strategy included in the progress review briefing book (training of health professionals) focused on ethnic-minority adolescents (U.S. Department of Health and Human Services, Public Health Service, 1993), although ethnic-minority adolescents could clearly benefit from implementation of many of the strategies proposed (e.g., expansion of Medicaid).

Office of Minority Health (OMH). In the absence of a functioning departmental level Office of Adolescent Health, researchers and advocates interested in the federal role in the health of ethnic-minority adolescents might naturally turn to OMH as a center of activity. The OMH, however, does not focus on specific age groups (G. Buggs, personal communication, 1992).

The OMH was created within the DHHS's Office of the Assistant Secretary of Health in 1985 to implement the recommendations of the Secretary's Task Force on Black and Minority Health (Payne & Ugarte, 1989). These recommendations included stimulating the development of innovative programs to improve the health status of minority populations and advocating a national strategy to address the health needs of minorities (Payne & Ugarte, 1989; U.S. Department of Health and Human Services, Office of the Secretary, 1985). But OMH was criticized in 1990 because it did not have "specific goals or objectives . . . or short- and long-term strategic plans for its objectives" related to any of the ethnic-minority groups it purported to help (U.S. Congress, General Accounting Office, 1990). In response, the U.S. Congress statutorily established an OMH, to be headed by a deputy assistant secretary for minority health, and authorized an increase in funding to $25 million per year for fiscal years 1991 through 1993 (Public Law 101-527). Far fewer funds were actually appropriated, however ($15.3 million in fiscal year 1993, $20.9 million in fiscal year 1994).

Some projects funded by OMH have focused on adolescents, including programs designed to reduce teenage pregnancy, reduce the risk of alcohol and other drug problems among high-risk, urban Latino youth, and provide AIDS education to American Indian high school students and adults using Native healing principles and techniques. Additional HIV education and prevention programs directed at Black and Latino adolescents and adults have also been funded, as has a special initiative on minority males (Bowles & Robinson, 1989; U.S. Department of Health and Human Services, n.d.; U.S. Department of Health and Human Services, Public Health Service, Office of the Assistant Secretary for Health, Office of Minority Health, 1990). The Minority Male Grants program funds conference grants, coalition development grnts, and coalition intervention grants to address health and social problems that affect adolescent minority males (e.g., HIV infection and sexually transmitted diseases, homicide, teenage fatherhood, delinquency) (U.S. Department of Health and Human Services, n.d.). In addition to these programs, minority adolescent males may eventually be affected by several OMH data collection and tracking activities under development. These include a critical review of the status and trends in the health and quality of life of minority populations (which would result in an update of the 1985 secretary's report on minority health) and the Minority Health Tracking System (which is to contain information on PHS grants and contracts related to minority health). Nevertheless, the fact remains that no federal agency focuses on the overall health of minority adolescents.

Administration for Children and Families (ACF)

The ACF consists of the Administration for Children, Youth, and Families (ACYF), the Administration on Developmental Disabilities, the Office of Child Support Enforcement, the Office of Community Services, the Office of Family Assistance, the Administration for Native Americans, and the Office of Refugee Resettlement (see Table 7.1). The ACF is the product of the reorganization of several DHHS social-welfare agencies formerly under the jurisdiction of the Office of Human Development Services and the Family Support Administration (Office of the Federal Register, 1993; U.S. Congress, Office of Technology Assessment, 1991a, 1991c). Comprehensive counts of ACF services specifically for adolescents cannot be readily provided.

The Office of Family Assistance affects a great number of poor adolescents, as it oversees the AFDC program. In fiscal year 1987, 33% (2.5 million) of the children receiving AFDC benefits were adolescents ages 10 through 18 (U.S. Congress, Office of Technology Assessment, 1991c). Another 121,000 adolescents, 85% of whom were females, received AFDC benefits as heads of households.

Some ACYF programs include the Child Abuse Prevention and Treatment Program, drug abuse prevention for youth gangs programs, the administration of the Runaway and Homeless Youth Act, and Child Welfare Services training and research and demonstration programs. The Children's Bureau in ACYF provides federal support for child-welfare services and provides Independent Living Formula Grants to states that help adolescents in foster care make transitions into the work world (U.S. Department of Health and Human Services, Office of Human Development Services, 1989).

Child-welfare training opportunities are designed to increase the number of minorities entering the field of social work in this area. Funds are provided for traineeships and in-service training to historically Black colleges and universities and to colleges controlled by Indian tribes or serving Indian reservations. These training programs are important because of the widely acknowledged need for "culturally competent" health services for ethnic-minority adolescents. Other programs specifically oriented to ethnic-minority adolescents include the Family and Youth Services Bureau's programs to prevent substance abuse among runaway and homeless Native American adolescents. These projects are expected to incorporate Indian tribal values and languages and develop a positive cultural and family identity (54 FR 15092-15106).

The ACF's Administration for Native Americans (ANA) targeted the problem of drug- and alcohol-abuse prevention in the late 1980s (see Fleming, Manson, & Bergeisen, in this volume, for a more complete discussion of federal programs for American Indian and Alaska Native adolescents).

The Office of Refugee Resettlement has several programs that serve thousands of adolescents. For example, between 1979 and 1989, there were more than 8,500 new enrollees in the Unaccompanied Minor Refugee Program. In addition, the Transition Program for Refugee Children provides funds for the special educational needs of refugee children and adolescents (U.S. Department of Health and Human Services, Family Support Administration, Office of Refugee Resettlement, 1989).

U.S. DEPARTMENT OF EDUCATION

In 1989, the U.S. Department of Education had a budget of approximately $22 billion and was responsible for 187 programs spanning six different offices (U.S. Department of Education, 1989). It is impossible to determine total expenditures on adolescents, because most U.S. Department of Education funds are distributed to state and local educational agencies that determine their own priorities.

Schools can play a role in either exacerbating or ameliorating the considerable number of health problems adolescents bring with them every day (U.S. Congress, Office of Technology Assessment, 1991b). As illustrated in the DHHS HSHC effort, policymakers interested in improving adolescent health are increasingly turning to the schools as a potential site and source of intervention (Carnegie Corporation of New York, 1989; Dryfoos, 1994; National Commission on the Role of the School and the Community in Improving Adolescent Health, 1990; U.S. Congress, Office of Technology Assessment, 1994). The U.S. Department of Education and DHHS show signs of working together to make the schools both healthier institutions and sites for providing health education and services, although no one discounts how difficult such a task might be (U.S. Department of Health and Human Services, 1993). Congress has recently encouraged Department of Education involvement in school health by providing for an Office of Comprehensive School Health Education.

In addition to its potential role in helping implement school health programs, the Department of Education is responsible for various education and training programs, some of which are specifically intended to help children and adolescents who are socioeconomically disadvantaged or from ethnic-minority groups. The well-demonstrated association between levels of educational completion and health status suggests that these programs can also help enhance the health of Americans in adolescence and later in life. The Department of Education also administers the provisions of the Drug Free Schools and Communities Act (Public Law 99-570 and subsequent amendments) and the Safe and Drug Free Schools and Communities Act (Public Law 103-382), the largest federal program addressing drug abuse prevention, with $598 million in appropriations in fiscal year 1993 (U.S. Congress, Office of Technology Assessment, 1994). The educational *research* program of perhaps most direct potential relevance to ethnic-minority and poor adolescents may be the National Institute on the Education of At-Risk Students, which the Department of Education was directed to form as a result of the Goals 2000: Educate America legislation of March 1994.

The education and training programs administered by the Department of Education include $8 billion (in 1995) in grant programs authorized by Title I and administered by the Office of the Assistant Secretary for Elementary and Secondary Education (U.S. Congress, Library of Congress, Congressional Research Service, 1989a). The programs are designed to meet the educational needs of educationally disadvantaged children from prekindergarten through secondary school (i.e., children performing below their appropriate grade level, children of migrant workers, children with physical disabilities, and neglected or delinquent children under state care). A 1988 law (Public Law 100-297) providing funds for compensatory education for secondary school students lacking basic skills and at risk of dropping out of school was particularly significant for low-income adolescents because Title I services have historically been focused on pupils enrolled in kindergarten through grade six. More recently, the Improving America's Schools Act of 1994 (Public Law 103-382) authorized grants to state education agencies to improve the education of young people at high risk of school dropout because they are involved in the juvenile-justice system, pregnant, or parenting. The 1994 law also authorized the provision of health and social services if those services could be expected to improve the adolescents' educational achievement and reduce the risk of dropping out. In general, Public Law 103-382 continuously emphasized the need to focus services on minority and other students likely to be underserved by the education system.

U.S. DEPARTMENT OF AGRICULTURE

The U.S. Department of Agriculture (USDA) administers a wide range of programs related to farms, nutrition, food, hunger, rural development, and the environment. Several USDA food assistance programs can potentially help poor adolescents meet their nutritional needs, including the Food Stamp Program, the National School Lunch and Breakfast Programs, and the Special Supplemental Food Program for Women, Infants, and Children (WIC). The USDA also funds and administers 4-H, a program that may be particularly useful to poor adolescents living in rural areas, and the USDA's Extension Service has focused on developing an agenda to better serve youth at risk (U.S. Department of Agriculture, Extension Service, 1989).

The USDA's Food and Nutrition Service also administers a food distribution program for low-income Indians living on or near reservations (U.S. Department of Agriculture, Food and Nutrition Service, 1989). Participating agencies receive monthly distributions of food from local warehouses. How many Indian adolescents benefit from this program is not known. However, because many American Indians are at high risk for obesity, diabetes, and other problems that may be affected by diet, the negative effects of the types of high-fat commodities made available through the food distribution program may outweigh any potential benefit (U.S. Congress, Office of Technology Assessment, 1991c).

U.S. DEPARTMENT OF JUSTICE

The Office of Juvenile Justice and Delinquency Prevention (OJJDP) in the U.S. Department of Justice focuses on problems related to delinquency among adolescents in general rather than among any particular group of minority adolescents.

However, OJJDP has funded several research projects on minorities in the juvenile-justice system to determine the extent to which processing decisions are influenced by the ethnic background of the adolescent offender (see Taylor & Katz, in this volume). The OJJDP has also provided funding for Proyecto Esperanza, a project implemented by the National Coalition of Hispanic Health and Human Services Organizations (COSSMHO), whose goal is to assess family strengthening and crisis intervention programs for Hispanic families and to design model programs to prevent child abuse and reduce the incidence of running away within Hispanic families (Kumpfer, 1989).

Legislation in 1992 directed the OJJDP to improve coordination among federal, state, and local agencies (including schools and recreation facilities), to emphasize community-based programs and services, and to take those initiatives that would help adolescents in racial and ethnic groups disproportionately likely to become involved with the juvenile-justice system (cf., Fleming, Manson, & Bergeisen; Katz & Taylor, in this volume). Through the OJJDP, the Office of Justice Program in the U.S. Department of Justice is working with Columbia University's Center on Addiction and Substance Abuse to help six cities rescue their high-risk preadolescents from the interrelated threats of poverty and drugs through the Strategic Intervention for High-Risk Youth Program, which serves a coordinating function (U.S. Department of Health and Human Services, n.d.).

U.S. DEPARTMENT OF HOUSING AND URBAN DEVELOPMENT

The U.S. Department of Housing and Urban Development (HUD) did not respond to OTA's 1989–1990 survey because it had no relevant programs. Since that survey, however, Congress has directed HUD to support midnight-basketball programs, and, most recently, training and partnership grant assistance, in public and assisted housing (Public Law 103-227), but it did not appropriate funds for such studies..

U.S. DEPARTMENT OF LABOR

The U.S. Department of Labor (DOL) has responsibility for fostering U.S. workers' welfare, improving working conditions, and promoting opportunities for employment. Within DOL, the Employment and Training Administration (ETA) is the agency most directly supporting activities affecting adolescents. In program year 1989, funding for adolescents and young adults ages 14 and older was estimated to account for 58% ($2.2 billion) of the ETA budget. The ETA administers programs for economically disadvantaged youth under Titles II-A (training grants), II-B (summer youth employment), II-C (year-round youth training services), IV-B (Job Corps) of the 1982 Job Training Partnership Act, as amended, and the School-to-Work Opportunities Act (Public Law 103-239) targeting ethnic-minority and poor adolescents.

CORPORATION FOR NATIONAL AND COMMUNITY SERVICE (FORMERLY ACTION)

The Corporation for National and Community Service is an independent (non-cabinet) agency formed in May 1944 that administers several federal domestic volunteer service programs providing human services to disadvantaged, poor, and elderly Americans, as well as opportunities for national and community service and national service educational awards.

ACTION's Office of Domestic Operations had sponsored a number of efforts that affected adolescents as volunteers or as beneficiaries (ACTION. 1989). These programs included adult-volunteer, youth-serving programs such as the Foster Grandparent Program and programs engaging adolescents as volunteers, such as the Student Community Service Program.

In fiscal year 1988, the Foster Grandparent Program served about 70,000 young people, including about 25,500 ages 6 through 12 and 15,400 ages 13 through 20. Typically, the youths served by the program are at risk of drug or alcohol use, are in the delinquent detention system, are pregnant or parenting, or are mentally, physically, or emotionally disabled. Also in fiscal year 1988, 244 Volunteers in Service to America projects focused on youth. As of 31 August 1989, fifteen VISTA projects involving sixty-six volunteers were focusing on juvenile health, including the prevention of adolescent pregnancy, substance abuse, suicide, and violence.

The Student Community Service Program, begun in 1987, funded projects that enable high school and college students to work as volunteers to help eliminate poverty-related problems. As of 1 October 1989, ACTION was funding 121 Student Community Service projects; the estimated budget for the Student Community Service Program was $893,000 in fiscal year 1990. In 1988, an estimated 28,000 students provided more than

850,000 hours of community service in various settings, such as Head Start programs, juvenile diversion programs, shelters, and soup kitchens.

ACTION estimated that its fiscal year 1990 budget request for adolescents was about $16 million. In contrast, a 1994 Senate Appropriations Committee report recommended a budget of $610 million for the Corporation for National and Community Service (U.S. Congress, Senate, 1994). At least $55 million of the amount recommended by the Senate would be directly relevant to children and adolescents from kindergarten through twelfth grade as part of the Learn and Serve America programs that are integrated with school curricula.

Conclusions

Many U.S. executive branch agencies and legislative committees have jurisdiction over programs related to adolescent health and related issues. On the basis of reports from federal agencies, OTA estimated that in fiscal year 1989 the federal government spent at least $12 billion on adolescent health, broadly defined. The bulk of the federal funds is spent on services for economically disadvantaged adolescents (e.g., $3,322 million for Medicaid; $4,000 million for Chapter 1 and other elementary and secondary education purposes; $7.1 million for the school-lunch program). Relatively few dollars are spent on so-called discretionary purposes such as basic research and innovative demonstration programs. The OTA analysis of federal policy related to adolescents and other reports of the late 1980s and early 1990s concluded that federal efforts related to adolescent development and health had been dismally inadequate and often shortsighted and that poor and ethnic-minority adolescents are likely to suffer the most from inattention (Feldman & Elliott, 1990; Irwin & Millstein, 1987; National Academy of Sciences, 1989).

There has been considerable improvement since the release of the OTA and other documents on adolescent health (e.g., the ADD HEALTH study; support for and evaluation of school-based health services; the Minority Youth Service Initiative; national service initiatives directed at elementary- and school-age children and adolescents). At a rather basic level, the fact that services to ethnic-minority youth are identifiable in a recent federal report on prevention activities suggests that more attention is being paid to these adolescents' needs at the federal level (U.S. Department of Health and Human Services, n.d.). However, OTA's analysis, much of which was summarized and updated in this chapter, continues to suggest several shortcomings at the federal level, both related to adolescents generally and to poor and ethnic-minority adolescents in particular.

No executive administration has fully responded to directives from Congress to address issues of fragmentation, inappropriate focus, and lack of visibility for adolescent health issues. Although there are now several actual or proposed focal points for coordination (the Adolescent Health Branch in the HRSA's MCHB, integration of school and health between the Department of Education and DHHS, collaboration between NICHD and OMH, and several PHS interagency working groups), a proposal to create an office of adolescent health where there was an AFL program was not supported by Congress or AFL, and there is still no central locus for a strong federal role in addressing adolescent health issues. For example, the Adolescent Health Branch in HRSA's MCHB has no authority cutting across even the myriad DHHS programs.

The OTA speculated that a central locus for adolescent issues could take many forms, from a new cabinet-level federal agency, to an agency within DHHS, to an interagency, interdepartmental coordinating body of some type (U.S. Congress, Office of Technology Assessment, 1991a). The mission of such an office would be to see that the nation had a coherent youth and adolescent policy. For example, the research agenda of the executive branch might be much improved by establishing a permanent council or councils to provide ongoing advice to federal agencies on research directions in adolescent health. Such a group could invigorate federal activities in data collection related to adolescent health by publishing periodic reports on the health status of U.S. adolescents. Such reports could include information on a comprehensive range of health status measures, utilization of the range of health services, providers, and settings likely to be used by adolescents, the availability and utilization of recreational facilities and outlets, volunteer and paid work activities, and other environmental risk and protective factors (e.g., family structure, abuse, neglect). Congress could frame a request for such data in such a way that health-related findings for specific age, gender, ethnic, income, regional, and residential groups are highlighted.

It may not be easy to take comprehensive, coordinated, strong action on adolescent health issues, which cut across so many agencies and interest groups and touch so many social hot buttons—such as whether federal assistance should be targeted (e.g., to ethnic minorities or the poor) or universal (e.g., Skocpol, 1992) and the appropriate lines between individual and government, parental and societal, responsibilities. No matter which programmatic approach Congress decides to take—or not take—a guiding principle underlying any policy should be the importance of providing a prolonged sympathetic and supportive environment for all adolescents, regardless of socioeconomic status, ethnicity, or residence. Such a change in policy orientation is essential to help adolescents face a crucial turning point in their lives and may also be essential to the future well-being of the nation (U.S. Congress, Office of Technology Assessment, 1991a).

References

ACTION. (1989). [Response to 1989 Office of Technology Assessment questionnaire regarding adolescent health initiatives.] Washington DC: Author.

American Psychological Association. (1994, May/June). Adolescent health study funded. *Psychological Science Agenda, 7* (3), 5.

Bergeisen, L. (1989). *Physical health of Indian adolescents—Draft.* (Available from U.S. Congress, Office of Technology Assessment, Washington DC)

Bowles, J., & Robinson, W. (1989). PHS grants for minority group HIV infection education and prevention efforts. *Public Health Reports, 104,* 552–559.

Carnegie Corporation of New York. Carnegie Council on Adolescent Development. Task Force on Education of Young Adolescents. (1989). *Turning points: Preparing American youth for the 21st century.* Washington DC: Author.

Cross, T., Bazron, B., Dennis, D., & Isaacs, M. R. (1989). *Towards a culturally competent system of care: A monograph on effective services for minority children who are severely emotionally disturbed.* Washington DC: CASSP Technical Assistance Center, Georgetown University Child Development Center.

Dryfoos, J. (1994). *Full-service schools: A revolution in health and social services for children, youth, and families.* San Francisco: Jossey-Bass.

Family Planning Perspectives. (1991). Documents: U.S. Supreme Court considers new Title X regulations. *Family Planning Perspectives, 23,* 38–40.

Feldman, S. S., & Elliott, G. (Eds.) (1990). *At the threshold: The developing adolesFeldman, S. S., & Elliott, G. (Eds.). (1990). At the threshold: The developing adolescent.* Cambridge: Harvard University Press.

Gittler, J. D., Quigley-Rick, M., & Saks, M. J. (1990). *Adolescent health care decision-making: The law and public policy.* (Contract paper). (Available from Carnegie Council on Adolescent Development and Carnegie Corporation of New York, New York)

Holden, C. (1991). New center to study therapies and ethnicity. *Science, 251,* 748.

Hutchins, V., & Walch, C. (1989). Meeting minority health needs through special MCH projects. *Public Health Reports, 104,* 621–626.

Irwin, C. E., Jr., & Millstein, S. (1987). Biopsychosocial correlates of risk-taking behaviors during adolescence. *Journal of Adolescent Health Care, 7,* 825–935.

Isaacs, M. R., & Benjamin, M. P. (1991, December) *Towards a culturally competent system of care. Volume 2: Programs which utilize culturally competent principles.* Washington DC: CASSP Technical Assistance Center, Center for Child Health and Mental Health Policy, Georgetown University Child Development Center.

Kumpfer, K. (1989). *Office of juvenile justice and delinquency prevention: Effective parenting strategies for high-risk youth and families: Phase one assessment report.* (Research Report No. 3). Salt Lake City: Social Research Institute, University of Utah.

Miike, L. (1989, December) *Health and related services for Native Hawaiian adolescents.* (Contract paper). (NTIS No. PB91-154 385/AS)

Morgan, D. (1995, August 3). "Family planning funds restored." *Washington Post,* p. A1.

National Academy of Sciences. Institute of Medicine. National Research Council. (1989). *Social policy for children and families: Creating an agenda.* Washington DC: National Academy Press.

National Center for Education in Maternal and Child Health. (1993a). *Adolescent health: Abstracts of active projects, FY 1992 and FY 1993.* Arlington VA: Author.

National Center for Education in Maternal and Child Health. (1993b, May). *Maternal and Child Health Bureau adolescent health activities.* McLean VA: Author.

National Commission on the Role of the School and the Community in Improving Adolescent Health. National Association of State Boards of Education, & American Medical Association. (1990). *Code blue: Uniting for healthier youth.* Alexandria VA: National Association of State Boards of Education.

Office of the Federal Register, National Archives and Records Administration. (1993). *The United States government manual 1993/1994.* Washington DC: U.S. Government Printing Office.

Ooms, T., & Herendeen, T. O. (1990, July 20). *Evolving state policies on teen pregnancy and parenthood: What more can the feds do to help?: Background briefing report.* (Available from the Family Impact Seminar of the American Association for Marriage and Family Therapy, Research and Education Foundation, Washington DC)

Payne, K., & Ugarte, C. (1989). The Office of Minority Health Resource Center:

Impacting on health-related disparities among minority populations. *Health Education, 20* (5), 6–8.

Skocpol, T. (1992). *Protecting soldiers and mothers: The politics of social provision in the United States, 1870–1920*. Cambridge: Harvard University Press.

Spencer, M., & Dornbusch, S. (1990.) Minority youth in America. In S. S. Feldman & G. Elliott (Eds.), *At the threshold: The developing adolescent* (pp. 123–146). Cambridge: Harvard University Press.

U.S. Congress. General Accounting Office. (1990, June). *Minority health: Information on activities of HHS's Office of Minority Health.* (GAO/HRD-90-140FS). Washington DC: Author.

U.S. Congress. Library of Congress. Congressional Research Service. (1989a, January). *Education for disadvantaged children: Major themes in the 1988 reauthorization of Chapter 1*. Washington DC: Author.

U.S. Congress. Library of Congress. Congressional Research Service. (1989b, March 20). *Teenage pregnancy: Issues and legislation*. Washington DC: Author.

U.S. Congress. Library of Congress. Congressional Research Service. (1992, December). *Federal programs for children and their families*. Washington DC: Author.

U.S. Congress. Office of Technology Assessment. (1991a, April). *Adolescent health. Volume 1: Summary and policy options* (OTA-H-468). Washington DC: U.S. Government Printing Office.

U.S. Congress. Office of Technology Assessment. (1991b, November). *Adolescent health. Volume 2: Background and the effectiveness of selected prevention and treatment services* (OTA-H-466). Washington DC: U.S. Government Printing Office.

U.S. Congress. Office of Technology Assessment. (1991c, June). *Adolescent health. Volume 3: Crosscutting issues in the delivery of health and related services* (OTA-H-467). Washington DC: U.S. Government Printing Office.

U.S. Congress. Office of Technology Assessment. (1994). *Technologies for understanding and preventing substance abuse and addiction*. Washington DC: U.S. Government Printing Office.

U.S. Congress. Senate Committee on Appropriations. (1994, July 14). *Report 103-311* [Report to accompany H.R. 4624, a bill making appropriations for the Departments of Veterans Affairs and Housing and Urban Development, and for sundry independent agencies]. Washington DC: Author.

U.S. Department of Agriculture. Extension Service. (1989, May). *Youth: The American agenda: A report of the National Initiative Task Force on Youth at Risk*. Washington DC: Author.

U.S. Department of Agriculture. Food and Nutrition Service. (1989). [Response to 1989 Office of Technology Assessment questionnaire regarding adolescent health initiatives]. Washington DC: Author.

U.S. Department of Education. (1989). [Response to 1989 Office of Technology Assessment questionnaire regarding adolescent health initiatives]. Washington DC: Author.

U.S. Department of Health and Human Services. (1993). *Healthy People 2000 progress review: Adolescents and young adults* (briefing book). Washington DC: Author.

U.S. Department of Health and Human Services. (n.d.). *Prevention '93/'94*. Washington DC: Author.

U.S. Department of Health and Human Services. Family Support Administration. Office of Refugee Resettlement. (1989). *Refugee Resettlement Program: Report to Congress*. Washington DC: U.S. Government Printing Office.

U.S. Department of Health and Human Services. Office of Human Development Services. (1989). [Response to 1989 Office of Technology Assessment questionnaire regarding adolescent health initiatives]. Washington DC: Author.

U.S. Department of Health and Human Services. Office of the Secretary. Secretary's Task Force on Black and Minority Health. (1985, August). *Report of the Secretary's Task Force on Black and Minority Health*. Washington DC: U.S. Government Printing Office.

U.S. Department of Health and Human Services. Public Health Service. Alcohol, Drug Abuse, and Mental Health Administration. Office for Substance Abuse Prevention. (1990). *Breaking new ground for youth at risk: Program summaries*. (DHHS Pub. No.89-1658). Washington DC: U.S. Government Printing Office.

U.S. Department of Health and Human Services. Public Health Service. Health Resources and Services Administration. (1989). [Response to 1989 Office of Technology Assessment questionnaire regarding adolescent health initiatives]. Washington DC: Author.

U.S. Department of Health and Human Services. Public Health Service. Health Resources and Services Administration. (1994, June). *Request for Proposal No. HRSA 240-OA-27 (4)*. Rockville MD: Author.

U.S. Department of Health and Human Services. Public Health Service. Health Resources and Services Administration. Bureau of Health Care Delivery and Assistance. (1989). [Response to 1989 Office of Technology Assessment questionnaire regarding adolescent health initiatives]. Washington DC: Author.

U.S. Department of Health and Human Services. Public Health Service. National Institutes of Health. National Institute on Child Health and Human Development. (1993). *NIH research targeting the needs of adolescents*. Bethesda MD: Author.

U.S. Department of Health and Human Services. Public Health Service. National Institutes of Health. National Institute of Nursing Research. (1993). *Health promotion for older children and adolescents: A report of the NINR priority expert panel on health promotion*. Bethesda MD: Author.

U.S. Department of Health and Human Services. Public Health Service. Office of the Assistant Secretary for Health. Office of Minority Health. (1990). *Minority Community Health Coalition demonstration grants*. Washington DC: Author.

U.S. Executive Office of the President. Office of Management and Budget. (1994). *Budget for the United States government for fiscal year 1995*. Washington DC: U.S. Government Printing Office.

Yudkowsky, B., Cartland, J., & Flint, S. (1990). Pediatrician participation in Medicaid: 1978 to 1989. *Pediatrics, 85,* 567–577.

8

Policy Recommendations for Ethnic-Minority Adolescent Health Issues: A Paradigm Shift

Nancy Lois Ruth Anderson and Marjorie Kagawa-Singer

The present effort on behalf of the youth of our country can be described fairly generously as one of unconcern (Williams & Miller, 1992). A brief overview of some of the statistics reported in this volume shows:

• Adolescents make up the single largest population segment in the United States—31 million;
• 8.3 million youth live below the poverty line;
• one in ten youth in poverty live in inner-city areas that are pervasively poor:
  • greater than 40% are non-Hispanic Whites
  • greater than one third still belong to two-parent families;
• one third of all adolescents in poor and near-poor families in the United States are unprotected by health insurance. The United States and South Africa are the only industrial nations that do not have a national health-insurance plan.

Despite the fact that the federal government spends more than $11.3 billion annually on programs to benefit youth (see Kemp and Dougherty, in this volume), a young Black man in Harlem has a shorter life expectancy than a young Black man in Ethiopia because of poor health conditions and high-risk behaviors (McCord & Freeman, 1990).

We believe that the general lack of responsiveness to the problems of minority youth can be partially attributed to a dominant monocultural perspective. Therefore, we explore here an alternative multicultural paradigm. Such a paradigm offers greater flexibility and a richer theoretical rationale with which to develop more effective, culturally responsive programs and research agendas.

Barriers to Quality Health-Care Delivery for Ethnic Teenagers

In the United States today, funding for social and health programs tends to be guided by the reality of "limited good" in funding for social and health programs. Amid seemingly unlimited technical ability, we paradoxically have increasingly unmet needs for basic primary health services such as immunizations, health screening, preventive care, mental-health services, and prenatal care for adolescents. Four major barriers to adequate health care for our youth emerge from the issues covered by the authors in this volume: difficulty with access to health care, a quick-fix public mentality, fragmentation of services, and a lack of cultural responsiveness in the programs and by care providers.

Access. As described by Allen and Mitchell (in this volume), poverty is one of the greatest single health risk factors. Two million adolescents have no health insurance; those youth who are insured are often underinsured. Even those who have apparently adequate coverage are too often unable to obtain care because either facilities are not geographically accessible or there are too few practitioners who accept Medicaid coverage to provide the care.

Short-Term Solutions. Short public attention spans support a single-problem focus with quick effects; this approach, while politically popular, hampers the long-term, intensive efforts required to make a difference. In the last few years, for example, much attention, money, and professional and volunteer effort have been expended on the problems of AIDS and homelessness. Although the problems are growing, the public seems to be disenchanted, less interested, and turning toward the search for more responsive causes. Similarly, since teenage health and social problems appear recalcitrant to single-focus solutions, early public interest seems to be turning into frustration and resignation.

Fragmentation of Available Services. Many agencies and federal programs are directed toward youth welfare, but these agencies compete for the limited supply of both trained personnel and funds and even duplicate each other's efforts. Consolidation and coordination could vastly improve service delivery. Molly Coye, former director of the California State Department of Health Services, has described how a reconfigured public health-care system requiring relatively minor funding to improve data systems would simplify the complicated bureaucratic web that is supposed to function as a safety net for the indigent and the underinsured.

The problems delineated in earlier chapters are multifactorial and socially contextual. Effective solutions must consider the entire ecosystem within which such behavior occurs as suggested in the chapter by Katz and Taylor. A holistic approach to understanding, preventing, and treating high-risk behavior is needed rather than the more typical fragmented, symptom-management approach. The design of Hawaii's Native Hawaiian youth program described by Miike (in this volume) exemplifies this approach.

Cultural Responsiveness. Adolescents from all cultures go through comparable physical changes and learn similar developmental tasks. Considerable variation exists, however, between and within cultural groups in defining acceptable group parameters for adolescent behavior, degrees of responsibility that must be assumed, and desired adult roles. To be effective these cultural differences must be incorporated into the design of programs for adolescent health and in the training and practice of adolescent health practitioners.

Cultural responsiveness requires that adolescents be treated differently to achieve fair and equitable outcomes (Konner, 1991); a single design is insufficient. More accurate knowledge about the nature and influence of culture on adolescent behavior would enable us to provide more effective intervention programs.

Adolescence, Culture, and Ethnicity

Culture provides a blueprint that guides our behavior, helps us to determine our values and beliefs, and enables us to evaluate and make sense of our world (Herberg, 1989). Culture passes from the generation of our ancestors to future generations, linking past, present, and future through this heritage (Anderson, 1992a). In this context, *ethnicity* refers to the traditions, values, perceptions, and practices we share through identification with a group of individuals who have in common a geographic and/or racial origin, a language and dialect, a religious faith, or some combination of these (Spector, 1991). These definitions of culture and ethnicity provide the basis for the subsequent discussion of adolescents who live within two cultures: that of their ethnic group and that of the dominant Western society.

Adolescence is the transition between childhood and adulthood. In many cultures special rites and rituals signal the onset of puberty. These initiation ceremonies mark the beginning of specialized education concerning gender roles, community rules, and adult responsibilities of the group. Initiation rites are not universal, however. Among many ethnic groups, the interval of adolescence holds no special significance apart from growing up and taking on adult roles (Stone & Church, 1975).

In the modern Western world, we have come to expect teenagers to challenge authority and test rules. In mainstream Western society most people do manage to make their way through the perilous teen years and become productive adults. For adolescents who live outside the mainstream as a result of poverty, homelessness, or ethnic-minority status, however, these years often present additional challenges accompanied by deprivation, loneliness, alienation, and hopelessness.

ADOLESCENT GROWTH AND DEVELOPMENT FROM
THE WESTERN PERSPECTIVE

The adolescent passage is marked by the biologically universal rapid physical growth of primary and secondary sexual organs, corresponding psychosexual development, and body image changes. This stage is characterized by a pervasive search for identity, expressed in risk taking, limit-challenging behaviors, and increased reliance on peer-group relationships (Elliott & Feldman, 1990; Schuster & Ashburn, 1980). Western society expects adolescents to adapt to a new body image and new gender roles, become independent financially and emotionally and acquire its adult values and ethics (Erikson, 1968; Havighurst, 1953; Mercer, 1979).

These expectations, and the psychological events associated with adolescent passage, "are not a necessary counterpart of the physical changes of puberty" but rather "a product of an increased delay in assumption of adult responsibilities" in complex mainstream Western society (Stone & Church, 1975, p. 8). Many of these same expectations exist in many less technologically complex societies, but they are condensed into a shorter time frame. In the industrialized world, with its long educational process required for work preparation, the adolescent passage may last for eight or more years. This fact has led many investigators to subdivide adolescence into early, middle, and late substages, spanning from as early as age 10 to as late as the middle 20s, each with differing characteristics (Elliott & Feldman, 1990). This long interval between the onset of biological maturity and the full assumption of adult roles is relatively recent even in modern Western society (Stone & Church, 1975).

INFLUENCE OF CULTURE ON ADOLESCENT GROWTH AND DEVELOPMENT

Families are the primary source of training in a culture's values and way of life to develop self-confidence and trust. Most ethnic groups, however, define *family* more broadly than the nuclear or extended family definition recognized as the "legitimate" structure in mainstream U.S. culture. For minority teenagers, family tends to be more inclusive and constitutes a major source of strength.

In many traditional Native American tribes, for example, the family constellation was structurally open and included clusters of other family groups in several different households like a small village (Red Horse et al., 1978). Whenever a problem occurred for one family member, a natural network was already in place to help the individual cope with it. If a parent was unable to serve as a caretaker, grandparents, aunts and uncles, and cousins were readily available to carry out the parenting role (Red Horse et al., 1978). Adolescents who had difficulties with their biological parents could seek shelter and advice from other trusted adults. Furthermore, the adolescents themselves often engaged in necessary and valued work within the community.

Compadrazgo, a Filipino coparent ritual kinship or compadre system, is another example of extended ethnic family systems (Affonso, 1978). The network of parents, godparents, and family friends in many Filipino communities is reinforced by shared rituals, gatherings, and celebrations that bring members together. The compadre system provides adolescents with additional caring adults in their communal network and develops expanded kinship ties and reciprocal obligations which help foster adolescent self-esteem (Affonso, 1978). Affonso described her participation in this system: "As I grew older, especially during high school, I became resentful of my responsibilities to the chickens. I would always have to rush home after school to be sure the chickens were fed. When we had after-school functions, I would run home, feed the chickens, and then run back to school" (Affonso, 1978, p.129). Nevertheless, Affonso appreciated the praise she received and recognized how fulfillment of the needed childhood roles contributed positively to her development.

As Sandra Cisneros has described such roles, "Salvador whose name the teacher cannot remember, is a boy who is no one's friend, runs along somewhere in that vague direction where homes are the color of bad weather, lives behind a raw wood doorway, shakes the sleepy brothers awake, ties their shoes, combs their hair with water . . . Helps his mama, who is busy with the business of the baby" (Cisneros, 1991, p.10). Like Salvador, teenagers are responsible for taking care of younger siblings and do work essential for the economic and social welfare of the family, which contributes to adolescent growth and development (Mead, 1928; Whiting & Whiting, 1975). A sense of community, important work to do, and reciprocal networks of obligation and support all aid healthy transitions from childhood to adulthood.

Initiation rituals associated with puberty also help tie the adolescent to the community. Even when these ceremonies involve pain and humiliation, adolescents anticipate them positively because of the associated community solidarity and assigned status as an adult.

The extended network of ethnic-community ties provides both advantages and disadvantages for teenagers. The Filipino and American Indian kinship systems, and that of Native Hawaiians as described by Miike in this volume, demonstrate some of the advantages. Through consanguinal (blood), affinal (in-law), and compadre (coparent) ties, adolescents receive gifts, advice, love, and concern from many adults besides their biological parents. Thus, they have more alternatives and a greater variety of adult role-modeling behaviors. These advantages are continued after immigration if members of an ethnic group are able to retain their group identity.

The primary disadvantages for ethnic teenagers are discrimination, poverty, isolation, alienation associated with racism, and related sequelae such as mental and physical illness. The words of a 17-year-old Southern Cheyenne boy express the crisis of identity he feels between his native culture and the world he must live in: "I think differently at home. My people don't think like the white man. For us, things happen when other things happen. I think in two different ways: the Indian way and the white man's way. Sometimes—like when I think that maybe so many bad things have happened to my family because my mother angered a witch—it's like I use white man's thinking, but it's about Indian things. So I wonder just who am I?" (Allen, 1973, p.374).

Many aspects of culture can be lost in the process of acculturation into mainstream society. These losses leave holes in the fabric of everyday family and group life that are poorly filled by the dominant culture. Adolescents become confused if they feel they must choose one or the other. While the implicit message is to relinquish one's ethnic identity and take on that of the standard White culture, complete assimilation is often prevented by discrimination. In a pluralistic society, bi- or multiculturalism should be recognized and fostered for the strengths and options it provides.

The acculturation process in many ethnic families is initiated first among the children and teenagers who must adapt to the expectations and mores of the dominant culture expressed in school rules and in their interactions with teachers and peers. These children often have to lead double lives: one in school and one at home. They frequently speak different languages, eat different foods, and interact with others in radically different ways at home and at school.

American Indian children who were forced to attend federal boarding schools, for example, were forbidden to speak their native language or practice their indigenous religion at these schools. On their return home, these children often had to face ritual cleansing to "rid them of their white man's ways" (Allen, 1973, p.372). The more fully these Plains Indians students learned "White man's ways," the more likely they were to assume an identity that was seen by their tribe as negative and disloyal to their heritage. Thus, they straddled two cultures and were comfortable or welcome in neither, risking "dead-end acculturation without assimilation" (Allen, 1973, pp.372–373).

Other ethnic adolescents face similar dilemmas. Their discomfort or alienation may lead to emotional despair, alcohol and drug use, and even suicide to dull the confusion and pain. These teenagers may need assistance to recognize that the choices are not to live in one culture or another but rather to develop an ability to function effectively in many cultural worlds.

They can learn to be culturally as well as linguistically fluent and enrich their identities as they gain a sense of self-worth through these increased skills.

THEORETICAL APPROACHES TO ADOLESCENCE

Policies that have guided development of the health-care infrastructure in the United States are largely based on beliefs and premises originating from restrictive or outdated theories that fail to value the importance of ethnic identity.

Psychoanalytic Theory. Early psychological theories of adolescence were greatly influenced by Freud, whose psychoanalytic theory posited that the adolescent passage (the genital stage, begun at puberty) revived the issues of infantile sexuality and eventually resolved the Oedipus complex (Blos, 1980; Deutsch, 1944; Freud, 1905/1953). Adolescent problems were thought to arise from an inability to find socially acceptable outlets for their sexual drives (Rappaport, 1972).

Developmental and Social Theories. Many clinicians and theorists found that classical psychoanalytic theory did not adequately explain many aspects of teenage behavior. Consequently, subsequent theories moved in directions more developmental or sociological.

Erikson (1968), in a more psychosocial version of psychoanalytic theory, suggested that healthy teenagers successfully pass through adolescence when they achieve a solid sense of identity, of who they are in relationship to their world. Levine (1980) claimed that two basic psychosocial needs dominate adolescence: the need for a belief system, an intense belief in something relevant, and the need for a sense of belonging, a sense of community.

Jessor and Jessor (1977) developed a model to explain adolescent problem behavior using an approach that linked social, developmental, and personality psychology. This theory was grounded in the belief that problem behavior is an expression of social-psychological relationships between three systems: the personality system, the perceived environment system, and the behavior system. According to this model, behavior is connected with "its conceptual determinants in the personality and the perceived environment," and problem behavior is viewed as an expression of "opposition to conventional society" (Jessor & Jessor, 1977, p. 37).

Social-learning theories posited that teenagers learned socially acceptable and age-appropriate behaviors through a modeling process (Bandura, 1977). Mastering these tasks results in the recognition of personal efficacy (Bandura, 1977). Schinke and Gilchrist (1984) extrapolated from this theoretical base to propose that life-skills counseling that helped young people solve problems increased their sense of social and personal competence. Their active intervention approach incorporated six components: age-appropriate and topic-relevant information; problem-solving strategies and practice; development of the inner voice for positive self-instruction; practice with adaptive coping strategies; choice of effective personal verbal and nonverbal communication style; and building of an interpersonal support system (Schinke, Botvin, & Orlandi, 1991; Schinke & Gilchrist, 1984). Many current programs for adolescents are based on this approach.

This progression of theories demonstrates an evolution of thinking that focuses on an instructional path to guide adolescent growth and development. Such models reflect the desire of mainstream society to actively predict, direct, and control adolescent behavior. Power and control remain in the hands of adult experts; the positive contributions of diverse ethnic and cultural identity are not actively considered. Instead, ethnic identity is implicitly viewed as a deficiency or barrier by the dominant culture (see Taylor & Katz, in this volume). Underlying these developmental models is the belief that expert knowledge and power can be used to guide and direct the behavior of others.

Theory of Power Utilization. The seminal questions in a multicultural society are these: Who holds the power? How is it used? How is it viewed by those who are manipulated by the agents enacting the power? French and Raven (1968) defined power in terms of influence exerted on an individual by a social agent to effect behavior, attitude, or value change. An agent whose goal is to influence change in another person employs one or more of five power bases: reward power, or positive reinforcement; coercive power, usually associated with the threat of punishment; legitimate power, given as a behavioral prescription through the culture by a trusted agent; expert power, through the specialized knowledge of the agent; and referent power, through identification with a respected agent (French & Raven, 1968).

We argue that the consistent use of coercive power, through the exercise of force and punishment, and expert power, through the use of knowledgeable agents, has dominated the approach to treatment and prevention of adolescent problems in Western society. Referent power, which depends more on mutual respect and participation, is often ignored. The results of emphasis on coercive- and expert-power tactics that exclude minorities from participation in mainstream policy decision making are reported in preceding chapters.

Culture-based Models. Dissatisfaction with the limitations of theories based on the biomedical model has led anthropologists who study health-related phenomena to explore more holistic and culturally sensitive theoretical constructs. Ecological models that combine cultural, environmental, and biological concerns became central to the development of medical anthropology (Alland, 1966; McElroy, 1990; Wellin, 1978; Wiley, 1992).

As McElroy pointed out: "To be truly integrative in design means more than doing a little ethnography as a supplement to collecting biological data. . . . Integrative thinking means *rethinking* basic assumptions, asking new questions, challenging existing theories, and forging new methods. It means moving flexibly between biological and cultural realms in an era that rewards specialization" (McElroy, 1990, p.244). McElroy described a biocultural model that integrates research methods to focus equally on sociocultural, biological, and environmental data collection and analysis, thus providing a much broader perspective on human health-related behavior.

Kleinman (1980) provided another such approach. The individual is at the center of his models of general and clinical reality. He argued that the health-care delivery system is a system of symbolic meanings that evolve within social institutions and patterns of interpersonal interactions. "In every culture, illness and the responses to it, individuals experiencing it and treating it, and the social institutions relating to it are all systematically interconnected. The totality of these interrelationships is the health care system" (Kleinman, 1980, p.24).

The nature of these interrelationships is depicted in Figure 8.1. As can be seen, the *person* is located at the center of three concentric spheres of psychological and biological processes. These processes incorporate both *psychological reality* (the inner world of the individual) and *biological reality* (the infrastructure of the organism) (Kleinman, 1980). The *social world* surrounding the person comprises the person's perceived social reality, in-

Figure 8.1. Types of reality

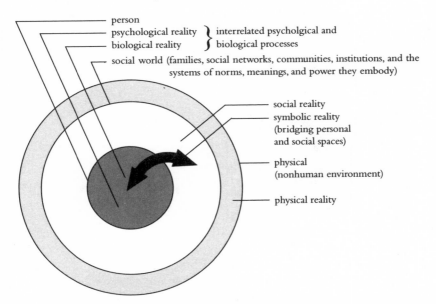

person
psychological reality } interrelated psycholgical and
biological reality   } biological processes
social world (families, social networks, communities, institutions, and the
        systems of norms, meanings, and power they embody)

social reality
symbolic reality
(bridging personal
and social spaces)

physical
(nonhuman environment)

physical reality

Source: Arthur Kleinman. (1980). *Patients and healers in the context of culture: An exploration of the borderland between anthropology, medicine and psychiatry* (p. 106). Berkeley: University of California Press.

cluding families, social networks, communities, institutions, and systems of norms and meanings, as well as the power they generate. Kleinman identified the transactional world as the place where everyday life occurs and social roles receive definition through negotiation and performance. Transactions between the person and the social world occur through the use of recognized symbols or *symbolic reality*, which forms a bridge linking social reality with the psychological and biological reality within the person. The outermost sphere is the *physical environment*, which incorporates *physical reality*. Physical reality refers to the material structures and spaces of the nonhuman, physical environment (Kleinman, 1980).

Kleinman (1980) used a second set of three concentric spheres to explain illness and illness behaviors as depicted in Figure 8.2. The *sick person*, and his or her *psychobiological reality of symptoms*, is at the core surrounded by the *clinical world*. Within this world, *clinical reality* refers to the beliefs, expectations, norms, and behaviors associated with illness and the delivery of health care. Communicative transactions occurring in the clinical world

Figure 8.2. Clinical reality

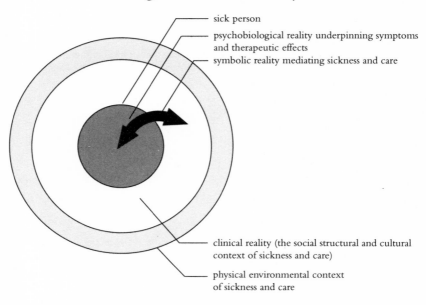

sick person

psychobiological reality underpinning symptoms and therapeutic effects

symbolic reality mediating sickness and care

clinical reality (the social structural and cultural context of sickness and care)

physical environmental context of sickness and care

Source: Arthur Kleinman. (1980). *Patients and healers in the context of culture: An exploration of the borderland between anthropology, medicine and psychiatry* (p. 106). Berkeley: University of California Press.

constitute symbolic reality and are primarily involved with the mediation of sickness and health care. In this model, the outermost sphere is the *physical environmental context of sickness and care* (Kleinman, 1980).

The Application of Culture Theory. Within biocultural models, such as Kleinman's, the teenager as an individual and as a member of an ethnic group is given a legitimate social position. The perspective of teenagers becomes a central focus. If health practitioners were to view culture and ethnic-group identity as an asset, they could assess adolescent behavior from a positive perspective within the teenage social world; this approach could reduce the need for coercive power and could channel expert power toward more effective collaborative efforts between teenagers and clinicians.

A holistic assessment begins with the teenager's physical and psychological development (Kleinman, 1980). This biological reality of the adolescent's personal inner world interacts with his or her social world, and its significance is filtered through ethnic and cultural symbols.

THE INFLUENCE OF ETHNICITY ON SOCIAL SUPPORT
IN ADOLESCENCE

Ethnic kinship patterns and belief systems influence the behaviors of individuals and families during the process of acculturation into the larger society around them, and the manner in which ethnic members seek and give help is often rooted in traditional kinship structure and values, as illustrated by many of the authors in this volume. Social support must be understood within this context (Jacobson, 1987), which implies that the particular meaning of support for both the giver and the receiver and the context in which help is sought and provided may vary from one group to another.

As an example, Sudarkasa (1988) traced African American kinship relationships back to cultural patterns of early African family structure organized around a core consisting of "adult siblings of the same sex or by larger same-sex segments of patri- or matrilineages" (p. 31). In-marrying spouses and children from conjugal relationships formed the outer group. All lived together in a communal compound, and wives and husbands often lived in separate dwellings within the compound. Children, frequently grouped according to same-gender and age mates, were socialized within the extended family. Adolescents had available numerous trusted adults for nurturance and support.

Thus, while Black family structure has changed considerably from the cultural patterns of early African families, "the persistence of some features of African family organization among contemporary Black American families has been documented" (Sudarkasa, 1988, p. 39). During the intervals of slavery and subsequent emancipation, when African families were purposefully separated, the need for ethnic support networks was even greater and resulted in many creative variations of these traditional kinship systems. Stack (1974), for example, documented successful networks of material and emotional support shared among sisters and brothers, as well as extended networks that included neighbors and friends. Although this reliance on the consanguinal rather than the conjugal family unit has been interpreted as unstable by some investigators, others (e.g., Sudarkasa, 1988) regard it as a reflection of kinship traditions and a source of strength.

Regardless of the quality and availability of support at home, teenagers also look to peers for emotional support. Peer-group support may be found at school, within the neighborhood, and in youth gangs. Peer-group support may be beneficial when freely sought and received or detrimental when it involves coercive power or control.

Teenagers may willingly join a neighborhood youth gang, knowing they must adhere to gang control and surveillance, because the economic and group solidarity benefits outweigh the perceived price. Often the coercive aspects of gang membership become more prominent later. According to Horowitz (1990), there are two primary explanations as to why teenagers join gangs: they make a conscious and rational decision to join (Sanchez-Jankowski, 1991) or are pushed into gangs by their poverty or minority group status (Vigil, 1988). A somewhat different perspective emphasizing the need to escape was offered to one of the authors by a teenager in juvenile detention: "It started out when I was 11 . . . (when I tried) to get away from my problems . . . (by) eating a lot and (drinking) alcohol. I didn't have family love . . . and then time progressed and before I knew it . . . I started gangbanging . . . then I started smoking . . . and experimenting with drugs and stuff . . . (because of the homies) . . . then I ended up (on the street) being a prostitute. You know, it's just like the domino effect . . . it just keeps on going" (Anderson, 1992b).

Thus, social support can be either a positive force for adaptation or a negative force leading to trouble and pain. Regardless of the nature of the support network and the individual teenager's inner strengths, the social, political, and economic policies of the dominant culture still remain.

Overview of Critical Issues for Ethnic Adolescents
HEALTH-RELATED POLITICAL AND ECONOMIC ISSUES

Each of the preceding chapters identifies social, political, and economic forces that are determining factors for the future of today's teenagers. Both material and cultural changes have contributed to increasing problems for U.S. adolescents (Fuchs & Reklis, 1992). Among the indicators of these problems are the nearly tripled rates of suicide and homicide, increased rates of births to unwed mothers, rising poverty rates, tripled rates of child abuse, and lowered proficiency test scores of junior and senior high school students. The number of married women in the labor force has also more than tripled in the last thirty years (Fuchs & Reklis, 1992). This trend, coupled with the paucity of affordable quality day care, leaves many children and adolescents unattended and unguided during the day.

The impact of teenage pregnancy is felt by all but is likely to be particularly difficult for minority teenagers and their families. Most researchers agree that the consequences of adolescent pregnancy render teenage mothers at increased risk for educational, health, social, and economic problems in the future (Furstenberg, 1976; Hayes, 1987). A recent study reported that 37% of homeless families receiving public assistance in New York City had a baby born before the mother reached 18 (Weitzman, 1989).

Interestingly, the outlook for teenage parents may not be as bleak as these statistics imply. For some ethnic groups, pregnancy at a young age carries no stigma. Continued love and material and emotional support enable some teenage mothers to overcome barriers and manage to become both successful parents and individuals (Furstenberg, Brooks-Gunn, & Morgan, 1987).

Policy Gaps

We submit that the current myopic focus on short-term solutions to the complex problems of adolescent health has a high probability of failure in the long term. Funding priorities are currently directed toward single problems (e.g., teen substance abuse, adolescent pregnancy, and juvenile delinquency). The lack of significant improvement in these problems produces frustration and despair on the part of funding agencies. The result is that poverty and ethnicity are often used as both explanations for problems and justification for failure to intervene with comprehensive prevention and treatment programs. The approach to adolescent high-risk behaviors then becomes punitive (Reuter, 1992). Reuter suggested, for example, that the war on drugs be less "hawk"-like and more "owl"-like by placing major emphasis on prevention and treatment rather than only on tough enforcement (Reuter, 1992).

The present punitive approaches to adolescent high-risk behavior have not led to solutions and may have exacerbated the problems. As suggested by the present authors and the Office of Technology Assessment report on adolescent health (1991a, 1991b, 1991c), longer-range efforts directed to prevention and treatment would have a greater likelihood of saving future tax dollars and lives.

TARGETING CHILDHOOD HEALTH

High-risk adolescent acting-out behaviors do not suddenly emerge with puberty; their antecedents can be seen in childhood. For example, child abuse has been frequently implicated as a primary cause of subsequent runaway, substance-abuse, teen pregnancy, and other high-risk adolescent behaviors (Boyer & Fine, 1992; Dodge, Bates, & Pettit, 1990; Morris & Bihan, 1991; Polit, White, & Morton, 1990).

The term "child abuse" is generally used to cover a broad age span and range of behaviors—it refers to the physical, emotional, and sexual abuse of youths from infancy through adolescence. Placement of youth in foster care has been a major intervention strategy for abusive families. Issues that arise with foster care, however, present another example where programmatic gaps exist for both these young people and their parents (Hochstadt et al., 1987; Schor, 1989). First, there are too few qualified foster parents. Lack of adequate reimbursement for foster parents and problem complexity explain a large part of the paucity of good quality foster homes (Schor, 1989). Failed placements may result in further abuse and trauma (Molin, 1988; Schor, 1989; Stepleton, 1987; Woolf, 1990). Difficulties with placement are often intensified for adolescents since they often have a longer history in foster or institutional care. Many teenagers respond to continued foster care by running away and thereby become entangled in the juvenile-justice system. And the cycle continues.

RECOMMENDATIONS FOR EARLY INTERVENTION

Early intervention is needed for ethnic families who need assistance in dealing with social, economic, and physical- or mental-health problems and to prevent abuse and homelessness before they occur. The primary target for programmatic and funding efforts should center on establishing a "family friendly" atmosphere in which families can learn coping strategies and develop knowledge about childrens' growth and development.

Prevention of health problems and the empowerment of ethnic teenagers begin with ensuring equal access to educational and employment opportunities. Although strides have been made, we are still a long way from achieving this goal.

A logical starting point would be to provide adequate child care for all working families. This achievable primary intervention strategy would help to avoid some of the family crises that result when overstressed working parents must rely on inadequate or nonexistent care for their children. Impoverished ethnic-minority families currently have the fewest-available quality choices for day care (Hayes, Palmer, & Zaslow, 1990).

Examples of Effective Programs

Effective programs are cost-effective, eliminate or delay the onset of adolescent high-risk behaviors, prevent subsequent illness, and reduce the negative economic and social consequences of illness for teenagers and their families. Several such programs are worth noting here.

PREVENTION EFFORTS

A well-funded exemplary program is Homebuilders, a project initiated in Tacoma, Washington, that has proven that intensive coordinated help given to families at the time of crisis can prevent foster-care placement (Schorr & Schorr, 1989). Homebuilders provided in-home intensive family therapy and assisted families in repairing their own problems and regaining control of their own lives. While the initial amount expended ($2,600) for a single family may seem high, it is cheaper than long-term foster care ($3,600), group care ($19,500), or psychiatric hospitalization ($67,500). One year after completion of the Homebuilders program, 90% of those who would have been put in foster homes were still living at home (Schorr & Schorr, 1989). The question is why we continue to resort to costly tertiary interventions when primary prevention programs have proven their cost-effectiveness and their ability to save priceless human lives.

Recent focus on the prevention of adolescent high-risk behavior has resulted in many programs that target preteen and early-adolescent age groups. One such program, Postponing Sexual Involvement, was initiated in Atlanta in 1983 by the Henry W. Grady Memorial Hospital (Howard & McCabe, 1990). This program targeted 13–15-year-old boys and girls (many low-income minority students) with a public-school-based family-planning program. Older teenagers taught the younger ones how to resist peer pressure and postpone sexual involvement.

The results were extremely successful. As the authors noted: "By the end of eighth grade, students who had not participated in the program were as much as five times more likely to have begun having sex than were those who had the program" (Howard & McCabe, 1990). The state of California initiated a statewide program in April 1992 based on this curriculum (Education Now and Babies Later, or Project ENABL).

Another primary prevention program targets preteens (ages 10–13) and their parents. This program, Reaching Adolescents and Parents (RAP), was developed by the American Red Cross and is offered in community- and school-based settings. It includes active participation by parents during some segments of the course. Program goals include teaching about puberty and human reproduction, increasing decision-making and communication skills, facilitating family communication, and delaying the onset of sexual activity among the preteen program participants (American Red Cross, 1990).

Similar projects, such as DARE (Drug Abuse Resistance Education), target pre- and early-teen groups with programs designed to prevent adolescent substance abuse and gang involvement. One such community-based program, Making the Right Connections (MTRC), sponsored by the Sisters of St. Joseph Ministerial Services, reaches out to children in grades two through eight with an intensive six-week cooperative summer program. Started during the summer of 1989, this program has been successfully conducted in South Central Los Angeles for four years. The curriculum includes conflict resolution, community building, values clarification, gang and drug awareness, and multicultural art activities.

School-based clinics have been effective in numerous states across the country (Dryfoos, 1988; Kirby, Waszak, & Ziegler, 1991). Some school-based clinics have also included a special focus on pregnancy prevention and the prevention of substance abuse, HIV/AIDS, or sexually transmitted diseases. Overall evaluation of the effectiveness of school-based clinics is complicated by the fact that program services, organizational structure, and data-collection methods vary widely among programs (Dryfoos, 1988; Kirby et al., 1991).

The Mysteries Program, begun at a number of middle and secondary schools in the Southern California area, is a program designed to develop character, community, and spirit. It allows students to express personal authenticity and independence and to function cooperatively in the face of competing needs.

The program format is based on the Native American Indian council for problem resolution. Problems presented always relate to adolescence. Three basic rules are followed: speak only in turn, speak briefly, and speak from the heart. The participants are also taught the art of listening, skills for conflict resolution, stress management, group problem solving, and effective communication. Workshops for teachers are being held annually. The program, designed eight years ago, is now conducted regularly in schools all over the globe (Kessler, 1990).

Researchers identified several specific components from a variety of programs that have a positive impact on teenage participants. These components include life-skills training (Schinke & Gilchrist, 1984; Schinke et

234

al., 1991) peer support and counseling (Rind, 1992), mentoring (Hamburg, 1992; Levine, 1992), and habilitation (providing conditions which encourage learning and responsible behaviors [Morrison, 1990]). Traditional service delivery, self-esteem building, values clarification, and decision-making experience have also been found useful. A number of mediating factors influence program outcomes, including comprehensiveness of the program, a sense of control, a stable family life, intent and realistic potential for attending college, and economic self-sufficiency (Furstenberg et al., 1987; Horwitz et al., 1991; Miller et al., 1992).

Recommended Future Policy

HOLISTIC, CONTEXTUALLY BASED PROGRAMS

The approach advocated in this chapter for policy, program development, and research is an adolescent-centered paradigm that places adolescent development within a social, political, economic, and cultural context and builds on available strengths. Because of its emphasis on prevention, this paradigm, though rarely utilized, would be both psychologically effective and more cost-effective. Cultural responsiveness may also be of particular significance for ethnic teenagers, and its important elements are discussed in the concluding parts of this chapter.

CULTURALLY RESPONSIVE PROGRAMS

Sue (1991) has recommended that culturally responsive programs have four elements: inservice training about culture and health for psychotherapists; more recruiting and training of ethnic health-care practitioners; the establishment of specific ethnic services; and the creation of new, effective therapies and delivery systems.

There is ample evidence that African Americans, American Indians, Asian Pacific Americans, and Latino Americans are severely underrepresented among psychologists, nurses, and physicians (Howard et al., 1986). We need to know how the ethnic match between therapist and client affects outcomes.

Similarly, the outcomes of care in service centers designed and staffed by ethnic members have not been evaluated or compared with mainstream service centers. We do know, however, that, compared with population percentages, Asian Pacific Americans and Latinos have lower use rates for physical- and mental-health services and African Americans have higher use rates than the national average (Sue, 1977). Paradoxically, even with this higher utilization by African Americans, their health outcomes were as poor or worse than those of the Asian or Latino groups. Services that are effective in countering such negative results remain to be provided on a large-scale basis.

EMPOWERMENT FOR TEENAGERS AND FAMILIES: PLANNING FOR THE FUTURE

While many good programs have been established, they are often the victim of government and private-agency budgetary axes. Downsizing, restructuring, and streamlining for greater efficiency make sense when resources are limited, but they must be balanced by helping people intervene actively on their own behalf.

Planning interventions that start with and build from the strengths of an individual is an often-recommended cost-effective strategy that is rarely employed. The fundamental shift in approaching adolescent health problems must begin by recasting adolescence in a more positive, less negative light. Such a change would encourage care providers and policymakers to explore alternative intervention strategies using less punitive measures. When teenagers run away from a court-ordered placement, for instance, this behavior is legally classified as a status offense with attendant negative labeling and outcomes. Running away, however, could alternatively be viewed as an adaptive response to abuse and may be the only recourse open to a teenager. This changed perspective would lead to a much different intervention strategy.

Ethnicity often provides a basis for within-group solidarity as well as a history and a blueprint for behavioral expectations. Even when adolescents turn more to peers than parents for social and emotional contact, they still appreciate and frequently restate family values. When teenagers in juvenile detention, for example, were asked how decisions about pregnancies are made, they responded with such statements as "In my family we keep our babies and take care of them" (Anderson, 1990). These teenagers fully expected that their pregnancy would be a family matter and that the family would provide the solutions.

Adolescents throughout the country are demonstrating that they have the courage, strength, and fortitude to rise above the incredible odds of poverty, violence, abuse, abandonment, discrimination, and failed family resources, and to survive in an alien world. Mainstream and corporate

America may not always approve of the nature of some routes to adolescent survival, but survival it is. If we want them to survive in more acceptable ways, then we must provide the resources for them to do so. Even more important, we must find ways to use their survival skills to good purpose and help teens direct their innate strengths toward productive and effective outcomes.

One of our best resources for helping adolescents is the power of the person. Teenagers look to parents and other significant adults for guidance. The teenagers Anderson works with in juvenile detention are searching for adult role models they can respect, those who offer honest respect to them, listen, and understand. During focus group discussions about decisions concerning substance use or abuse among detained teenagers, conversation often centers on prevention and treatment programs (Anderson, 1992b). The teenagers frequently commented that good programs were led by adults who "really understand and listen and try to help us" (Anderson, 1992b) and that "adults say we should give them respect (as their elders), but they don't respect us; they treat us like criminals, they call us criminals" (Anderson, 1990).

For many reasons, it is difficult for many adults to really listen to and respect teenagers. In many cities and villages, alienated teenagers have become the adversaries of frightened adults. Fear has clouded our vision.

Programs serving adolescents need to increase input from teenagers themselves. When agencies or organizations attempt to institute change based on their own perceptions without eliciting the teenagers' perceptions and goals and involving them in the design and implementation of the program, behavior change rarely happens. Instead, the long-range impact may result in increased mistrust for mainstream efforts by adolescents.

Referent power, according to French and Raven (1968), is based on the identification the individual has with the agent of social change and on the quality of their relationship. Respecting relationships are built through active involvement and participation where the individual and the change agent are equal partners in a joint endeavor.

Teenagers thrive, learn, grow, and develop new skills and understanding when they are given the opportunity to participate in planning and enacting new programs. The reason peer counselors are such effective change agents is because of their shared worldview and team approach. Adolescents can and should be trusted to work effectively on their own behalf, al-

237

though they are typically not consulted by policymakers. We can no longer afford to continue making this costly error. Teenagers and their families deserve to participate in charting their future.

We can also no longer procrastinate in initiating much-needed policy and programmatic changes. The physical- and mental-health needs of minority adolescents are urgent. As Konner (1991) poignantly noted:

Adolescence [is] a tumultuous phase of childhood with a sense of paradox and hope. . . . Adolescents are facing the fact that we will not take care of them always, and they know that taking care of themselves will involve hard work and hard choices. Understandably, they resent this. Yet somehow, most children sail the rough seas of adolescence without running aground or going under. With a steady wind behind them in the form of a nurturing childhood, and some adult help in charting a safe course through the teenage years, only a small minority should founder. But this sea is unforgiving and the dangers are grave ones; we are losing far too many as it is and we need to become more serious about preventing those losses (p. 389).

References

Affonso, D. D. (1978). The Filipino American. In A. L. Clark (Ed.), *Culture/childbearing/health professionals* (pp. 128–153). Philadelphia: Davis.

Alland, A. (1966). Medical anthropology and the study of biological and cultural adaptation. *American Anthropologist, 68,* 40–51.

Allen, J. R. (1973). The Indian adolescent. *American Journal of Orthopsychiatry, 43,* 368–375.

American Red Cross. (1990). *Reaching adolescents and parents (RAP).* American National Red Cross. Washington DC.

Anderson, N. L. R. (1990). Pregnancy resolution decisions in juvenile detention. *Archives of Psychiatric Nursing, 4,* 325–331.

Anderson, N. L. R. (1992a). Transcultural nursing. *Kitasato International Journal of Nursing Science, 1,* 47–55.

Anderson, N. L. R. (1992b, September). *Resolutions and risk taking in juvenile detention.* Invited presentation at the Clinical Research with Stigmatized Populations conference, Brentwood Division Department of Veterans Affairs, Los Angeles.

Bandura, A. (1977). *Social learning theory.* Englewood Cliffs NJ: Prentice-Hall.

Blos, P. (1980). Modifications in the classical psychoanalytical model of adolescence. *Adolescent Psychiatry, 7,* 6–25.

Boyer, D., & Fine, D. (1992). Sexual abuse as a factor in adolescent pregnancy and child maltreatment. *Family Planning Perspectives, 24* (4), 4–19.

Cisneros, S. (1991). *Woman hollering creek*. New York: Random House.

Deutsch, H. (1944). *The psychology of women: A psychoanalytic interpretation* (Vol. 1). New York: Gruen & Stratton.

Dodge, K. A., Bates, J. E., & Pettit, G. S. (1990). Mechanisms in the cycle of violence. *Science, 250,* 1678–1683.

Dryfoos, J. G. (1988). School-based health clinics: Three years of experience. *Family Planning Perspectives, 20,* 193–200.

Elliott, G. R, & Feldman, S. S. (1990). Capturing the adolescent experience. In S. S. Feldman & G. R. Elliott (Eds.), *At the threshold: The developing adolescent* (pp. 1–13). Cambridge: Harvard University Press.

Erikson, E. H. (1968). *Identity: Youth and crisis*. New York: Norton.

French, J. R. P., & Raven, B. (1968). The bases of social power. In D. Cartwright & A. Zander (Eds.), *Group dynamics: Research and theory* (3d ed., pp. 259–269). New York: Harper & Row.

Freud, S. (1953). Three essays on the theory of sexuality (the transformations of puberty). In J. Strachey (Ed.), *Standard Edition* (Vol. 7, pp. 125–245). London: Hogarth, 1953. (Originally published 1905).

Fuchs, V. R., & Reklis, D. M. (1992). America's children: Economic perspectives and policy options. *Science, 255,* 41–46.

Furstenberg, F. F. (1976). *Unplanned parenthood: The social consequences of teenage childbearing*. New York: Free Press.

Furstenberg, F. F., Brooks-Gunn, J., & Morgan, S. P. (1987). Adolescent mothers and their children in later life. *Family Planning Perspectives, 19,* 142–151.

Hamburg, D. A. (1992). Interventions for education and health in very poor communities. *Proceedings of the American Philosophical Society, 136,* 333–346.

Havighurst, R. J. (1953). *Human development and education*. New York: Logmans, Green.

Hayes, C. D. (Ed.). (1987). *Risking the future: Adolescent sexuality, pregnancy, and childbearing* (Vol. 1). Washington DC: National Academy Press.

Hayes, C. D., Palmer, J. L., & Zaslow, M. J. (Eds.). (1990). *Who cares for America's children: Child care policy for the 1990s*. Washington DC: National Academy Press.

Herberg, P. (1989). Theoretical foundations of transcultural nursing. In J. S. Boyle & M. M. Andrews (Eds.), *Transcultural concepts in nursing care* (pp. 3–65). Glenview IL: Little Brown.

Hochstadt, N. J., Jaudes, P. K., Zimo, D. A., & Schachter, J. (1987). The medical and psychosocial needs of children entering foster care. *Child Abuse and Neglect*, *11*, 53–62.

Horowitz, R. (1990). Sociological perspective on gangs: Conflicting definitions and concepts. In C. R. Huff (Ed.), *Gangs in America* (pp. 37–54). Newbury Park CA: Sage.

Horwitz, S., Klerman, L. V., Kuo, H. S, & Jekel, J. F. (1991). School-age mothers: Predictors of long-term educational and economic outcomes. *Pediatrics*, *87*, 862–868.

Howard, A., Pion, G. M., Gottfredson, G. D., Falttau, P. E., Oskamp, S., Pafafflin, S. M., Bray, D. W., & Burstein, A. G. (1986). The changing face of American psychology: A report from the Committee on Employment and Human Services. *American Psychologist*, *41*, 1311–1327.

Howard, M., & McCabe, J. B. (1990). Helping teenagers postpone sexual involvement. *Family Planning Perspectives*, *22*, 21–26.

Jacobson, D. (1987). The cultural context of social support and support networks. *Medical Anthropology Quarterly*, *1*, 42–62.

Jessor, R., & Jessor, S. L. (1977). *Problem behavior and psychosocial development: A longitudinal study of youth.* New York: Academic Press.

Kessler, S. (1990). The mysteries program. *Holistic Education Review*, *3* (4), 10–19.

Kirby, D., Waszak, C., & Ziegler, J. (1991). Six school-based clinics: Their reproductive health services and impact on sexual behavior. *Family Planning Perspectives*, *23* (1), 6–16.

Kleinman, A. (1980). *Patients and healers in the context of culture.* Berkeley: University of California Press.

Konner, M. (1991). *Childhood.* Boston: Little, Brown.

Levine, B. (1992, February 16). For the love of a child. *Los Angeles Times*, pp. E1, E7.

Levine, S. V. (1980). Adolescents, believing, and belonging. *Adolescent Psychiatry*, *7*, 41–51.

McCord, C., & Freeman, H. P. (1990). Excess mortality in Harlem. *New England Journal of Medicine*, *332*, 173–177.

McElroy, A. (1990). Biocultural models in studies of human health and adaptation. *Medical Anthropology Quarterly*, *4*, 243–265.

Mead, M. (1928). *Coming of age in Samoa.* New York: Morrow.

Mercer, R. T. (1979). *Perspectives on adolescent health care.* New York: Lippincott.

Miller, B. C., Card, J. J., Paikoff, R. L., & Peterson, J. L. (1992). *Preventing adolescent pregnancy.* Newbury Park CA: Sage.

Molin, R. (1988). Treatment of children in foster care: Issues of collaboration. *Child Abuse and Neglect*, *12*, 241–250.

Morris, P. A., & Bihan, S. M. (1991). The prevalence of children with a history of sexual abuse hospitalized in the psychiatric setting. *Child and Adolescent Psychiatric and Mental Health Nursing*, 4, 49–54.

Morrison, M. A. (1990). Addiction in adolescents [Special issue]. *Western Journal of Medicine*, 152, 543–546.

Polit, D. F., White, C. M., & Morton, T. D. (1990). Child sexual abuse and premarital intercourse among high-risk adolescents. *Journal of Adolescent Health Care*, 11, 231–234.

Rappaport, L. (1972). *Personality development: The chronology of experience*. Glenview IL: Scott Foreman.

Red Horse, J. G., Lewis, R., Feit, M., & Decker, J. (1978). Family behavior of urban American Indians. *Social Casework*, 69, 67–72.

Reuter, P. (1992). Hawks ascendant: The punitive trend of American drug policy. *Daedalus*, 121, 15–52.

Rind, P. (1992). Peer support to keep teenagers alive and well. *Family Planning Perspectives*, 24, 36–40.

Sanchez-Jankowski, M. (1991). *Islands in the street: Gangs in American urban society*. Berkeley: University of California Press.

Schinke, S. P., Botvin, G. J., & Orlandi, M. A. (1991). *Substance abuse in children and adolescents: Evaluation and intervention*. Newbury Park CA: Sage.

Schinke, S. P., & Gilchrist, L. D. (1984). *Life skills counseling with adolescents*. Baltimore: University Park Press.

Schor, E. L. (1989). Foster care. *Pediatrics in Review*, 10, 209–215.

Schorr, L. B., & Schorr, D. (1989). *Within our reach*. New York: Doubleday.

Schuster, C. S., & Ashburn, S. S. (1980). *The process of human development*. Boston: Little, Brown.

Spector, R. E. (1991). *Cultural diversity in health and illness* (3d. ed.). Norwalk CT: Appleton & Lange.

Stack, C. B. (1974). *All our kin*. New York: Harper & Row.

Stepleton, S. S. (1987, March–April). Specialized foster care: Families as treatment resources. *Children Today*, 27–31.

Stone, L. J., & Church, J. (1975). Adolescence as a cultural invention. In A. H. Esman (Ed.), *The psychology of adolescence, essential readings* (pp. 7–11). New York: International University Press.

Sudarkasa, N. (1988). Interpreting the African heritage in Afro-American family organization. In H. P. McAdoo (Ed.), *Black families* (2d ed.) (pp. 27–43). Newbury Park CA: Sage Publications.

Sue, S. (1977). Community mental health services to minority groups: Some optimism, some pessimism. *American Psychologist, 32*, 616–624.

Sue, S. (1991). Ethnicity and mental health: Research and policy issues. Paper presented at the SPSSI Presidential Address, San Francisco, article forthcoming in *Journal of Social Issues*.

U.S. Congress. Office of Technology Assessment. (1991a). *Adolescent health: Volume 1. Summary and policy options.* (OTA-H-468). Washington DC: U.S. Government Printing Office.

U.S. Congress. Office of Technology Assessment. (1991b). *Adolescent health: Volume 2. Background and the effectiveness of selected prevention and treatment services.* (OTA-H-466). Washington DC: U.S. Government Printing Office.

U.S. Congress. Office of Technology Assessment. (1991c). *Adolescent health: Volume 3. Crosscutting issues in the delivery of health and related services.* (OTA-H-467). Washington DC: U.S. Government Printing Office.

Vigil, J. D. (1988). *Barrio gangs: Street life and identity in Southern California.* Austin: University of Texas Press.

Weitzman, B. C. (1989). Pregnancy and childbirth: Risk factors for homelessness? *Family Planning Perspectives, 21* (4), 175–183.

Wellin, E. (1978). Theoretical orientations in medical anthropology: Change and continuity over the past half-century. In M. H. Logan & E. E. Hunt, Jr. (Eds.), *Health and the human condition* (pp. 23–30). Belmont CA: Wadsworth.

Whiting, B. B., & Whiting, J. W. M. (1975). *Children in six cultures: A psychocultural analysis.* Cambridge: Harvard University Press.

Wiley, A. S. (1992). Adaptation and the biocultural paradigm in medical anthropology: A critical review. *Medical Anthropology Quarterly, 6*, 216–236.

Williams, B. C., & Miller, C. A. (1992). Preventive health care for young children: Findings from a 10-country study and directions for United States policy. *Pediatrics, 89* (Suppl. 5), 981–998.

Woolf, G. D. B. (1990). An outlook for foster care in the United States. *Child Welfare, 69* (1), 75–81.

The Contributors

LaRue Allen is professor and chair in the Department of Applied Psychology at the New York University School of Education. She received her A.B. in social relations from Harvard University and her Ph.D. in psychology from Yale University. Her research interests include prevention of psychopathology in high-risk populations, the role of families in the development of ethnically diverse children, sociocultural influences (including gender and social class) on the development of social competence, and humor responsiveness as a measure of adaptive behavior.

Hortensia Amaro is professor of social and behavioral sciences in the School of Public Health at Boston University. She received her doctorate in development and social psychology in 1982 from the University of California at Los Angeles. She is founder and past president of the Latino Health Institute of Massachusetts and founder of the Multicultural AIDS Coalition and the National Hispanic Psychological Association. Her research has focused on epidemiological studies and community-based interventions for substance abuse and HIV among women and on Hispanic health issues.

Nancy Lois Ruth Anderson is associate professor at the UCLA School of Nursing and principal investigator for the School of Nursing Health Center, which serves a homeless population in Los Angeles at the Union Rescue Mission. An anthropologist and a nurse practitioner, she conducts her research and clinical practice with youth and their families in juvenile detention and community-based settings. Her research program and publications focus on adolescent risk behaviors.

Lois Bergeisen is currently a senior staff associate in the Division of Minority Health, Education, and Prevention at the Association of American Medical Colleges (AAMC). Before joining the AAMC, she was a contractor with the Office of Technology Assessment (OTA) on its adolescent health study. She also served as project director for the Minnesota Adolescent Health Survey and the Indian Adolescent Health Survey. Ms. Bergeisen has completed doctoral coursework in both sociology and health-services research at the University of Minnesota.

Richard Cervantes received his B.A. in business administration and psychology and M.A. and Ph.D. in clinical psychology from Oklahoma State University. Following his educational training, he was employed as a staff psychologist at the Didi Hirsch Community Mental Health Center in Culver City, California. From 1984 to 1989, he was an assistant research psychologist at the Spanish Speaking Mental Health Research Center at UCLA. From 1988 to 1990, he was assistant professor and coordinator of community/clinical track at the California School of Professional Psychology. Currently, he is assistant professor of clinical psychiatry and behavioral sciences at the University of Southern California Medical School.

Denise Dougherty was program director of the Education and Human Resources Program (EHR) at the U.S. Congress OTA. Before becoming program director, she was a senior associate and project director in OTA's Health Program. Her special interest is in the appropriate application of scientific research standards to the information used in public policy debates. She received a Ph.D. in social psychology from Boston University in 1987.

Candace M. Fleming (Kickapoo/Oneida/Cherokee) was raised on the Northern Cheyenne Reservation in southeastern Montana. She received a B.A. in psychology and music history from Wellesley College in 1973 and a Ph.D. in clinical psychology from the University of North Carolina at Chapel Hill in 1979. In 1987, she joined the staff of the National Center for American Indian and Alaska Native Mental Health Research as an Alcohol

Research Scholar. Since 1992, she has served as a codirector for the Healthy Nations Program, funded by the Robert Wood Johnson Foundation.

Marjorie Kagawa-Singer is a nurse and anthropologist and assistant professor in the School of Public Health and Asian American Studies Center at UCLA. She received her master's degree in nursing from UCLA School of Nursing and her master's and doctorate in anthropology from UCLA. She has published in various journals on a variety of issues in cross-cultural health care and multicultural issues in cancer care. She has also lectured extensively on the influence of culture on patient and family responses to chronic diseases as well as the dynamics involved in multicultural staff interactions.

Phyllis A. Katz received her Ph.D. from Yale University in clinical and developmental psychology. She has taught at New York University and City University of New York and is currently the director of the Institute for Research on Social Problems in Boulder, Colorado. Her research has focused on children's gender-role development and racial attitude acquisition. She is founding editor of *Sex Roles: A Journal of Research* and editor-elect of the *Journal of Social Issues*.

Kerry B. Kemp was managing editor at the U.S. Congress OTA. Before holding this position, she worked as an analyst or as a writer or editor on a wide range of OTA studies—including federal vaccine and immunization policies, young children's health, strategies for medical technology assessment, the commercialization of biotechnology, technology and handicapped people, Medicare's prospective payment system, life-sustaining technologies and elderly people, AIDS, osteoporosis, and adolescent health. She has also worked as a freelance writer and publications consultant. She was also the administrator of the National Rural Housing Coalition and worked as a writer and editor at Americans for Democratic Action. She has a B.A. in political sciences from Middlebury College.

Spero M. Manson (Pembina Chippewa) is professor, Department of Psychiatry, and director, National Center for American Indian and Alaska Native Mental Health Research, at the University of Colorado Health Sciences Center. He also serves as program codirector of the Robert Wood

Johnson Foundation's Healthy Nations Initiative, which assists Indian and Native communities in their struggle to reduce harm due to substance abuse. He received his Ph.D. in medical anthropology from the University of Minnesota in 1978.

Miriam Messinger has worked for the last eight years in the areas of youth and community health. She has been involved in research and program evaluation efforts on health issues and projects affecting young people. She has coordinated peer leadership and youth advocacy programs in Boston for youth of color and White youth and currently coordinates a statewide program in Massachusetts on the health promotion needs of lesbian, gay, and bisexual youth. She received her M.A. in public health from Boston University in 1955.

Lawrence Miike holds a degree in medicine from the University of California, San Francisco, and a law degree from the University of California, Los Angeles. He is currently director of the Department of Health, State of Hawaii. Based in Washington DC from 1972 to 1989 and subsequently in Hawaii, he has been involved in a broad array of both national- and state-level health-policy issues.

Christina M. Mitchell is a research psychologist at the National Center for American Indian and Alaska Native Mental Health Research, University of Colorado Health Sciences Center and assistant professor of psychiatry, University of Colorado. Her areas of interest include adolescent development among ethnic-minority youth and culturally relevant and appropriate interventions to prevent mental disorder and promote well-being. She received her Ph.D. from Michigan State University.

Elena O. Nightingale is a scholar-in-residence at the National Research Council and the Institute of Medicine of the National Academy of Sciences, adjunct professor of pediatrics at Georgetown University, adjunct professor of pediatrics at George Washington University, and a lecturer in social medicine at Harvard University. She recently retired from her positions as special adviser to the president and senior program officer after eleven years with the Carnegie Corporation at New York. She received an A.B. degree in zoology from Barnard College, a Ph.D. in microbial genetics from Rockefeller University, and an M.D. from New York University School of Medicine.

Stanley Sue is professor of psychology and director of the National Research Center on Asian American Mental Health at UCLA. The center is funded by the National Institute of Mental Health to conduct research on Asian Americans. He received his B.S. degree from the University of Oregon and his Ph.D. from UCLA. For ten years, he was a faculty member at the University of Washington.

Ruby Takanishi has been executive director of the Carnegie Council on Adolescent Development, an operating program of the Carnegie Corporation of New York, since its inception in 1986. She previously served as director of the Office of Scientific Affairs for the American Psychological Association, first executive director of the Federation of Behavioral, Psychological, and Cognitive Sciences, the American Psychological Association's officer for children, youth, and families, and a legislative assistant in the U.S. Senate. Her research and policy interests center on child and adolescent development and their linkage to education and public policies for children, youth, and families. She was an American Association for the Advancement of Science–Society for Research on Child Development Congressional Science Fellow. She received her A.B. and Ph.D. degrees from Stanford University and an A.M. degree from the University of Michigan. She has held faculty positions at UCLA, Yale University, and Teachers College, Columbia University.

Dalmas A. Taylor received his B.A. in psychology from Western Reserve University in 1959, M.S. from Howard University in 1961, and Ph.D. from the University of Delaware in 1965. He also received a Certificate for Educational Management in 1980 from Harvard Business School. He has served as director of the Afro-American Studies Program at the University of Maryland, followed by positions as associate dean for research in the graduate school, assistant vice chancellor for academic affairs, and director of the graduate program in social psychology at the university. After completing a one-year position as Distinguished Fellow for Policy at the American Psychological Association, he was appointed provost at the University of Texas at Arlington.

Judith H. M. Vanderryn is currently on the psychology staff at the Denver Veterans' Affairs Medical Center, where she works in intensive inpatient treatment for veterans with severe posttraumatic stress disorder (PTSD). She is a past member of the cross-cultural training team at the University of Colorado, where she received her Ph.D. in 1993. Her research experience and interests focus on PTSD treatment, interventions to decrease bias and stereotyping, and the nature and development of racial identity among Whites.

Nolan Zane is associate professor in the Counseling/Clinical/School Psychology Program and Asian American Studies Program at the University of California, Santa Barbara. He also is coprincipal investigator of the National Research Center on Asian American Mental Health and currently serves as the leader of the center's research program on treatment process and outcomes. His research interests include the development and evaluation of culturally responsive treatments for Asian and other ethnic-minority clients, change mechanisms in treatment, program evaluation of substance-abuse and mental-health programs, and the cultural and physiological determinants of addictive behaviors among Asians. He received his Ph.D. from the University of Washington in 1987.

Author Index

Aase, J. M., 121, 139
Abbey, P., 24, 31
Aber, J. L., 3, 4, 31, 58, 74
Ackerson, L. M., 122, 136, 138
ACTION, 209, 212
Aday, L. A., 101, 105
Adler, N., 1, 26
Affonso, D. D., 221, 222, 238
Aguiar, M., 104, 105
Aiken, L., 14, 27
Alcohol, Drug, and Mental Health
  Administration, 144, 163
Aldwin, C. M., 1, 27
Alland, A., 226, 238
Allen, D. V., 46, 78
Allen, E. A., 38, 67, 68, 73
Allen, J. R., 223, 238
Allen, L., 3, 4, 10, 11, 27, 31, 192, 218
Allen, W. R., 77
Amaro, H., 9, 46, 83, 84, 87, 94, 95, 99,
  104, 105, 106, 115
American Academy of Pediatrics
  Committee on Adolescence, 7, 27
American Alliance for Health, 122
American Council on Education, 82, 106
American Indian Health Care Association,
  131, 137
American Psychiatric Association, 120
American Psychological Association, 197

American Red Cross, 234, 238
Andersen, R. M., 101, 105
Anderson, N. L. R., 219, 230, 236, 237, 238
Andrade, S. J., 99, 106
Aneshensel, C. S., 93, 106
Annalora, D. J., 125, 138
Apospori, E., 12, 34
Apssori, E., 97, 98, 115
Arroyo, W., 99, 106
Asian American Subpanel to the President's
  Commission on Mental Health, 161, 163
Asian/Pacific Task Force on High Blood
  Pressure Education and Control, 148, 163
Asian Week, 142, 163
Astone, N. M., 9, 18, 30
Attneave, C. L., 122, 137
Avant, R. F., 157, 166
Azzara, C. V., 6, 29

Bachman, J., 97, 110
Bachrach, C. A., 101, 111
Baisden, K., 90, 111
Baker, E., 98, 109
Baker, L. G., viii, x
Balance, M. F., 105, 106
Balentine, M., xv, xvi
Balka, E. B., 98, 106
Bandura, A., 225, 238
Bane, M. I., 2, 3, 27

Bang, K. M., 90, 106
Baron, A. E., 121, 122, 136, 138
Barringer, C., 119, 138
Barringer, H., 172, 185
Barrish, C., 101, 111
Bates, J. E., 231, 239
Bazron, B., 22, 28, 200, 212
Bean, F. D., 80, 106
Beauvais, F., 123, 137
Becerra, R. M., 93, 106
Bechtold, D. W., 120, 122, 127, 137, 139
Beckman, R., 93, 109
Beiser, M., 122, 137
Bell, R. M., 65, 74
Benjamin, M. P., 200, 213
Bennet, F. C., 119, 137
Benson, P., 4, 34
Berenson, G. S., 91, 115
Bergeisen, L., v, xix, xxvi, 46, 118, 119,
   120, 129, 137, 188, 205, 208, 212
Berkman, B., xxiii, xxvi
Beschner, G., 73
Betsey, C. L., 59, 77
Bettes, B. A., 98, 106
Biernoff, M. P., 127, 139
Bihan, S. M., 231, 241
Blendon, R., 14, 27
Blos, P., 224, 238
Blount, W. R., 12, 27
Blum, R. W., 2, 5, 7, 24, 27, 32, 118, 119,
   120, 137
Blumenthal, S., 7, 27
Boggiano, A. K., 49, 76
Bonner, J., xv, xvi
Botvin, G. J., 98, 106, 109, 225, 234, 241
Bower, B., 105, 115
Bowler, S., 94, 106
Bowles, J., 203, 212
Bowman-Terrell, M., 11, 12, 28
Boyce, T., 1, 26
Boyd, N., 66, 67, 73
Boyer, C. B., 9, 27, 95, 109
Boyer, D., 231, 239
Boykin, A. W., 58, 73
Boyle, G. J., xxiii, xxiv, xxvi
Bray, D. W., 235, 240

Brindis, C., 93, 94, 106
Brink, K. L., 13, 23, 34
Brisbane, F. L., 66, 67, 73
Britt, D., 10, 27
Brogan, D., 51, 76
Bromet, W., 11, 27
Bromley, S., viii, x
Bronfenbrenner, U., 40, 44, 73
Brook, J. S., 98, 106
Brookins, G. K., 77
Brooks-Gunn, J., 9, 25, 27, 231, 239
Brown, E. F., 126, 137
Brown, S. S., 44, 45, 74
Brown, T. R., 146, 163
Brunswick, A. F., 43, 56, 62, 73
Bryant, J., 75
Buggs, G., 203
Bureau of Census, U.S. See U.S. Bureau of
   Census
Burgos, W., 12, 28
Burhansstipanov, L., xxi, xxvi
Burnam, M. A., 102, 110
Burstein, A. G., 235, 240
Burt, M., 59, 77
Burton, R. V., 54, 73
Butler, J., 13, 27

Caetano, R., 100, 107
Califano, J. A., Jr., 56, 74
Campion, E., xxiii, xxvi
Cantor, P., 7, 27
Caplan, N., 147, 163
Caples, V., 4, 31
Card, J. J., 235, 240
Carnegie Commission, xxiii, xxvi
Carnegie Corporation, 70, 74, 205, 212
Carroll, M., 90, 106
Carter, J. H., 4, 33, 45, 46, 74
Carter-Pokras, O. D., 89, 90, 107
Cartland, J., 192, 216
Castro, F. G., 102, 108
Centers for Disease Control, 46, 52, 59, 62,
   74, 87, 88, 92, 93, 94, 95, 96, 101, 107,
   108, 118, 148, 149
Cervantes, R. C., 9, 46, 99, 102, 106, 108
Chamie, M., 19, 28

Chang, W., 153, 155, 163
Chan-Sew, S., 159, 163
Chapa, J., xiii, xvii, 81, 82, 83, 108
Chapman, J. M., 149, 164
Chavez, E. L., 98, 108
Chavez, G., 89, 107
Chesney, M. A., 1, 26
Chesney-Lind, M., ix, x
Cheung, F. M., 146, 155, 163, 165
Chew, T., 147, 148, 163
Children's Defense Fund, 42, 45, 74
Chitwood, D. D., 23, 28
Chitwood, J. S., 23, 28
Chung, R.-C. Y., xxii, xxvi
Church, J., 220, 221, 241
Cisneros, S., 222, 239
Clark, L., xv, xvi
Clark, P. I., 97, 110
Clinchy, B. M., 105, 106, 108
Cluz-Collins, M., 21, 30
Cochran, W., 62, 77
Cockerham, W. C., 123, 137
Coe, R., 15, 29
Coffman, G., 99, 106
Cohall, A. T., 95, 110
Cohen, D., 96, 110
Cohen, R. J., 23, 31
Cohen, S., 1, 26
Colp, C., 90, 108
Comer, J. P., 39, 74
Comstock, B., 16, 33
Connell, J. P., 58, 74
Conrad, D., 24, 29
Conway, G. A., 94, 113
Coombs, R. H., 11, 12, 28
Corin, E., 96, 113
Corwin, S., 125, 137
COSSMHO. See National Coalition of
   Hispanic Health and Human Service
   Organizations
Costa, L. A., 95, 113
Costello, E. J., 11, 28
Coulter, E., 1, 31
Council on Scientific Affairs, 84, 108
Cranston, V. A., 125, 138
Crawford, J. H., 16, 30

Crawford, S. L., 95, 113
Cromwell, R. E., 99, 108
Cromwell, V. L., 99, 108
Crosby, F., viii, x
Cross, A. W., 4, 34
Cross, T., 22, 28, 200, 212
Crowley, M. F., 148, 166
Cypress, B., 154, 167

D'Angelo, L. J., 94, 106
Daniels, R., 144, 164
Davids, A., 96, 110
Davidson, S. M., 14, 31
Davies, M., 10, 32, 100, 113
Davis, S. M., 95, 109
Decker, J., 221, 241
Dembo, R., 12, 27, 28, 52, 53, 55, 74
Dennis, D., 200, 212
Dennis, K., 22, 28
Desenclos, J. C. S., 85, 86, 109
DesJarlais, D., 12, 28
Deutsch, H., 224, 239
Development Associates, 124, 125, 138
Deykin, E., 11, 34
Diaz-Guerrero, R., 99, 109
Dick, R. W., 121, 122, 136, 138
DiClemente, R., 95, 109
Dillon, H., 15, 28
DiSarno, N. J., 119, 138
Dise-Lewis, J. E., 128, 138
Dixon, R. A., 7, 29
Dodge, K. A., 231, 239
Dohrenwend, B. S., 11, 29
Doi, T., xxiii
Dondero, T. J., 94, 114
Donnerstein, E., 53, 75
Donovan, P., 70, 74
Dopkins, S. C., 100, 113
Dornbusch, S., 188, 214
Dougherty, D., xv, 3, 14, 128, 138, 217
Dovidio, J. F., viii, x
Dressler, C. M., xxi, xxvi
Droter, D., xxiii
Dryfoos, J. G., 24, 28, 205, 212, 234, 239
Dui, Q. L., 147, 163
Durant, R. H., 93, 109

Dusenbury, L., 98, 106, 109

Echemendia, R., 167
Edgerton, R. B., 102, 110
Edwards, R., 98, 108, 123, 137
Eisenberg, J., 47, 77
Eiskovits, Z., 53, 76
Eisman, S., 19, 28
Ellickson, P. L., 65, 74
Elliot, D. S., 53, 75
Elliott, G. R., xv, xvi, 210, 212, 220, 221, 239
Ellwood, D. T., 2, 3, 27, 28
Emans, S. J., 18, 28
English, A., 61, 74
Epstein, N., 68, 74
Erickson, R. V., 146, 150, 164
Erikson, E. H., 47, 70, 75, 220, 224, 239
Erikson, P. I., 95, 111
Escobar, J., 102, 110
Espin, O., 100, 109
Evans, J., 194, 195, 196
Evans, R., 147, 164
Evans, R. I., 12, 28
Exner, T. M., 95, 113
Ezzatti, T. M., 91, 109

Fagan, J., 13, 32
Fairchild, H., 53, 75
Falttau, P. E., 235, 240
Family Planning Perspectives, 201, 212
Farrington, D. P., 52, 55, 75
Faundez, A., 105, 109
Fawcett, N., 95, 113
Fawzy, F. I., 11, 12, 28
Federle, K. H., ix, x
Feit, M., 221, 241
Feldman, S. S., xv, xvi, 210, 212, 220, 221, 239
Feshbach, N. D., 53, 75
Fielder, E. P., 93, 106
Fielding, J., 15, 28
Finder, E. J., 157, 165
Fine, D., 231, 239
Fingerhut, L., 103
Fink, R., 5, 31

Fischler, R., 127, 138
Fishman, C., 147, 164
Fishman, G., 53, 76
Flegal, M. K., 91, 109
Fleming, C. M., 46, 122, 138, 205, 208
Flemming, G. V., 101, 105
Flint, S., 192, 216
Foley, J., 24, 28
Folkman, S., 1, 26
Ford, K., 93, 95, 109, 112
Forke, C. M., 9, 21, 33
Forrest, J. D., 19, 28
Forslund, M. A., 123, 124, 125, 137, 138
Foster, H., 14, 31
Foster, L. W., xxiii, xxvi
Franklin, D. L., 8, 9, 18, 29
Franklin, L., 16, 33
Franz, W. B., 157, 166
Freedman, J. L., 53, 75
Freeman, H. P., 14, 27, 217, 240
Freire, P., 104, 105, 109
French, J. R. P., 225, 237, 239
Frerichs, R. R., 149, 164
Freud, S., 224, 239
Frey, D. L., ix, x
Friedman, A., 73
Friedman, A. S., 22, 29
Frisancho, A. R., 89, 109
Frisone, G., 23, 31
Fuchs, V. R., 230, 239
Fujino, D., 146, 147, 150, 167
Furstenberg, F. F., 8, 29, 231, 235, 239

Gaertner, S. L., viii, ix, x
Galambos, N. L., 7, 29
Gallagher, S. S., 6, 29
Garbarino, J., 7, 16, 17, 29
Garfinkel, I., 2, 29
Garland, A. F., 6, 29
Gelles, R. J., 16, 33
General Accounting Office, 83, 110
Gergen, P. J., 90, 106, 107
Gersten, J., 47, 77
Gibbs, J. T., 42, 45, 49, 50, 57, 62, 73, 74, 75, 78
Gil, A. G., 12, 34, 97, 98, 115

Gilchrist, L. D., 225, 234, 241
Gilliam, G., 7, 16, 17, 29
Giordano, J., 166
Gittler, J. D., xvi, xvii, 192, 212
Glickman, N. W., 22, 29
Glidden, C., 152, 166
Goering, J., 15, 29
Goldberger, N. R., 105, 106
Goldfield, A., 96, 112
Gong-Guy, E., 146, 164
Gonzalez, A. M., 99, 115
Goodman, E., vii, viii, x, 95, 110
Goodman, P., 11, 29
Gordon, P., 153, 155, 165
Gornemann, I., 95, 106
Gottfredson, G. D., 235, 240
Gottleib, M. I., 119, 141
Gottlieb, A. A., 7, 9, 32
Gould, M., 11, 29
Gould-Martin, K., 151, 164
Goulet, L., 96, 112
Grace, E., 18, 28
Graham, G., 4, 29
Greenberg, B. S., 53, 75
Gregory, S. J., 97, 110
Grembowski, D., 24, 29
Griego, T., 148, 164
Grossman, B., 96, 110
Groves, B. M., 96, 110
Gruen, R. S., 95, 113
Guarnaccia, P. J., 90, 91, 110
Guggenheim, P., 23, 33
Gunter, E., 89, 107
Gutierrez, E., 100, 110
Guttman, E., 53, 76
Guyer, B., 6, 29
Guzman, P., 167

Haffner, S. M., 91, 114
Haggerty, R. J., 14, 32
Haignere, C. S., 10, 32, 95, 113
Hall, E., 54, 75
Hamburg, B. A., 98, 106
Hamburg, D. A., xvi, xvii, 235, 239
Hammond, W. R., 6, 29

Hampton, R. L., 7, 29, 46, 75
Hanks, G. A., 125, 138
Harmon, B., 118, 119, 120, 137
Harris, D. E., 146, 163
Harris, L., 118, 119, 120, 137
Harris, M. B., 95, 109
Harris, M. I., 91, 109
Harris, V. W., 125, 138
Harsha, D. W., 91, 115
Hauser, S., 63, 70, 78
Hausman, A., 6, 29
Havighurst, R. J., 220, 239
Hawaii, state of, 169, 171, 172, 173, 174, 175, 178, 181, 186
Hawley, L., 11, 29
Hayes, C. D., 231, 232, 239
Hayes-Bautista, D. E., xiii, xvii, 80, 87, 110
Hayman, C. R., 94, 113
Haynes, S. G., 91, 109
Health Resources Administration, 101, 110
Heath, R. W., 172, 173, 175, 186
Hedin, D., 24, 32
Heelas, P., xxiii
Heeren, T., 99, 106
Hein, K., 9, 27, 62, 75
Heiss, A. L., 16, 30
Helfer, R., 127, 138
Henderson, R., 95, 113
Hepner, R., 4, 30
Herberg, P., 219, 239
Herendeen, T. O., xix, 188, 213
Hessler, R. M., 155, 164
Hewitt, N., 21, 30
Heyman, P. W., 4, 34
Hiat, A. B., 127, 139
Hibicht, J. P., 5, 30
Hidalgo, H. A., 90, 91, 115
Hill, C. J., 16, 30
Hill, H., 39, 74
Hill, I., 44, 66, 75
Hill, R., 67, 75
Hindelang, M. J., 12, 13, 30
Hirschi, T., 12, 13, 30
Hoang, G. N., 146, 150, 164
Hochstadt, N. J., 232, 239
Hogan, D. P., 9, 18, 30

Holden, C., 198, 213
Hollingshead, A. B., 3, 11, 30
Holmes, K. K., 10, 30
Holmes, M. D., 94, 110
Holzer, C. E., 96, 99, 114
Honey, E., 62, 75
Hongo, R., 176, 183, 185
Hops, H., 49, 50, 76
Horikawa, H., 146, 165
Horowitz, R., 230, 240
Horton, J. M., 125, 138
Horwitz, S., 235, 240
Hough, R. L., 102, 110
Houstin-Hamilton, A., 62, 75
Howard, A., 235, 240
Howard, M., 233, 240
Howie, V. M., 119, 138
Huang, K., 146, 163
Huang, L. N., 42, 50, 75
Hui Malama Ola Na'Oiwi, 180, 185
Huizinga, D., 53, 75
Huston, A. C., 53, 75, 76
Hutchins, V., 194, 213
Hymbaugh, K. J., 121, 139

Indian Center (Lincoln, Nebraska), 126, 138
Institute of Medicine, 26, 30
Irwin, C. E., Jr., 210, 213
Isaacs, M. R., 200, 212, 213

Ja, D. Y., 150, 153, 155, 165, 166
Jacobs, D. F., 12, 31
Jacobson, D., 229, 240
Jaffe, L., 93, 111
James-Ortiz, S., 98, 106, 109
Jaramillo, P. T., 99, 115
Jaudes, P. K., 232, 239
Jay, M. S., 7, 9, 32
Jekel, J. F., 235, 240
Jemmott, J. B., 21, 30
Jemmott, L. S., 21, 30
Jenks, E., 147, 164
Jensen, G. F., 125, 138
Jessor, R., xxiv, 65, 72, 76, 224, 240
Jessor, S. L., 72, 76, 224, 240
Joe, T., 13, 30

Johnson, A. W., xxiii
Johnson, D. B., 169, 173, 174, 186, 187
Johnson, F., 155, 165
Johnston, L., 96, 97, 110
Johnston, P., 24, 31
Jones, D. Y., 5, 30
Jones, E. E., 51, 65, 76
Jones, T., 53, 78
Jordan, J. D., 114
Juarez, R. Z., 91, 109

Kagawa-Singer, M., xxii, xxiii, xxvi
Kahn, R. L., 1, 26
Kaiser Permanente Center for Health Research, 175, 184, 185
Kalichman, S. C., 20, 30
Kamehameha Schools/Bernice Pauahi Bishop Estate, 174, 176, 177, 178, 185
Kaplan, A. G., 114
Karnavas, B. A., 91, 114
Karno, M., 102, 110
Karon, J. M., 10, 30
Kasper, J. A., 101, 111
Kato, P. M., 93, 111
Katz, P. A., 9, 13, 49, 54, 70, 75, 78, 192, 208, 219, 225
Kavanagh, K., 49, 50, 76
Kazdin, A. E., 11, 30
Keemer, J. B., 86, 87, 111
Kelling, G. L., 55, 79
Kelly, G. D., 92, 113
Kelly, J. A., 20, 30
Kemp, K., 3, 14, 217
Kempe, C., 127, 138
Kenney, A. M., 24, 30
Kerkman, D., 53, 76
Kerner, J. F., 98, 106, 109
Kessler, S., xxiv, 234, 240
Khalid, H., 9, 21, 33
Kilner, L., 63, 70, 78
Kim, B. L. C., 146, 151, 152, 155, 156, 159, 164
Kim, K. K., 148, 164
Kim, S. C., 157, 164
Kinzie, J. D., 150, 153, 155, 164, 165
Kirby, D., 24, 30, 234, 240

Kirkman-Liff, B., 14, 27
Kisker, E. E., 24, 31
Kitagawa, E. M., 9, 18, 30
Kitano, H. H., 144, 146, 152, 164
Klein, K., 18, 28
Kleinman, A. M., 153, 155, 164, 226, 227, 228, 240
Kleinman, D. V., 87, 112
Klerman, G., 11, 34
Klerman, L. V., 235, 240
Kligfeld, M., 23, 31
Knowler, W. C., 91, 109
Koh, E., 4, 31
Kohrs, M. B., 148, 164
Konner, M., xxii, 219, 238, 240
Koopermen, C., 10, 32
Koopman, C., 95, 100, 113
Korchin, S. J., 51, 65, 76
Kreiss, L., 10, 30
Krisberg, B., 53, 76
Kromer, M. E., 90, 91, 115
Kronick, R., 174, 184, 185
Kumpfer, K., 208, 213
Kuo, H. S., 235, 240
Kutner, N. G., 51, 76

Ladner, J. A., 59, 60, 76
Lamb, M. E., 54, 75
Landsverk, J. A., 102, 110
Langer, T., 47, 77
Lau, B. W. K., 155, 163
Laub, J. H., 53, 78
Lavizzo-Mourey, R., 83, 115
Leadbeater, B. J., 93, 111
Leahy, W., 15, 34
Lear, J., 14, 31
Lee, D. H., 91, 114
Lee, E., 155, 164
Leighton, C. K., 100, 112
Leon, A. C., 98, 111
Leong, F. T. L., 144, 146, 152, 165
Lescohier, I., 6, 29
Lesser, I. M., 157, 165
Levine, B., 235, 240
Levine, S. V., 224, 240
Lew, L., 155, 166

Lewis, D. O., 23, 31, 33
Lewis, R., 221, 241
Lewit, E. M., viii, x
Library of Congress, 189, 201, 206, 214
Lieberman, J., 90, 108
Lin, K. M., 157, 165
Lin, W.-S., 149, 167
Linares, L. O., 93, 111
Lindsey, D., viii, x
Lin-Fu, J. S., 145, 165
Linskey, A. O., 96, 99, 114
Litt, I. F., 10, 31
Little, T. D., 12, 31
Liu, W. T., xix, xxvii, 63, 77, 146, 165
Lock, A., xxiii
Los Angeles County Department of Mental Health, 146, 165
Lundman, R. J., 55, 77

MacAskill, R., 51, 78
Madsen, W., 99, 111
Maes, E. F., 149, 164
Magaña, J. R., 105, 111
Maiden, N., 4, 30
Majidi-Ahi, S., 11, 27
Mak, H., 24, 31
Mann, J. J., 98, 111
Manson, S. M., 46, 116, 120, 121, 122, 127, 136, 137, 138, 139, 205, 208
Maran, S., 96, 110
Marcia, J. E., 48, 70, 77
Margullis, C., 155, 166
Marin, B., 100, 111
Marin, G., 100, 111
Markides, K. S., 100, 111
Marks, Q., 100, 111
Marsella, A. J., 153, 155, 165
Marston, A. R., 12, 31
Martin, A. D., 20, 31
Martin, C., 96, 112
Martorell, R., 90, 111
Marzuk, P. M., 98, 111
Maslow, A. H., 72, 77
Mason, H. R. C., 100, 111
Matthieu, M., 95, 113
Maurer, J. D., 86, 87, 111

May, P. A., 121, 122, 123, 125, 139
Mayfield, J., 184
Mays, V., 62, 77
McAdoo, H. P., 65, 77
McCabe, J. B., 233, 240
McConahay, J. B., ix, x
McCord, C., 217, 240
McDill, E. L., 82, 112
McElroy, A., 226, 240
McGee, Z. T., 6, 33
McGoldrick, M., 165
McGraw, S. A., 95, 113
McKinlay, J. B., 95, 113
McKinney, H., 146, 166
McLanahan, S. S., 2, 29
McManus, M. A., 14, 31, 89, 112
McNassor, D., 176, 183, 185
Mead, M., 222, 240
Melton, G. B., viii, ix, x
Mendoza, F. S., 90, 111
Mercer, R. T., 220, 240
Merola, J., 18, 28
Merzel, C., 43, 73
Messeri, P., 43, 73
Messinger, M., 9, 46
Meyer, M., 4, 32
Meyer-Bahlburg, H. F. L., 95, 100, 113
Mezan, P., 96, 112
Michelman, D. F., 9, 21, 33
Miike, L., xix, 188, 213, 219, 222
Milazzo-Sayre, L., 51, 78
Milgrom, P., 24, 29
Miller, B. C., 235, 240
Miller, C. A., 1, 31, 94, 113, 217, 242
Miller, J. B., 114
Miller, M. A., 91, 114
Millstein, S. G., xv, xvii, 10, 31, 70, 77, 210, 213
Mitchell, C. M., 3, 4, 31, 192, 218
Moen, P., 2, 31
Molin, R., 232, 240
Monzon, C. M., 157, 166
Moore, D. S., 95, 111
Moore, K. A., 8, 29, 59, 77
Morales, A., 74
Morales, E., 95, 100, 109, 111

Moran, D., 90, 108
Morgan, D., 201, 213
Morgan, E. B., 98, 111
Morgan, S. P., 8, 29, 231, 239
Morishima, J. K., 144, 145, 149, 152, 155, 158, 166
Morris, P. A., 231, 241
Morrison, M. A., 235, 241
Morton, T. D., 231, 241
Mosca, J., 96, 112
Mosher, W. D., 101, 111
Moss, A. J., 89, 101, 102, 114
Mueller, C. W., 3, 31
Mullins, M. R., 16, 30
Murase, T., 155, 165
Murphy, D. A., 20, 30
Murphy, I., 14, 27
Murray, J. P., 53, 75
Myers, H., 167
Myers, R. E., 124, 138

Nadar, P., 4, 32
Nakasaki, G., 146, 147, 150, 167
Na Pu'uwai, 179, 186
Nathan, A., 96, 112
National Academy of Sciences, 210
National Assembly of School-Based Health Centers, 195
National Center for American Indian and Alaska Native Mental Health Research, 122, 123, 127, 128, 139
National Center for Education in Maternal and Child Health, 194, 213
National Center for Health Statistics, 46, 77, 83, 85, 103,112, 144, 154
National Coalition of Hispanic Health and Human Service Organizations (COSSMHO), 104, 114
National Commission on the Role of the School and the Community in Improving Adolescent Health, 205, 213
National Institute on Drug Abuse, 39, 56, 77
Native American Rehabilitation and Training Center, 121
Natriello, G., 82, 112

Nelson, S., 15, 28
Nesheim, M. C., 5, 30
Netting, F. E., xxiii
New, J. C., xxiii
New, P. K., 155, 164
Newacheck, P. W., 89, 112
Newberger, E. H., 7, 29
Ng, J., 145, 165
Ngin, K., 151, 164
Nightingale, E. O., xv, xvii
Nikias, M., 5, 31
Ninan, O. P., 23, 33
Nisbett, R. E., 49, 78
Nock, S. L., 3, 32
Nolan, M. F., 155, 164
Nopshitz, J. D., 99, 106
Norris, A. E., 93, 95, 109, 112
Novello, A. C., 87, 112

O'Connell, J. C., 120, 121, 139
O'Dowd, M. A., 96, 112
Oetting, E. R., 98, 108, 123, 137
Office of Management and Budget, 83, 112
Office of the Federal Register, 191, 204, 213, 205
Ogbru, B., 155, 164
Ogbu, J. U., 39, 41, 42, 77
O'Grady, K. E., 95, 112
O'Hagan, P., 172, 185
Ohlin, L. E., 55, 75
Okada, L., 14, 32
Ollendick, T. H., 76
O'Malley, P., 97, 110
Ooms, T., xix, 188, 213
Orlandi, M. A., 225, 235, 241
Orr, L., 95, 113
Orr, M. T., 19, 28
Ortiz, I. E., 13, 23, 34
Oskamp, S., 235, 240
Otto, D., 89, 113
Oviatt, B. E., 125, 137
Owan, T. C., 165, 166
Owen, R. G., 95, 113
Oyama, N., 169, 173, 174, 186, 187

Padilla, E. R., 95, 112

Pafafflin, S. M., 235, 240
Paikoff, R. L., 235, 240
Palank, C. L., xxiv, xxvi
Pallas, A. M., 82, 112
Palmer, J. L., 232, 239
Panem, S., 77
Pappas, J., 90, 108
Paradise, J. L., 119, 139
Parcel, G., 4, 32
Parcel, R. L., 3, 31
Park, M. K., 91, 114
Paulson, J. A., 6, 32
Pauly, M., 14, 32
Payne, K., 203, 214
Peake-Raymond, M. P., 129, 139
Pearce, J. K., 165
Pendergrast, R., 93, 109
Peralta, V., 146, 165
Perez-Stable, E. J., 91, 100, 109, 111
Perlmutter, M., 54, 75
Petersen, A. C., xv, xvii
Petersen, L. R., 94, 113
Peterson, J. L., 8, 29, 235, 240
Pettit, G. S., 231, 239
Pfeffer, C., 7, 32
Phelps, L., xxiii
Phillips, G. T., 91, 115
Piaget, J., 70, 78
Piasecki, J. M., 127, 139
Pierce, H. B., 52, 78
Pion, G. M., 235, 240
Pirkle, J., 89, 107
Pleck, J. H., 60, 61, 78, 100, 112
Pless, I. B., 14, 32
Plett, J. D., 172, 173, 175, 186
Plotkin, S. L., 9, 21, 33
Ploussard, J. H., 119, 138
Poland, R. E., 157, 165
Polit, D. F., 231, 241
Portes, A., 80, 112
Powell, G., 74
Powers, S., 63, 70, 78
Prihoda, T. J., 90, 91, 115
Prinz, R. J., 76
Prizzia, R., 146, 165
Pumariega, A. J., 96, 99, 114

Putnam, R. D., viii, xi

Quality Education for Minorities Project, xiii, xvii
Quigley-Rick, M., xvi, xvii, 192, 212
Quintero-Salinas, R., 96, 99, 114

Raboin, R. M., 123, 137
Raines, B. E., 12, 28
Rapoport, R. N., 25, 32
Rappaport, L., 224, 241
Raven, B., 225, 237, 239
Ray, L. A., 100, 111
Raymond, E. V., 129, 139
Razin, A. M., 96, 112
Rebach, H., 98, 113
Red Horse, J. G., 221, 241
Redlich, F. C., 11, 30
Reed, R. J., 58, 78
Regier, D., 102, 110
Reinarman, C., 13, 32
Reisine, S., 24, 32
Reklis, D. M., 230, 239
Renaud, C., 96, 113
Resnick, M., 24, 32, 118, 119, 120, 137
Reuter, P., 231, 241
Revenson, T. A., 1, 27
Rice, M. L., 53, 76
Richardson, J. L., 100, 111
Rickert, V. I., 7, 9, 32
Rind, P., 235, 241
Roberson, M. K., 13, 23, 34
Roberts, R. E., 96, 113
Robins, L., 7, 32
Robinson, D. O., 46, 78
Robinson, W., 203, 212
Robyn, A. E., 65, 74
Rodriquez, I., 96, 112
Romero, A., 74
Rosario, M., 95, 100, 113
Rosauer, R., 61, 78
Rosenberg, H. M., 86, 87, 111
Rosenstein, M., 51, 78
Rossi, P. H., 3, 32
Rotheram–Borus, M. J., 10, 32, 95, 100, 113
Rousseau, C., 96, 113

Rubin, W., 181
Rubinstein, E. A., 53, 75
Ruch-Ross, H., 4, 34
Ruiz, M. S., 100, 111
Rumbaut, R. G., 80, 112
Runyan, C., 7, 27
Russo, N. F., xxii, 49, 78
Ruuska, S. H., 119, 137
Ryan, A. S., 89, 109

Saks, M. J., xvi, xvii, 192, 212
Saldivar, L., 90, 111
Salinas, L., 92, 113
Sampson, R. J., 53, 78
Sanchez-Jankowski, M., 230, 241
Sandefur, G. D., 3, 33
Sanders-Phillips, K., xxiv
Sarnet, J. M., 121, 139
Sasao, T., 150, 167
Sata, L. S., 146, 165
Saxe, L., viii, x
Sceftel, S., 96, 112
Schachter, J., 232, 239
Schiller, B. R., 1, 33
Schink, W. O., xiii, xvii
Schinke, S. P., 225, 234, 241
Schmeidler, J., 12, 28
Schor, E. L., 232, 241
Schorr, D., 233, 241
Schorr, L. B., 233, 241
Schulberg, H., 11, 27
Schuster, C. S., 220, 241
Schwartz, I., 53, 76
Schwartz, J., 89, 113
Scott, C. S., 95, 113
Scott-Jones, D., 8, 33
Seidman, E. S., 3, 4, 31
Seymore, C., 93, 109
Shainline, A., 68, 74
Shanok, S. S., 23, 31, 33
Shapiro, S., 5, 31
Shear, C., 11, 29
Sheley, J. F., 6, 33
Sheon, A. R., 94, 106
Sherman, R., 119, 137
Shifman, L., 95, 113

Shon, S. P., 150, 153, 165
Shore, J. H., 120, 137
Shu, R., 146, 166
Signorella, N., 54, 78
Sikkema, K. J., 20, 30
Silva, A., 102, 115
Silvern, L. E., 49, 76, 78
Simmons, J., 16, 33
Simms, M. C., 59, 77
Simon, J. M., 11, 12, 28
Simoni, J., 100, 111
Simpson, J. W., 91, 115
Singer, J., 13, 27
Singer, R. D., 12, 31
Skocpol, T., 212, 214
Slap, G. B., 9, 21, 33
Smith, D. E., 18, 28
Smith, K. W., 95, 113
Snider, D. E., Jr., 92, 113
Snow, L. F., 68, 78
Sobhan, M., 96, 113
Sokol-Katz, J. S., 98, 115
Sonerstein, F. L., 60, 61, 78, 100, 112
Spears, H., 21, 30
Spector, R. E., 220, 241
Spencer, M., 188, 214
Spencer, M. B., 58, 74, 77
Squires, B. D., 125, 139
Srinivasan, S. R., 91, 115
Stack, C. B., 229, 241
Stajic, M., 98, 111
Stanlon, K., 148, 167
Staples, R., 53, 78
Stark, A., 11, 29
Stark, N. M., 157, 166
State of Hawaii. *See* Hawaii, state of
Steele, C. M., 49, 78
Stein, K. M., 146, 163
Stepleton, S. S., 232, 241
Stern, M. P., 91, 109, 114
Stewart, J. L., 119, 139
Stitt, K., xv, xvi
Stiver, I. P., 114
St. Louis, M. E., 94, 113
Stoddard, J. J., 89, 112
Stone, L. J., 220, 221, 241

Stoyer, J., 119, 138
St. Peters, M., 53, 76
Straus, J. H., 125, 138
Straus, M. A., 16, 33
Stroup-Benham, C. A., 100, 111
Strunin, L., 10, 33
Sturz, E. L., 25, 33
Sudarkasa, N., 229, 241
Sue, D. W., 146, 166
Sue, S., 144, 145, 146, 149, 152, 155, 158,
  166, 235, 236, 242
Suitor, W., 148, 166
Sullivan, J., 4, 33
Sumaya, C. V., 92, 114
Surendar, C. M., 23, 33
Surrey, J. L., 105, 114
Sutherland, J. E., 157, 166
Swaim, R. C., 98, 108
Swain, S. O., 60, 61, 78
Swanson, J. W., 96, 99, 114
Syme, S. L., 1, 26
Szapocznik, J., 104, 114
Szasz, M., 125, 139

Talamo, R. C., 24, 31
Tardiff, K., 98, 111
Tarule, J. M., 105, 106
Taylor, D. A., 9, 13, 70, 76, 208, 219, 225,
  238
Taylor, S. S., 127, 139
Tereszhiewicz, L., 61, 74
Thomas, M. A., 65, 74
Thompson, J., 51, 78
Thu, N. D., 149, 167
Tienda, M., 80, 106
Timbers, D., 102, 110
Tinsley, H. E. A., 155, 167
Tommasello, A., 96, 98, 114
Torres, A., 19, 28
Towers, R. L., 56, 79
Tracey, T. J., 152, 166
Tracy, P. E., 55, 79
Trevino, F. M., 89, 100, 101, 102, 111, 114
Trowbridge, F., 148, 167
Troxler, R. G., 91, 114
Tuckson, R. V., xxiv

Tung, T. M., 153, 154, 166
Tuthill, J. W., 4, 34
Twork, R., 148, 164
Tyler, F. B., 96, 98, 114
Tyler, S. L., 96, 98, 114

Ugarte, C., 203, 214
Ulbrich, P. M., 98, 113
Ungemack, J. A., 99, 115
University of Hawaii–Manoa, 182, 187
University of Minnesota, 121, 126, 127, 130, 140
University of Nebraska–Lincoln, 138
U.S. Advisory Board on Child Abuse and Neglect, ix
U.S. Bureau of Census, 1, 3, 33, 39, 79, 81, 107, 116, 137, 142, 143, 166
U.S. Congress, Committee on Ways and Means, 1, 3, 9, 34
U.S. Congress, General Accounting Office, 203, 214
U.S. Congress, House of Representatives, xv, xvii
U.S. Congress, Joint Economic Committee, 59, 79
U.S. Congress, Library of Congress, 189, 201, 206, 214
U.S. Congress, Office of Technology Assessment, xiii, xv, xvi, xvii, 3, 5, 7, 8, 9, 10, 13, 14, 15, 16, 18, 19, 20, 21, 22, 26, 63, 79, 120, 122, 123, 127, 128, 129, 139, 140, 169, 170, 173, 174, 183, 186, 188, 189, 190, 192, 195, 196, 200, 201, 202, 203, 205, 206, 207, 210, 211, 212, 214, 231
U.S. Congress, Select Committee on Children, Youth and Families, 43, 57, 79
U.S. Congress, Select Committee on Hunger, 45, 79
U.S. Congress, Senate, Select Committee on Indian Affairs, 126, 127, 140
U.S. Congress, Senate Committee on Appropriations, 210, 214
U.S. Department of Agriculture, 207, 214
U.S. Department of Education, 205, 215
U.S. Department of Health and Human Services, 83, 114, 116, 117, 118, 122, 126,

129, 130, 140, 144, 173, 184, 186, 195, 199, 200, 202, 203, 204, 206, 208, 210, 215
U.S. Department of Justice, 52, 79
U.S. Department of the Interior, Bureau of Indian Affairs, 126, 131, 140
U.S. Executive Office of the President, 194, 202, 216

Valencia, R. R., 81, 82, 83, 108
Van Deusen, J. M., 157, 166
Vasquez, M. T. J., 99, 115
Vaughn, R. D., 9, 20, 34
Vega, W. A., 12, 34, 83, 84, 87, 97, 98, 115
Velez, C. N., 99, 115
Ventura, S. J., 90, 111
Vermund, S. H., 94, 106
Vigil, J. D., 230, 242
Villanueva-King, O., 146, 165
Vincenzi, H., 47, 79

Wagner, N., 155, 166
Walch, C., 194, 213
Waldmann, E., 155, 163
Walker, D. K., 4, 34
Wallerstein, N., 105, 115
Walter, H. J., 9, 20, 34
Walter, J., 15, 34
Wan, T., 14, 32
Warheit, G. J., 12, 34, 97, 98, 106, 115
Warren, R. C., 83, 115
Waszak, C., 234, 240
Waszak, C. D., 70, 74
Wax, M. L., 125, 140
Wax, R. H., 125, 140
Weaver, J. L., 151, 166
Webber, L. S., 91, 115
Wechsler, J. G., 125, 141
Weibel, O. J., 123, 140
Weinstein, H., 23, 33
Weis, J. G., 12, 13, 30
Weisman, A. D., xxiii, xxviii
Weitzman, B. C., 231, 242
Wellin, E., 226, 242
Wells, V., 11, 34
Wenger, M., 13, 27

Werner, D., 105, 115
Westendorp, F., 13, 23, 34
Whitaker, R., 99, 106
White, A. B., 8, 33
White, C. M., 231, 241
White, J. L., 65, 66, 79
Whiteman, M., 98, 106
Whiting, B. B., 222, 242
Whiting, J. W. M., 54, 73, 222, 242
Whitmore, J. K., 147, 163
Wichlacz, C. R., 126, 141
Widaman, K. R., 12, 31
Wilcox, B. L., 53, 75
Wiley, A. S., 226, 242
Williams, B. C., 217, 242
Williams, D. R., 83, 115
Wilson, C. C., xxiii
Wilson, J., 39, 79
Wilson, J. Q., 55, 75, 79
Wilson, W. L., 2, 6, 11, 34
Winter, W., 13, 27
Wirt, R., 96, 110
Wise, P. H., 87, 112
Wohlford, P., 167
Wolf, W., 123, 137
Wolfgang, M. E., 55, 79
Womble, M., 66, 67, 73
Wood, P. R., 90, 91, 115
Woods, D. W., 174, 187
Woods, E. R., 18, 28
Woolf, G. D. B., 232, 242
Wright, J. C., 53, 76
Wright, L. D., 6, 33

W. T. Grant Foundation Commission on
    Work, Family and Citizenship, 2, 34
Wunsch-Hitzig, R., 11, 29
Wyatt, G. E., xxii, 8, 35, 60, 79
Wylie, W. G., 14, 31

Yamamoto, J., 74, 102, 115
Yasuda, K., 146, 147, 150, 167
Ye, G.-S., 149, 167
Yee, B. E. K., 149, 167
Yip, R., 148, 167
Young, W. R., 125, 141
Yu, E. S. H., xix, xxvii, 63, 77, 145, 154,
    167
Yudkowsky, B., 192, 216
Yuen, R. K. W., 155, 167
Yung, B., 6, 29

Zane, N., 146, 147, 150, 155, 167
Zapata, J. T., 99, 115
Zaslow, M. J., 232, 239
Zauber, A., 98, 109
Zellman, G. L., 65
Zhang, Y., 96, 98, 114
Ziegler, J., 234, 240
Zigler, E., 6, 29
Zillman, D., 75
Zimmerman, C., 105, 108
Zimmerman, R. S., 12, 34, 97, 98, 115
Zimo, D. A., 232, 239
Zinkus, P. W., 119, 141
Zuckerman, B., 96, 110
Zuckerman, D., 53, 74

Subject Index

abortion, 60, 118; funding, 61, 192, 201

abuse, child, 7, 16–17, 204, 231, 232; alcohol- and drug-related, 55–56; American Indian, 126–27, 132; Black, 46; rate of, 230; reporting of, 17–18, 126

abuse, sexual, 8, 60, 100; American Indian, 126, 127; Black, 46

accidents, 6, 117, 145, 154; automobile, 5, 39, 43, 56, 87, 119, 134

acculturation, 223, 229; health care utilization and, 155; Latinos, 98–99, 100; substance use and, 98–99

ACF. *See* Administration for Children and Families

acting-out behavior, 52, 231

ACTION, 190, 209–10

ACYF. *See* Administration for Children, Youth, and Families

ADAMHA. *See* Alcohol, Drug Abuse, and Mental Health Administration

adaptive behaviors, 39–42

ADD HEALTH, 197, 210

Administration for Children and Families (ACF), 190, 193, 204–5

Administration for Children, Youth, and Families (ACYF), 193, 204

Administration for Native Americans (ANA), 193, 204, 205

Administration on Developmental Disabilities, 204

adolescence: cultural influences on, 49, 221; definition of, xxi, 1; as developmental period, xxii, xxiv, 47, 70, 220–22; strengths of, xxii, 236; theories of, 220, 224–25, 226, 228

Adolescent and School Health Programs (ASHP), 199

Adolescent Family Life Act of 1981, 61

Adolescent Family Life Program, 18

Adolescent Health Branch (MCHB), 211

Adolescent Health project, xv–xvi

Adolescent Pregnancy Prevention, Office of, 18

adolescents: input from, 237–38; population of, 217

adoption, 66

AFDC. *See* Aid to Families with Dependent Children

AFL. *See* American Family Life Program

African Americans. *See* Black Americans

aggressive behavior, 52, 53–54

AIDS, 9–10, 19–20; Asians and, 152, 162; associated health risks, 10, 46; Blacks and, 62; as cause of death, 36, 62, 85; drug use and, 57; education, 20, 21, 104, 199, 203, 234; ethnicity and, 10, 85, 94; hemophilia and, 10; homosexuals and, 62, 95; Latinos and, 85, 94–95, 100, 203; public support and, 218; rate of, 9–10, 62, 95; safe sex and, 10, 20–21, 203

Aid to Families with Dependent Children (AFDC), 59, 204
Alcohol, Drug Abuse, and Mental Health Administration (ADAMHA), 144, 199–200
Alcoholics Anonymous, 67
alcohol use, 12, 55, 56, 71; abuse and, 55–56; by American Indians, 117, 119, 121, 123–24, 125, 126, 127, 128, 129–30, 131, 132, 134, 205; by Asians, 149, 150; by Blacks, 39, 56, 97; and fetal alcohol syndrome, 121; by Hawaiians, 171, 173; by Latinos, 97, 98, 100; parental, 127, 134; prevention of, 64, 67, 205; treatment of, 131, 134
alternative medicine: Asians and, 154; Blacks and, 65, 68; Hawaiians and, 176, 178, 179, 180, 182, 183, 184
American Bar Association, 196
American Family Life program, 211
American Indians, 116; abuse, 126–27, 132; accidents/injuries, 119, 134; AIDS education, 203; alcohol and, 117, 119, 121, 123–24, 125, 126, 127, 128, 129–30, 131, 132, 134, 205; anxiety and, 122–23; birth-rate, 118; child abuse and, 126–27, 132; collective interdependence among, 133; cultural influences, 132–34; data on, xxi; delinquency and, 124–25; demographics, 116; developmental disorders and, 120–21; diabetes and, 117, 118, 207; diversity among, 116, 132, 133; education and, 125, 131, 203; family, 125, 127, 133–34, 221, 222; health-care utilization, 15, 22, 128, 129, 130, 135; hearing impairments, 119, 121; identity problems, 124, 132, 133, 222–23; life expectancy, 117; mental health, xiii, 117, 120–22, 124, 129, 132; mortality, 117, 119, 122, 127, 145; nutrition programs, 207; obesity, 198, 207; pregnancy, 118, 119; runaways, 125, 126, 205; schools, 118, 125, 127, 128, 223; sexual behavior, 118–19; smoking, 120, 132, 134; socioeconomic status, 116; spirituality, 133; stress, 127, 128, 135; substance abuse, 123–24, 126, 128, 130, 131, 134, 205; Sun Dance, 132–33; unemployment rates, 116; urban health programs, 131; violence, 117, 120

American Psychological Association, 196
American Red Cross, 233–34
ANA. See Administration for Native Americans
anxiety, 122–23
APA. See Asian Pacific Americans
Argus community (Bronx), 25, 26
arrest records, 52–53
A/SAPB. See Alcoholism/Substance Abuse Program Branch
ASHP. See Adolescent and School Health Programs
Asian Pacific Americans (APA); acculturation, 143, 144, 150, 155, 156; AIDS, 152, 162; alcohol, 149, 150; alternative medicine, 154; Cambodian, 143, 146, 147, 156; communities, 151, 152; concepts of health, 152–53, 162; crime, 145; cultural factors, 150, 151–55; data on, xiv, 144, 156, 161, 162; delinquency, 145, 152; demographics, 142–43, 161; dental health, 146; diet, 147–48, 156; diversity among, 142, 143, 144, 145, 147, 156, 161; divorce, 145; education, 143, 145, 159, 160; family support, 147, 150, 158; growth stunting, 148; Guamanian, 142, 143; health-care organization, 157–59; health-care utilization, 151–52, 153, 154, 155, 162, 235; health status, xix, 145–46, 147, 148–49; Hmong, 143; identity issues, 147, 156, 162; immigrants, viii, 144, 146, 147–48, 149, 150, 156, 161–62; Indian (Asian), 142, 143, 150; intergenerational conflicts, 157, 162; Korean, 142, 143, 146, 147, 150, 151, 156; language problems, 151, 156, 160; Lao, 143, 146; mental health, 146, 149, 152, 153, 157; mental health services, 155, 157, 159, 160; mortality, 145; obesity, 148, 149; poverty, 143, 152; psychotropic drugs, 157; refugees, 145, 146, 148, 149, 156, 157; Samoan, 142, 143; shame/stigma, 151–52, 154, 157, 158, 160, 162; smoking, 149; somatization, 155; stereotypes, 145, 161; stress, 146, 149, 153, 157, 161–62; substance abuse, 144, 147, 150; Thai, 143, 146, 147; Tongan, 143, 146, 147; Vietnamese, 142, 143, 146, 147,

Asian Pacific Americans (APA) (*continued*)
149, 150; violence, 154. *See also* Chinese;
Filipinos; Hawaiians, Native; Japanese
Assistant Secretary for Planning and Evaluation, 190, 191
asthma, 89, 90–91, 103, 198
Atlanta (Georgia): Postponing Sexual Involvement program, 233
automobile accidents, 5, 39, 43, 56, 87, 119,
134

Baltimore survey of children, 4
barbiturate use, 150
barriers to health care: access, 14–15, 19, 24,
26, 188, 192, 218; fragmentation of services, 211, 218–19; short-term solutions,
218, 231
benefit programs, 2
BIA. *See* Bureau of Indian Affairs
bicultural staff, xxv, 102, 147, 161, 162
bilingual services, xxv, 82, 102, 147, 156,
157, 160, 161, 162
birth control. *See* contraception
birth rates, viii, 8; American Indian, 118;
Black, 59; Hawaiian, 173; non-marital,
18, 59, 173
Black Americans: adaptive behaviors, 39–
42; of African heritage, 229; birth rate, 59;
of Caribbean heritage, 37–38; data on,
xiv, 89; diversity of, 37, 38, 40; family, 3,
37, 54, 65–66, 71; health-care utilization,
43, 62, 63, 65, 68, 101, 235–36; health status, xv, 42–43, 45–46, 71, 89, 236; kinship, 229; life expectancy, 42, 217; mental
health, 47, 49, 50–51, 64; mortality, 42–
43, 145; population, 36–37, 38–39; poverty, 2, 3, 37; pregnancy rate, 8; religion,
65, 67–68, 71; social ecology, 40; stress,
39, 40, 50, 51; substance abuse, 39, 56, 68,
97; treatment bias, 22; urban vs. rural, 37,
38, 39
Black Job Corps, 62
BPHC. *See* Bureau of Primary Health Care
Bureau of Indian Affairs (BIA), 124, 126, 141,
128, 131–32; schools, 124, 127, 131, 132
Bureau of Primary Health Care (BPHC), 191,
193, 195

burn injuries, 6

Cambodians, 143, 146, 147, 156
cancer, 172, 184
cardiovascular disease, 45, 46, 91, 103, 145,
148, 172
Caribbean populations, 37–38
Carnegie Corporation, xiii–xiv, xv
Carnegie Council on Adolescent Develop-
ment, xvi
CBOS. *See* community-based organizations
CCDC. *See* Chinatown Child Development
Center
CDC. *See* Centers for Disease Control and
Prevention
Center for Mental Health Services (CMHS),
191, 193, 200
Center for Substance Abuse Prevention
(CSAP), 191, 193, 200
Centers for Disease Control and Prevention
(CDC), 193, 194, 198–99
Chapter I funds, 210
CHCS. *See* community health centers
Chicago Woodlawn Project, 8
child abuse. *See* abuse, child
Child Abuse Prevention and Treatment
Program, 204
Child and Adolescent Service System Pro-
gram, 200
child care, 159, 232
child development research, 49
childhood health, 231–32
Children's Bureau, 204
Child Welfare Services, 204
Chinatown Child Development Center
(CCDC), 159
Chinese: demographics, 144, 142, 143, 150;
in Hawaii, 172; health, concepts of, 153;
health care, 155, 159; health needs, 146,
147, 151, 156; mortality, 145; smoking, 149
cholera, 146
cholesterol levels, 91, 148–49
class, socioeconomic, 1; abuse and, 17; contraception and, 18; mental health and, 10,
11; mortality and, 145; sexual activity and,
8–9; substance abuse and, 12

clinics, 25; community-based, 157, 158; school-based, xxv, 18, 24–25, 69–70, 71, 190, 195, 210, 234; teen attitudes toward, 24
CMHS. *See* Center for Mental Health Services
cocaine, 56, 57, 64, 97, 98, 99, 123
Columbia University Center on Addiction and Substance Abuse, 208
community-based clinics, 157, 158
community-based organizations (CBOs), 22, 208
community-based paraprofessionals, 68–69, 71
community health centers (CHCs), 14
community networks, influence of, 151
compadrazgo (kinship system), 221–22
condoms, 19, 21, 93, 95, 100, 119
conduct disorder, 124
Consumer Product Safety Commission, 189
contraception, 9, 18–19; Blacks, 9, 201; class differences, 9, 18; condoms, 19, 93, 100; gender and, 60, 61; Latinos, 93–94, 95, 100, 101, 103; sex education and, 60–61
Corporation for National and Community Service, 209–10
Corporation for National Service, 189
COSSMHO. *See* National Coalition of Hispanic Health and Human Service Organizations
Coye, Molly, 219
crime, 39, 53, 55, 145, 172
criminal behavior, 52, 53, 54–55
crisis-oriented care, 15
CSAP. *See* Center for Substance Abuse Prevention
Cubans, 81, 82, 89–90, 93, 97, 101
cultural aspects of health care, 152–53
cultural bias: in diagnosis, 22, 49, 51, 53, 64; monocultural, 217
cultural competence, 26, 63, 157, 205; definition of, 200
cultural differences, 49; in illness, 153–54; in mental disorders, 47
cultural responsiveness, 218, 219, 235–36

culture-based models, 226–28

DARE program, 234
data, national health, 84
day care, 230
death, causes of. *See* mortality
decision-making experience, 235
delinquency, 12–13, 23, 53; American Indians, 124–25; Asians, 145, 152; Blacks, 54–55; definition of, 12; prevention of, 55, 207–8, 231; as response to stress, 124
dental health, 5, 16, 195; American Indians, 130; Asians, 146; Blacks, 62; insurance, 24; Latinos, 101
Department of Education, 189, 202, 205–7, 211
Department of Health and Human Services (DHHS), 18, 189, 190, 202, 203, 204, 205, 211
depression, 11, 68; American Indians, 120, 121–22; Asians, 146, 149, 153; Blacks, 47, 50–51; data on, 47; Latinos, 96; manic-, 50, 68; substance abuse and, 96, 121; suicide, 11, 50
developmental disorders, 120–21
DHHS. *See* Department of Health and Human Services
diabetes, 45; American Indians, 117, 118, 207; Hawaiians, 172–73, 184; Latinos, 85, 89, 91, 103
diagnosis, bias in, 22, 49, 51, 53, 64
diet, 4, 148; Asians, 147–48, 156; food distribution programs, 207. *See also* nutrition
Disadvantaged Minority Health Improvement Act of 1990 (HR 5702), 83–84
discrimination, viii, ix, 105, 222, 223. *See also* cultural bias; diagnosis, bias in; racism
Division of Maternal and Child Health, 194
Division of Maternal, Infant, Child, and Adolescent Health, 194
DOL. *See* Department of Labor
Door (multiservice program), 25, 26
drug abuse. *See* substance abuse
Drug Free Schools and Communities Act, 206

Earth Ambassadors, 135
eating disorders, xv
education, health, xxv; AIDS and, 20, 21,
104, 199, 203, 234; family emphasis in,
150; mental health, 159, 160; preventative,
xxv, 157, 234. *See also* sex education
education, participatory, 104
educational background: American Indians,
125, 131; Asians, 143, 145, 159, 160; Hawaiians, 172, 174, 177; Latinos, 82, 97,
203; non-marital births and, 18
Education Amendments Act, 131
Education Now and Babies Later (Project
ENABL), 233
effective environments, 39–40
Employment and Training Administration
(ETA), 208–9
empowerment, 105, 236
ENABL Project. *See* Education Now and
Babies Later
environmental health problems, 88–89, 103
ETA. *See* Employment and Training Administration
ethnicity, xxii, 11, 231; definition of, 219–
20; mental disorders and, 11, 49; social
support and, 229–30; strengths of, 236
ethnic minorities: classifications of, xxi;
data on, xv; population growth of, viii
exosystems, 40
Extension Service, 207

families, 2; American Indian, 125, 127, 133–
34, 221, 222; Asian, 147, 150, 158; Black,
3, 37, 54, 65–66, 71; cultural variations in,
221–22, 229; disruption of, 127; Hawaiian, 176, 222; involvement of, 64, 65, 150,
157, 158, 184; Latino, 82, 83, 99; single-
parent, 8, 37, 53, 54, 127; two-parent, 217
Family and Youth Services Bureau, 205
family counseling services, 157
family planning services: agencies and, 195,
200–201; Latino use of, 101
Family Support Administration, 204
federal programs, 188, 204, 211, 217; agencies, 191, 193; direct vs. indirect, 188
fetal alcohol effects (FAE), 121

fetal alcohol syndrome (FAS), 121
Filipinos: alcohol, 150; causes of death, 145;
compadrazgo (kinship system), 221–22; demographics, 142, 143, 150, 171; in Hawaii,
171, 173; health needs, 146, 147, 151
firearms, 6, 52, 57
fitness, 45
Food and Nutrition Service, 207
food stamps, 5, 45, 207
foster care, ix, 17, 121, 127, 204, 232, 233
Foster Grandparent Program, 209
4-H program, 207
Freud, S., 224
funding, health-care: agencies and, 194–95;
federal, 190, 210; focus of, 231; Omnibus
Budget Reconciliation Act of 1990, 192

Galveston (Texas) study, 4
gangs, 57, 104, 204, 230, 234
gender, 49, 54; disease patterns and, 46, 50,
90; mortality rates and, 43; substance use
and, 97, 98, 99
gender roles, 54; American Indian, 127; Latino, 99, 100, 103; socialization, xxi–xxii,
49, 54, 99, 100
genograms, 66, 71
Goals 2000: Educate America, 206
group homes, 17
growth patterns, 5
Guamanians, 142, 143
guns. *See* weapons

habilitation, 235
handicapped, programs for, 69
HANES. *See* National Health and Nutrition
Examination Surveys
Harlem Interfaith Counseling Service, 67
Hawaiians, Native, 168; alcohol and, 171,
173; birth rate, 173; child abuse, 172, 183;
Child and Adolescent Service System
Program, 178, 183; crime, 172; cultural
factors, 176–79, 180, 183; data on, 168,
169, 183; definition of, 168–69; demographics, 142, 143, 168–69, 170–71; diabetes, 172–73, 184; education, 172, 174,
177; family, 176, 222; health-care utiliza-

tion, 178–79; health insurance, 174–76, 179, 180; health services, 169, 178–83; health status, 171, 172–74; hearing impairments, 173, 174, 183; hypertension, 171; mental health, 178; mortality, 171, 172, 173; Native Hawaiian Health Care Act, 175–76, 179, 181, 183; obesity, 171, 173; Papa Ola Lokahi (service system), 176; payment for services, 180; physical impairments, 173–74; smoking, 171, 173; socioeconomic status, 171–72, 175; substance use, 181, 182; traditional healing, 176, 178, 179, 180, 182, 183, 184

HCFA. See Health Care Financing Administration

Head Start, 210

Head Start mothers, xxiv

health care, physical: barriers to, 14–15, 24, 26, 188, 192, 218; focus, 211; fragmentation of, 44, 211, 218–19; poverty and, 42; visibility of, 211

Health Careers Opportunity Program, 195

Health Care Financing Administration (HCFA), 190, 191

health-care professionals: insufficiency of, 15; minority, 162, 235; training, 63, 160–61, 235

health-care services, 157–58, 190

health-care utilization, 13, 102; acculturation and, 155; American Indian, 15, 22, 128, 129, 130, 135; Asian, 151–52, 153, 154, 155, 159, 160, 162, 235; Black, 43, 62, 63, 65, 68, 101, 235–36; Hawaiian, 178–79; insurance and, 24; Latino, 100–102, 103, 105, 235; socioeconomic class and, 23–24; welfare care, 24

health insurance, 14; adolescents without, 13–14, 217, 218; Hawaiian, 174–76, 179, 180

Health Promotion for Older Children and Adolescents, 197

Health Resources and Services Administration (HRSA), 191, 194, 195–96, 202, 211

Health Surveillance Program (HSP), 169

Healthy People 2000, 83, 202

Healthy Schools, Healthy Communities (HSHC), 195, 205

hearing impairment, 89, 173–74, 183, 198

hemoglobin E disorders, 146

hemophilia, 10

Henry W. Grady Memorial Hospital (Atlanta), 233

hepatitis, 145

heroin, 56, 57, 62, 97, 98

high blood pressure, 46, 91, 148, 157, 171

Hispanics. See Latinos

HIV. See AIDS

holistic approach, 219, 226, 228

Hollingshead–Redlich four-factor index, 3

Homebuilders, 233

homeless, 10, 20, 46, 195, 205; births among, 231; public support of, 218; substance abuse and, 55

home visitations, ix

homicide, 6, 43, 52, 85, 86; American Indians and, 117; drug/alcohol related, 55–56; weapons and, 6; Latinos and, 85, 86, 87; rate, 230. See also violence; weapons

homosexuals, 20, 62, 95, 100

Ho'ola Lahui Hawai'i, 184, 185

hopelessness, xxiii, xxiv

hospitalization, 101

housing conditions, 46

HRSA. See Health Resources and Services Administration

HUD. See Department of Housing and Urban Development

human resource development, 63, 161, 162

hypertension, 46, 91, 148, 157, 171

IAHS. See Indian Adolescent Health Survey

identity, xxiii, 48, 120, 124, 228; in adolescence, 47–49, 79, 220, 222–23, 224, 225, 228; negative, 48; protective, 49

IHS. See Indian Health Service

immigrants, vii, viii, 142, 146

Improving America's Schools Act of 1994, 207

Independent Living Formula Grants, 204

Indian Adolescent Health Survey (IAHS), 118, 119, 120, 122, 123, 126

Indian Adolescent Mental Health, 120

Indian Child Welfare Act, 132

Indian Health Care Improvement Act of 1976
Indian Health Service (IHS), 116, 118, 123, 128, 129, 130, 136, 191; as agency, 194; Alcoholism/Substance Abuse Program Branch (A/SAPB), 129–30, 140; Maternal and Child Health (MCH) Program, 129; Mental-Health Program, 129
Indians (Asian), 142, 143
Indian Self-Determination and Education Assistance Act of 1975, 130, 131
injuries. See accidents
institutionalization, 65
intervention, 232, 236

Japanese: alcohol, 150; demographics, 142, 143, 150, 171; in Hawaii, 171, 172; health needs of, 146, 147, 151, 156; mental health, 152, 153; mortality, 145
job programs, 25
Job Training Partnership Act, 209
juvenile-justice system, 16–17, 52, 208

kidney transplants, 51
kinship ties, 66; compadrazgo system, 221–22
Koreans, 142, 143, 146, 147, 150, 151, 156

language impairment programs, 198
Latinos: acculturation, 98–99, 100; AIDS, 85, 94–95, 100, 203; alcohol use, 97, 98, 100; Central and South American, viii, 81, 85, 96, 98; chronic conditions, 89–90, 103; contraception, 93–94, 95, 100, 101, 103; data on, xiv, 83–84, 90, 102; definition of, 80; demographics, 81; dental health care, 101; diabetes, 85, 89, 91, 103; education, 82, 97, 203; family, 82, 83, 99; gender norms, 99, 100, 103; health-care utilization, 100–102, 103, 105, 235; health risks, xix, 91, 92, 103; mental health, 86, 94–96, 105; mental health care, 102; mortality, 84–87, 88–92, 103; poverty, 82, 104; pregnancy, 93, 100, 103; programs, 203, 208; sexual behavior, 92–94, 95, 99, 100, 101, 103; smoking, 90–91, 97–98, 100; socio-cultural factors, 80, 83, 102–3; stereotypes, 80, 99, 103; substance use, 96–98, 99, 100, 103; superhealthy reputation, 80, 103; violence, 85, 86, 87, 88, 96. See also Cubans; Mexican Americans; Puerto Ricans
lead contamination, 88–89
Learn and Serve America, 210
leprosy, 146
life expectancy: American Indians, 117; Blacks, 42, 217; Whites, 42
life-skills training, 234

macrosystems, 40
MAHS. See Minnesota Adolescent Health Survey
Making the Grade project, 195
Making the Right Connections (MTRC), 234
malaria, 146
malnutrition, 4–5, 15, 45
manic-depression, 50, 68
marijuana use, 56, 64, 97, 98; American Indian, 123, 124; Black, 68; Latino, 99
Maternal and Child Health Bureau (MCHB), 191, 193, 194, 195, 196, 202, 211
Maternal and Child Health Program (MCH), 129
Medicaid, 14, 190, 192; abortion and, 192; eligibility, 14, 44, 63, 192; funding, 190–91, 210; physicians and, 15, 44, 218; prenatal care and, 44
mental health, 10–11; affective disorders, 50; American Indians, xiii, 117, 120–22, 124, 129, 132; Asians, 146, 149, 152, 153, 157; Blacks, 47, 49, 50–51, 64; class and, 10, 11; education and, 22, 159, 160; ethnicity and, 11, 47, 49; Hawaiians, 178; insurance, 22; Latinos, 86, 94–96, 105; professionals and, 62; psychosis, 49, 51, 64; rates of, 11, 63; schizophrenia, 50, 68, 152–53. See also depression
mental health care: access to, 17; American Indians and, 129; Asians and, 155, 157, 159, 160; Latinos and, 102
mental retardation, 55, 89, 120
mentoring, 235

mesosystems, 40

Mexican Americans, 81, 82; chronic conditions, 89, 90; health-care utilization, 15, 101; lead exposure, 88; mortality, 87; smoking, 97; substance use, 99

microsystems, 40

migrant health centers, 195

Minnesota Adolescent Health Survey (MAHS), 118, 120, 122, 128

minorities: native vs. foreign-born, viii; population, viii, xix; professional, 162, 204

Minority Health Tracking System, 204

Minority Male Grants, 203

Minority Youth Behavior Research, 197

Minority Youth Service Initiative, 210

Monitoring the Future Study, 96–97

monocultural bias, 217

mortality: adolescent, 42, 43; age-adjusted rates of, 145; American Indians, 117, 122, 127, 145; Asians, 145; Blacks, 42–43, 145; gender and, 43; Hawaiians, 171, 172; Latinos, 84–87, 88–92, 103; leading causes of, 5–6, 36, 43, 85, 117; legal intervention, 85, 86, 87; White, 42, 43, 145. *See also* suicide

motorcycle accidents, 119

MTRC. *See* Making the Right Connections

multicultural paradigm, 217, 223

multiservice centers, xxv, 25, 26

Mysteries Program, 234

NAHIC. *See* National Adolescent Health Information Center

NANACOA. *See* National Association for Native American Children of Alcoholics

National Adolescent Health Information Center (NAHIC), 196

National Adolescent Health Work Group, 196

National Association for Native American Children of Alcoholics (NANACOA), 134

National Association of Social Workers, 196

National Cancer Institute, xxi, 184

National Center for Health Services Research and Health Care Technology, 184

National Coalition of Hispanic Health and Human Service Organizations (COSSMHO), 104, 208

National Health and Nutrition Examination Surveys (HANES), 5

National Health Interview Survey, xxi, 89, 100, 101, 149

National Heart, Lung, and Blood Institute (NHLBI), 198

National Institute of Child Health and Human Development (NICHD), xv, 191, 193, 194, 196–97, 211

National Institute for Nursing Research (NINR), xv, 193

National Institute of Allergy and Infectious Diseases (NIAID), 198

National Institute of Diabetes and Digestive and Kidney Diseases (NIDDKD), 198

National Institute of Mental Health (NIMH), xv, 191, 193, 194, 196, 197

National Institute of Nursing Research (NINR), 191, 194, 196, 197

National Institute on Alcohol Abuse and Alcoholism (NIA), 191, 194, 196

National Institute on Deafness and Other Communication Disorders, 188

National Institute on Drug Abuse (NIDA), 144, 191, 194, 196

National Institute on the Education of At-Risk Students, 206

National Institutes of Health (NIH), xv, 191, 192, 194, 196, 197–98

National Medical Care Utilization and Expenditure Survey, 13

National School Lunch and Breakfast Programs, 207

National Survey of Family Growth, 7, 93, 101

National Survey on Drug Abuse, 56

National Transportation Safety Board, 189

Native American Rehabilitation and Training Center, 120, 121

Native Americans. *See* American Indians

needs of life, basic, xxiii

New Zealand family-group conferences, ix

NHLBI. *See* National Heart, Lung, and Blood Institute

NIA. *See* National Institute on Alcohol Abuse and Alcoholism

NICHD. *See* National Institute of Child Health and Human Development

nicotine. *See* smoking

NIDDKD. *See* National Institute of Diabetes and Digestive and Kidney Diseases

NIH. *See* National Institutes of Health

NINR. *See* National Institute for Nursing Research

non-marital births, 18, 59

nutrition, 4–5, 15, 45, 207. *See also* diet

OASH. *See* Office of the Assistant Secretary for Health

obesity, 4, 91, 198; Asians, 148, 149; Native Americans, 207; Native Hawaiians, 171, 173

ODPHP. *See* Office of Disease Prevention and Health Promotion

Office for Substance Abuse Prevention (OSAP), 200

Office of Adolescent Health, xv, 196, 202

Office of Child Support Enforcement, 204

Office of Community Services, 204

Office of Comprehensive School Health Education, 206

Office of Disease Prevention and Health Promotion (ODPHP), 191, 193, 200, 202

Office of Domestic Operations, 209

Office of Family Assistance, 204

Office of Human Development Services, 204

Office of Justice Program, 208

Office of Juvenile Justice and Delinquency Prevention (OJJDP), 207–8

Office of Management and Budget, race/ethnicity data standards, 83

Office of Minority Health (OMH), 191, 193, 194, 197, 200, 202–4, 211

Office of Population Affairs (OPA), 191, 193, 194, 200–202

Office of Refugee Resettlement (ORR), 193, 204, 205

Office of Technology Assessment (OTA), xiii–xiv, xv, xvi, xxv, 201, 210; adolescent health survey, 189; recommendations, 211, 231

Office of the Assistant Secretary for Elementary and Secondary Education, 206

Office of the Assistant Secretary for Health (OASH), 193, 200, 203

OJJDP. *See* Office of Juvenile Justice and Delinquency Prevention

OMH. *See* Office of Minority Health

Omnibus Budget Reconciliation Act of 1990, 192

OPA. *See* Office of Population Affairs

ORR. *See* Office of Refugee Resettlement

OSAP. *See* Office for Substance Abuse Prevention

OTA. *See* Office of Technology Assessment

otitis media, 46, 119, 121

outreach programs, 159–60, 162

paraprofessionals, 68–69, 71

parenting programs, 200

parents: aides for, 68, 69; attitudes of, 70; consent of, 19, 201; involvement of, 104, 184

peer counseling, 21, 235, 237

peer influence, 21, 60, 65, 98, 103, 220, 229; teaching resistance to, 64, 233

peer support, 235

persons in need of supervision (PINS), 16–17

pesticides, exposure to, 89

PHS. *See* Public Health Service

physicians, availability of, 15, 44, 192, 218

PINS. *See* persons in need of supervision

pneumonia, 145

police, 52; increase in, 55; legal intervention by, 85, 86, 87; stereotypes of, 53

Postponing Sexual Involvement, 233

Potential Life Lost, Years of (YPLL), 85–86

poverty, 2; definition of, 1, 189; demographics, xix, 1–3, 83, 188, 217; health and, 1, 4, 218; health care and, 17, 42; short- vs. long-term, 2; urban vs. rural, 3, 217; violence, 6

power utilization, theory of, 225–26

pregnancy, rates of, 8, 59; American Indian, 118; Black, 8; Latino, 93, 100, 103; White, 8

pregnancy, teenage, 8, 230–31; cultural attitudes toward, 231; education and, 8, 200; prevention programs, 18, 61, 199, 201, 231, 234; sexual abuse and, 8
prenatal care, 43–45, 118
prevention efforts, xxv, 64, 157, 233, 235, 237; aggressive, 159, 162
Project Alert, 65
Proyecto Esperanza, 208
psychopathology, 47, 51
psychosis, 49, 51, 64
psychotherapy, 51
psychotropic drugs, 157
Public Health Service (PHS), 190, 191, 192, 204, 211; agencies, 191, 193
Puerto Ricans: birth control, 93; demographics, 81, 82; health-care utilization, 101; health concerns, 88, 89, 90, 91; mortality, 85, 87; sexual behavior, 95; smoking, 97; substance use, 99
pulmonary disease, 145

racism, 26, 38, 50, 72. See also diagnosis, cultural bias in; discrimination
RAP. See Reaching Adolescents and Parents
rape, 55–56, 60
Rastafarianism, 68
Reaching Adolescents and Parents (RAP), 233
reality, types of, 226–27
recommendations on health care, xxiv–xxv, 211, 232–38
referent power, 237
Rehabilitation Act of 1973, 69
religion: American Indian spirituality, 133; Blacks and, 65, 67–68, 71
research, xxiv, 211
Research Center on the Psychobiology of Ethnicity, 198
Robert Wood Johnson Foundation, 14, 195
role models, 54, 72, 103
runaways, 7, 16, 17, 20, 124, 236; AIDS and, 10; American Indian, 125, 126, 205; programs for, 205, 208; Runaway and Homeless Youth Act, 204

Safe and Drug Free Schools and Communities Act, 206

SAMHSA. See Substance Abuse and Mental Health Services Administration
schizophrenia, 50; among Japanese, 152–53; Rastafarianism and, 68
school-based clinics, xxv, 18, 24–25, 69–70, 71, 210, 234; agency involvement in, 190, 195
school dropouts, 22, 57, 59, 98, 124, 207; American Indian, 118, 125; Asian, 143; Latino, 97
school failure (student), 57–58
school lunch programs, 45, 207, 210
schools, 48, 205, 206; American-Indian, 118, 125, 127, 128, 131, 132, 223; Black experiences in, 58; as community base, 69, 160; cultural sensitivity and, 58
School-to-Work Opportunities Act, 209
seat-belt use, 87, 119, 171, 173
Secretary's Task Force on Black and Minority Health, 83
security, components of, xxiii
SEER. See Surveillance, Epidemiology and End Results program
self-actualization, 72
self-care, xxiv
self-concept, 96, 124
self-destructive behavior, xxiv
self-esteem, xxiii, 38, 72, 235; American Indians, 124, 133; Latinos, 94–95, 105
SES. See socioeconomic status
sex education, 18, 21–22, 60–61, 233
sexual abuse, 8, 60, 100; American Indians, 126, 127; Blacks, 46
sexual behavior, 7–8; American Indian, 118–19; lack of change in, 95; Latino, 92–94, 95, 99, 100, 101, 103; peer pressure, 60; safe sex, 10, 20–21, 203. See also condoms; contraception
sexually transmitted diseases (STDs), 9, 19, 61–94; AIDS, 9–10, 57; condoms and, 19, 21, 95, 119; education about, 234; rates of, 9, 61, 62, 94; treatment/prevention of, 19–22, 104
sickle-cell anemia, 45–46, 89, 198
single-parent households, 37, 53, 54, 82, 111, 127; poverty and, 2, 3, 8, 54

Sisters of St. Joseph Ministerial Services, 234
skills acquisition, 48, 55
smoking: American Indians, 120, 132, 134; Asians, 149; Latinos, 90–91, 97–98, 100; passive, 90; prevention efforts, 64; teenage, 12, 56, 71
social class. See class, socioeconomic
social connectedness, decrease in, viii
social-ecological approach, 40
socialization, xxi–xxii, 49, 54, 99, 100
social morbidity, ix
social support, 229–30
socioeconomic status (SES), 3; abuse and, 16; AIDS and, 10; definition of, 3; delinquency and, 12–13; health-services utilization and, 23–24; mental disorders and, 10–11; suicide and, 6–7
South Cove Community Health Center (Boston), 158–59
Special Projects of Regional and National Significance (SPRANS), 194, 195
Spirit of the Rainbow Development Program, 135
SPRANS. See Special Projects of Regional and National Significance
STDs. See sexually transmitted diseases
Strategic Intervention for High-Risk Youth Program, 208
Strengthening Families Project, 104
stress, vii–viii; adolescence and, 70; American Indians, 127, 128, 135; Asians, 146, 149, 153, 161; Blacks, 39, 40, 50, 51; delinquency and, 124; posttraumatic, 149; sociocultural changes and, 127
Student Community Service Program, 209
subcultural differences. See cultural differences
substance abuse, 11–12, 22–23, 55–56; AIDS and, 57; American Indians, 123–24, 126, 128, 130, 131, 134, 205; Asians, 144, 147, 150; Blacks, 39, 55–57, 68, 97; class and, 12, 22, 23; depression and, 96, 121; fetuses exposed to, 55; gender and, 97, 98, 99; Hawaiians, 181, 182; homeless and, 55; Latinos, 96–98, 99, 100, 103; prevention

of, 204, 205, 206, 208, 231, 234; treatment of, 22–23, 57, 64, 130, 131; Whites, 56
Substance Abuse and Mental Health Services Administration (SAMHSA), 191, 194, 199
sudden death syndrome, 146
suicide, 6–7, 11, 16; American Indian, 117, 122; attempts, 122; Blacks, 39, 50; Latinos, 86, 96; rate, 6, 43, 50, 230; Whites, 43
Supplemental Food Program for Women, Infants, and Children (WIC), 4, 207
Surveillance, Epidemiology and End Results program (SEER), xxi
symptom-management approach, 219
symptoms, cultural influences, 153

Tacoma Homebuilders program, 233
Task Force on Black and Minority Health, 203
television: outreach programs and, 160; sexual activity on, 61; violence on, 53–54
Thais (Thailanders), 143, 146, 147
thalassemia, 146
Title I, 206
Title II-A (training grants), 209
Title II-B (summer youth employment), 209
Title II-C (year-round youth training), 209
Title IV-B (Job Corps), 209
Title X (family planning), 200–201
Title XX, 201
tobacco, 12, 56
Tongan population, 143, 146, 147
transactional models, 227
Transition Program for Refugee Children, 205
tuberculosis, 46, 92, 117, 145

Udry, Richard, 197
Unaccompanied Minor Refugee Program, 205
unemployment, 39, 116
United National Indian Tribal Youth (UNITY), 135
UNITY. See United National Indian Tribal Youth

University of New Mexico: Indian teen
centers, 135–36
U.S. Department of Agriculture (USDA),
190, 191, 207
U.S. Department of Education, 190, 191,
205–7
U.S. Department of Health and Human
Services, 191; Office of Adolescent
Health, xv
U.S. Department of Housing and Urban
Development (HUD), 191, 208
U.S. Department of Justice, 190, 191, 207–8
U.S. Department of Labor (DOL), 190, 191,
208–9

Vietnamese, 142, 143, 146, 147, 149, 150
violence, 6, 7; alcohol/drug related, 56, 57;
American Indians and, 120; Blacks and,
52; as cause of death, 43, 52, 85, 86, 88,
230; gender and, 54, 88; Latinos and, 85,
86, 87, 88, 96; poverty and, 6; television
and, 53–54; weapons and, 6, 52, 57, 88;
Whites and, 52. See also homicide;
weapons
VISTA programs, 209

weapons, 6, 52, 57, 88. See also homicide;
violence
welfare dependency, 9
white males, anger of, vii–viii
WIC. See Supplemental Food Program for
Women, Infants and Children
women: in labor force, 230. See also gender;
gender roles

Youth Risk Behavior Survey (YRBS), 84, 88,
96
YPLL. See Years of Potential Life Lost
YRBS. See Youth Risk Behavior Survey

In the Child, Youth, and Family Services series

Big World, Small Screen:
The Role of Television in American Society
By Aletha C. Huston, Edward Donnerstein,
Halford Fairchild, Norma D. Feshbach,
Phyllis A. Katz, John P. Murray,
Eli A. Rubinstein, Brian L. Wilcox,
and Diana M. Zuckerman

Health Issues for Minority Adolescents
Edited by Marjorie Kagawa-Singer,
Phyllis A. Katz, Dalmas A. Taylor,
and Judith H. M. Vanderryn

Home-Based Services for Troubled Children
Edited by Ira M. Schwartz and Philip AuClaire

Preventing Child Sexual Abuse:
Sharing the Responsibility
By Sandy K. Wurtele and
Cindy L. Miller-Perrin